D1708015

COUNTRY DOCTOR'S BOOK OF

FOLK REMEDIES & HEALING WISDOM

WRITERS

Paul Bergner

David J. Hufford, Ph.D.

CONSULTANT

Ara Der Marderosian, Ph.D.

ILLUSTRATOR

John Zielinski

Publications International, Ltd.

Louis Weber, C.E.O.
Publications International, Ltd.
7373 North Cicero Avenue
Lincolnwood, Illinois 60646

Manufactured in U.S.A.

8 7 6 5 4 3 2 1

ISBN: 0-7853-2831-9

Picture credits:

Front cover illustration: **Robert Crawford**

Back cover: **Archive Photos** (top); **Joan M. Rigal/Siede Preis Photography** (background); **SuperStock** (bottom).

Corbis-Bettmann: 5 (left), 48, 80 (top), 96, 102, 104, 127, 197; Grant Smith: 5 (right), 26; **FPG International:** 43; Steve Belkowitz: 4 (center), 80 (bottom); David Doody: 27; Richard Laird: 35; Ernest Manewal: 28; Barbara Peacock: 287; Ken Reid: 114; **International Stock:** Dario Perla: 116; **Positive Images:** Jerry Howard: 155, 156; Albert Squillace: 154; **SuperStock:** 64, 66, 75, 86, 115, 326; Lazaro Galdiano Museum, Madrid/Giraudon, Paris: 209; Hermitage Museum, St. Petersburg/ Leonid Bogdanov: 314; David Northcott: 242; Toledo Cathedral, Castille: 312.

Ara Der Marderosian, Ph.D., is professor of Pharmacognosy and Medicinal Chemistry and is Roth Chair of Natural Products at Philadelphia College of Pharmacy & Science. He has researched extensively in the areas of medicinal and poisonous plants, folkloric medicinal plants, hallucinogenic botanicals, herbal teas, ginseng, and medical foods.

Paul Bergner (Remedies) is editor of *Medical Herbalism* and is clinic director at the Rocky Mountain Center for Botanical Studies. He has published *The Naturopathic Physician* and *Clinical Nutrition Update* magazines and has written many books, including *The Healing Power of Minerals and Trace Elements* and *The Healing Power of Echinacea, Goldenseal, and the Immune System Herbs.*

David J. Hufford, Ph.D. (Introduction and Special Interests) is director of The Doctors Kienle Center for Humanistic Medicine and Academic Director of the Medical Ethnography Collection at Pennsylvania State University, College of Medicine. He also is professor of Medical Humanities, Behavioral Science, and Family & Community Medicine. Dr. Hufford serves on the editorial boards of several journals, including *Alternative Therapies in Health & Medicine.*

Additional contributing writers:

Alexandra F. Griswold, Ph.D., instructor, Department of Folklore and Folklife at the University of Pennsylvania

Bonnie O'Connor, Ph.D., professor, Community & Preventive Medicine, Medical College of Pennsylvania

Barbara Rieti, Ph.D., writer and researcher in the field of folklore

Joan L. Saverino, Ph.D., instructor, Department of Folklore and Folklife at the University of Pennsylvania

Editorial assistance: Gloria Bucco, president, Gloria Bucco & Associates

Contributing illustrator: Dan Krovatin

 # Contents 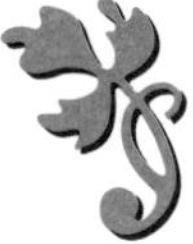

Remedies

Introduction 6
Acne 18
Allergies, Hives, and Hay Fever 22
Anxiety and Nervousness 30
Arthritis 38
Asthma 53
Bites and Stings 61
Bladder and Kidney Infections 69
Blood Purifiers and Blood Builders 82
Boils and Carbuncles 93
Breast Conditions 99
Burns and Sunburns 107
Catarrh 112
Cold and Flu 118
Colic 132
Constipation 141
Coughs 148
Depression 160
Diarrhea 170
Digestion 175
Ears 186
Eczema 193
Eyes 199
Fatigue 206
Fever 212
Foot Problems 222
Headaches 228
Hemorrhoids 239
Hiccups 248
Indigestion and Heartburn 252
Insomnia 258
Itching and Rashes 268
Menses 275
Mouth, Gums, and Teeth 289
Muscle Strains and Sprains 297
Nausea and Vomiting 303
Pain 309
Poison Ivy and Poison Oak 318
Pregnancy 324
Skin 332
Sore Throat 341
Sores and Chronic Skin Ulcers 351
Splinters 357
Wounds and Cuts 360
Bibliography 369
Index 373

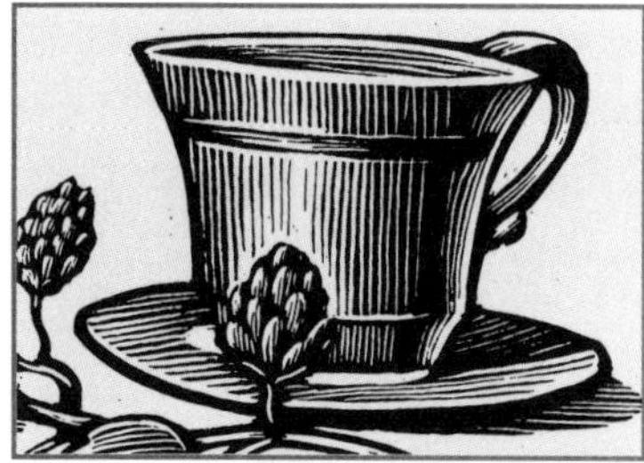

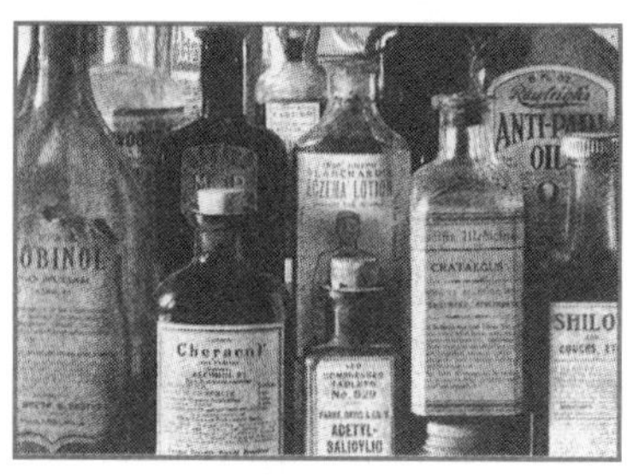

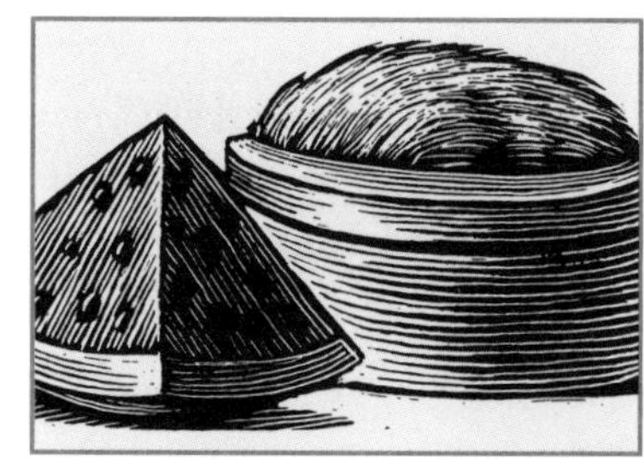

Special Interests

Animal Cures: Down on the Farm 26
Measuring Health 34
The Power of Amulets 42
Counterirritants: Like Cures Like 48
Magical Transference 58
Odors That Heal 64
Magic in Folk Medicine 74
Patent Medicines 80
Food for Thought 86
The Dead Lend a Hand 96
Powwow and the Pennsylvania Dutch 102
Wild Animal Magic 114
Birth Order and Healing Powers 120
American Indian Healing 126
Remedying Colic 134
Illnesses Unique to Folk Medicine 138
Asian-American Folk Medicine 144
Worms Be Gone! 150
Herbalism 154
Prayer vs. Magic 162
Aphrodisiacs and Love Potions 166
Finding the Balance 173
Medicinal Teas 178
Soul Loss and Lost Souls 182
The Calendar 188
Witchcraft 196
The Evil Eye 202
Sleep Paralysis 208
Jewish Folk Medicine in America 216
Rheumatism and Arthritis 225
Menstruation and Folk Medicine 232
Beating Headache 236
Fighting Cancer 242
Morning Sickness 250
African-American Folk Medicine 254
Curanderismo 260
Beliefs on Bedwetting 266
Unconventional Wart Cures 270
Healing Burns 273
The Bond Among Women 278
How Weather Affects Illness 283
Rootwork 287
Sties: Poor Behavior? 291
Baldness: Looking for a Cure 294
Italian-American Folk Medicine 300
Stopping Blood 307
Saints & Holy People 312
Poison Ivy 320
In Hopes of Fertility 326
Prenatal Influences 330
Sweating It Out 335
Falling Out 339
English Folk Medicine 346
Naturally Healthy Skin 353
Latino Folk Illnesses 362
New Age Folk Healing 366

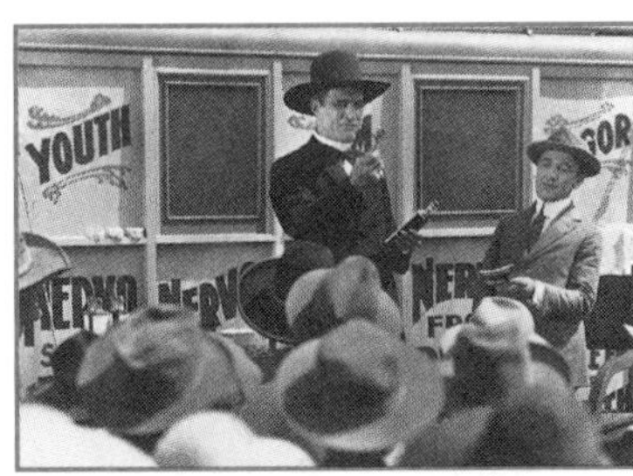

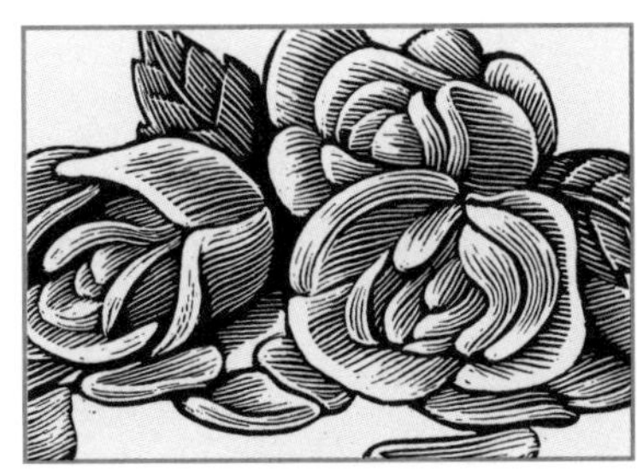

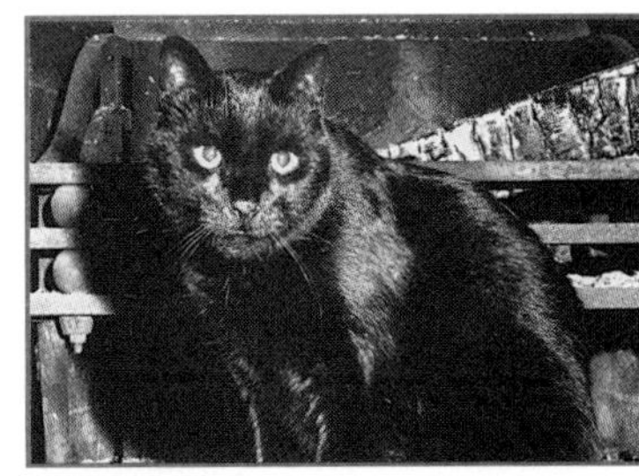

Defining Folk Medicine

"Folklore" is the traditional knowledge of ordinary people. Folk medicine, one kind of folklore, is made up of the ideas and practices of ordinary people concerning health and illness. In saying that folklore is "traditional," we emphasize that it has lasted through time—that it was not "born yesterday." But there is no hard and fast rule about how old something must be to be "folk." The jump rope rhymes of today's children—one kind of folklore—include some elements that are centuries old and others that have been newly created by the children who are using them. The same is true of folk medicine. Some of the remedies found in oral tradition in the United States today are truly ancient, such as the idea that health is influenced by heat and cold (as in the folk belief that getting chilled can cause one to "catch" a cold). Other items of contemporary folk medicine are quite new—for example, the odd belief that radon gas (produced by the decay of radium) is a remedy for lung ailments! This colorless and odorless gas has only been known since 1900, and its use as a health remedy has involved sitting in abandoned uranium mines. Of course, what is odd about this belief is that radon gas, which rises through the soil and can also accumulate in houses as well as mines, is actually a cause of lung cancer. So, the belief in radon as a remedy is not only recent—it is dangerous! However, this example is not meant to suggest that folk medicine is generally useless or dangerous—far from it, as we shall see.

Folklore includes a great variety of culture, from proverbs to quilt designs and from folktales to folk songs, as well as folk medicine. What all folklore has in common is that it is the property of ordinary people—that is, people who are not "officially" recognized as experts. For this reason, folklore tends to be passed on by word of mouth—what folklorists call "oral tradition." So while "classical" music is taught in music appreciation class, and popular music is heard on commercial recordings, folk songs are learned from those around us. (We learned to sing "Happy Birthday to You" or the songs that are popular around campfires, fires.) Sophisticated literature is taught in universities, and popular literature is found at bookstores, while folktales are told to children by their parents or, as in the case of many legends, told by friends. Official "bio-medicine" is taught in medical schools and passed on to the public by physicians—from the Surgeon General on down to your family doctor. Folk medicine is learned from parents and friends or provided by community folk practitioners, such as Mexican-American curanderas (page 260) or simply by a neighbor who knows a cure for warts. It would be a mistake to imagine that the boundaries between these forms of culture are always so clear and sharp. Folk songs have often become so popular that they reached the top of the music charts, and commercial popular music influences folk music throughout the United States. There is now, in fact, an entire category of commercial musicians called "folk singers"! In the same way, folk medicine has always influenced and been influenced by official medicine and commercial popular medicine. Many popular health books use "folk medicine" in the title. In these books, it is often impossible to determine what is folk medicine. What is the difference between the folk medicine actually collected from oral tradition and the old "regular medicine" from the last century? And what about the medical traditions of other cultures?

In folk medicine, as in language, religion, and all areas of culture, "purity" is rare. Culture develops through a mixing process, and the persistence of folk medicine and other kinds of folklore through the centuries demonstrates that, while this mixing does not always destroy traditions, it does constantly change them. In folk medicine what we see are trends, not absolutes. At the same time, it must be granted that the folk medicine traditions of people (for example, the American Indians) whose culture has been placed under great pressure by modern circumstances is sometimes threatened with being lost or changed beyond recognition.

Many people can respect most folklore—even if it is not from a tradition they identify with or actually appreciate. However, many do not have the same attitude toward folk medicine. Because folk belief is made up of things believed by ordinary people to be true, as opposed to what experts teach us to be true, it is often assumed that folk belief is mere superstition or false belief. Fortunately, in recent years, most people have begun to reconsider this attitude. After all, even the experts can be wrong. Folk medicine is very closely related to peoples' experience with their bodies and their minds and the world around them, and that experience is generally worth paying attention to! No one is an expert on your experience except you! Of course, as the "radon remedy" illustrates, ordinary people are sometimes wrong in ways that only an expert can best explain. Today, we are beginning to see more of a balance in the ways that we evaluate both expert and folk ideas concerning health.

FOLK MEDICINE, "QUACKERY," AND THE HISTORY OF MEDICINE

Because of the great practical importance of medical beliefs and practices—both official and folk—we'll start with the related issues of efficacy, risk, and quackery. What reasons might we have to believe that some folk medicine "really works" and that some does not? Why is the word "quackery" often used in connection with folk medicine, and when is the term appropriate? What risks may be associated with using folk medicine?

Official medicine generally assumes that it has accepted, or is in the process of accepting, every healing practice that has been shown to be effective. Medical history has always been intimately associated with folk medicine, and today official medicine actually defines folk and alternative medicines by exclusion. This very dominant position of official medicine, legally and in scientific terms, is a very new thing in Western culture. So we must begin with a little medical history.

Before the 20th century, the licensing of physicians was largely honorific, and it did not exclude unlicensed healers from practice. In 1760, New York City passed the first law for examining and exclusively licensing doctors, but that law was never enforced. In 1763, the physicians of Norwich, Connecticut, asked the colonial legislature for licensing "to distinguish between Honest and Ingenious physicians and the Quack or Empirical Pretender." The problem of competition was recognized as serious, but the request was denied. Following the American Revolution, medical societies organized and legislatures granted licensing, but these laws were powerless and ineffective. Americans have always been a fiercely independent lot, and the high value placed on individual choice was in direct conflict with the desire of medical professionals to control health care. As a result, folk medicine and a variety of popular forms of alternative medicine flourished openly. In fact, if we had been there in the mid-century, we would have had a hard time knowing just which practitioners were considered to be "regular" and which were "alternative."

Medical schools were, by and large, small businesses, and the quality of their graduates was very unreliable. Harvard was among the first of the medical schools to attempt reform. In 1869, Charles Eliot, the president of Harvard, said, "The ignorance and general incompetency of the average graduate of American Medical schools, at the time when he [is turned] loose upon the community, is something horrible to contemplate." Both the nature of the competition and the quality of medical education changed dramatically after Abraham Flexner, a young educator with a B.A. degree from Johns Hopkins, carried out a study of medical schools. His investigation was funded by the Carnegie Foundation for the Advancement of Teaching. Flexner made surprise visits to the schools and documented the often pathetic resources in laboratories, the lack of access to patients, the incompetent faculty, and the generally disreputable state of most American medical schools. His report, published in 1910, recommended that 100 of the 131 existing medical schools be closed, although 70 eventually survived. Flexner did not start the reform movement in medical education, but his report was a watershed event in the transformation of medicine. However, that reform not only improved the basics of education for "regular physicians," it also established a principle that many expected would eradicate the competition—including folk medicine. A whole new medicine, organized around "regular medicine" was to replace all separate medical sects.

The new medicine was to be objective and scientific. It was assumed that would mean that all treatments shown to work would be included and all those that were ineffective would be excluded. The Pure Food and Drug Act of 1906 and medical licensure soon consolidated the medical profession's political power. Using that power the profession actively worked to prevent others from practicing medicine without a license. Doctors labeled those who did not fit the medical model as "quacks," and their efforts to eradicate quackery were presented as public education and protection.

The word quack comes from the old Dutch word "quacksalver." The term became popular in the 1500s and described people who sold salves and ointments—and who generally made exaggerated claims for them. Some have suggested that the word is also derived in part from quicksilver, which is the element mercury. Mercury was a common ingredient in regular medicines of the day as well as in the home remedies sold by quacks.

By the 20th century, the term quack was not at all restricted to ointment sellers. Modern dictionary definitions are very specific about what the word means: people who pretend to have medical knowledge that they do not in fact have. In other words, quackery is fraud. Unfortunately, the term is used very loosely, so that it is often applied to all sorts of healers whose practices were believed to be ineffective. The implication seems to be that any intelligent adult should know that if a type of healing is not offered by a licensed doctor, then it is useless and therefore must be fraud. This sloppy use of the word merely serves to insult those with whom conventional medicine disagrees. But still worse, it "gives cover" to the real medical frauds, of whom there are many. After all, with no distinction made between charlatans and sincere folk healers, it is much harder to identify the charlatans.

THE EFFECTIVENESS OF FOLK MEDICINE

It has been shown that some folk medicine works—in the medical sense, that is. What's more, folk medicine is capable of serving goals that are broader and more complicated than those of modern medicine. Two recent examples come from women's folk health traditions. For many years, women have learned from other women that eating live culture yogurt helps to reduce vaginal yeast infections. In 1992, a study published in the *Annals of Internal Medicine* concluded that this practice is, in fact, effective. Similarly, women's oral folk tradition has long taught that drinking cranberry juice can prevent and treat urinary tract infections. In 1994, a study published in the *Journal of the American Medical Association* concluded that this tradition is also correct—cranberry juice does have this effect. Although there are prescription treatments available for both of these conditions, these folk remedies have the advantage of being inexpensive and without side effects. (They do not always work, however, and then prescription treatment may be necessary.) It is fascinating to consider that such widely known and practiced elements of folk medicine, used to treat very common medical problems, could have been ignored by conventional medicine for so long. Even now, after these studies, the use of these remedies has not become standard medical practice.

Prescription medications not only have their desired medical effects, but they also have side effects, some of which can be quite serious. The same is true for folk medicines. Many people have the mistaken idea that "If it's natural, it can't hurt me." Some of the most powerful poisons that we know of are found in nature. And every year, in addition to those individuals who are poisoned accidentally by plants, there are people who enter hospitals because plant remedies they prepared to treat medical conditions have in fact poisoned them. Poisoning can happen in several different ways.

Some plant medicines that are effective are simply too dangerous to use outside medical supervision. For example, the plant purple foxglove *(Digitalis purpurea)* contains digitalis, which has a powerful effect on the heart. Digitoxin and digoxin, the active ingredients of foxglove, have been used by physicians to treat some forms of heart disease since the 1920s. Digitalis was brought into medical use by William Withering, an English physician. He learned of the plant's use from an "old woman in Shropshire," a folk herbalist who had cured "dropsy" in individuals who doctors had given up on. (Dropsy is the accumulation of fluid in the body now known to be caused by congestive heart failure.) The Shropshire herbalist and other folk healers around the world had long used foxglove in this way, but the difference between a therapeutic dose and a toxic does is very narrow and a poisonous overdose can be rapidly fatal. So, today, most herbalists recommend against using the plant outside of medical supervision. The plant leaf is still available, and some physicians are willing to prescribe it—as opposed to pills of synthetic digitalis or digoxin—for those who insist on natural treatment.

The deadly reaction to poisoning doesn't always occur quickly. Some popular plants in folk medicine have turned out to cause health problems when used over time. For example, comfrey is a plant that has been widely used as a medicine, but laboratory studies have shown that, with chronic use, it can lead to liver damage or even liver cancer. This kind of effect, something that develops slowly over time, is difficult for folk healers to recognize. Today, most herbalists and all medical authorities recommend against the internal use of comfrey.

A third way that plant medicines can become dangerous is through adulteration. This can happen either by accident or intentionally. Accidents happen when someone gathering herbs in the wild unintentionally picks the wrong plant or happens to grab two plants at once, one intended and the other not noticed. Also, many plants have poisonous parts that need to be separated from the edible or medicinal portions. Because many commercially available herbs come from outside the country and the products are not regulated, sometimes herbal medicines contain enough plant poison to cause sickness or even death. Even more alarming is the fact that some herbal medicines coming from outside the country have been found to have pharmaceutical drugs added to them. It seems that some marketers feel that these hidden drugs will improve sales by making the effects of the medicine more immediately noticeable. Either directly or through interaction with prescribed medication, such adulterated herbs can cause serious illness or death.

All three of these dangers are greatest for infants or very sick people with a low body weight. These dangers have been most frequently associated with commercially available herbal medicines. These risks are not enormous, but they are real. It seems prudent, therefore, to learn about plant medicine before you try herbal remedies. Watch for unexpected side effects and discontinue the herbal remedy if side effects occur. And, for infants, it would be wise in general to avoid the use of most herbal products.

FOLK MEDICINE AND SPIRITUALITY

In addition to herbs, folk medicine places a strong and consistent emphasis on spiritual matters, and many folk remedies involve rituals and prayers of various kinds. Some people call such practices "superstition." Some strongly religious people find the spirituality of folk medicine to be primitive or even wicked— for example, those whose tradition does not use ritual may find the religious rituals of folk medicine to be similar to "black magic." Others reject the spirituality of folk medicine as superstition because they reject all spiritual belief. These skeptics often say that belief in prayer and other spiritual activities is irrational, because it lacks any possible evidence.

In 1988, a cardiologist named Randolph Byrd, M.D., published an article in the *Southern Medical Journal* in which he described a study that measured the effect of prayer on a large group of patients who had suffered heart attacks. Many psychologists and medical researchers over the years have shown that praying can powerfully effect those who do it, and this has generally been explained in terms of positive mental effects. But Byrd did not study people praying for themselves. He divided almost 400 patients into an experimental group and a control group. (Neither the patients nor their doctors and nurses had any way of knowing how the groups were divided until after the study was completed.) Dr. Byrd gave the first names of the patients in the experimental group to people in prayer groups. Each prayer group had been in existence, praying for others, for a substantial period of time. The members of these groups agreed to pray regularly for the people who were assigned to them. In the end, Dr. Byrd found that the patients who received prayer did better than those who did not. They were not miraculously healed, but they recovered with fewer complications and setbacks, and this difference was highly significant statistically. Today, some medical researchers consider it proven that prayer can have a direct effect on health, while others do not. Additional studies have been undertaken to try to confirm Byrd's findings. At any rate, there is now some evidence for the efficacy of prayer.

How do studies like Dr. Byrd's relate to the spiritual dimensions of folk medicine? Some would say not at all, because they do not recognize the forms of prayer used by folk healers as valid. For example, Pennsylvania German "powwow doctors" use secret prayers and bits of scripture, repeated in a formulaic way, to heal (see page 102). Some religious people believe that only spontaneous prayer is effective, and that such ritual prayer is wrong. Perhaps some forms of prayer are more effective than others, but we do not have research demonstrating that. What we have are the beliefs of various traditions being pitted against each other. But if Dr. Byrd's study shows that prayers offered at a distance, by strangers, can help a person get well, then the efficacy of spiritual folk medicine needs to be carefully reconsidered. No one today is in a position scientifically to show that one spiritual folk healing technique is more or less effective than another—it is enough to be able to say that some effectiveness for this kind of healing is starting to be documented.

MORE THAN CURING ILLS

Whether or not spiritual folk medicine or a particular plant medicine "works" in the medical sense, these healing efforts aim to do more than remedy purely physical ills. They help to find meaning in illness, to bring a sense of control at a time when people feel most out of control, and to help create and maintain a sense of community.

The explanations that folk traditions give for why sickness occurs serve several purposes. First, spiritual belief requires a belief that the universe is not simply composed of random events. Belief in God, held by the vast majority of Americans (over 90 percent by most surveys), requires that the universe be in some sense orderly. Second, and of almost equal importance, is the belief that, in order to cure, you need to know "why" something occurred. For example, if illness is caused by a hot-cold imbalance (page 173), health can be regained through proper foods and medicines. If a patient suffers from "soul loss" (page 182), his soul can be called back. With the establishment of universal regularity there comes a sense of control, not absolute control that can guarantee health, but at least the feeling that one is engaged in fighting a recognizable enemy.

A sense of community can be fostered by folk medicine. Mexican Americans who practice the curanderismo tradition are, at the same time, showing their allegiance to the traditional values and beliefs of their culture. Women have learned traditional remedies, such as the use of cranberry juice and yogurt in healing, through community with other women.

FOLK MEDICINE AND CULTURAL AUTHORITY

Folk tradition has long existed in tension with official medicine. An important source of that tension, and a large part of the difference between the two, involves cultural authority. Cultural authority is the power to make statements about how the world works—about the real nature of the world—and have those statements accepted. Throughout history, in most parts of the world, it was life experience that gave people cultural authority. Religious status and a few other factors, such as the family into which a person was born, could also influence one's authority. In folk medicine, the knowledge of remedies is learned orally, representing the accumulated knowledge of past generations, and the evaluation of the treatment is done by the patient's observations of what seems to help.

In the 19th century, as science and technology began the rapid change that now characterizes our modern world, the structure of cultural authority changed. Scientific discoveries increasingly revealed important but invisible things about the world, from invisibly small bacteria to radiation. It became more and more obvious that we could not know everything important about the world with unaided senses. Too many things you could not see might make you sick. As a result of this growing division between everyday experience and scientific knowledge, which was strongly supported by the apparent advantages that technology could deliver, modern society shifted. An unspoken agreement developed in which the experts in science and technology were given cultural authority and the right to govern their own institutions.

The internal control of experts over the definition of their own expertise includes the opportunity to set the limits on the area to which their expertise applies. The result is that the scope of expert cultural authority has grown consistently in modern society. Of course, that means that, at the same time, the scope of authority based on life experience, and not technical training, has decreased. The best medical care has come to be understood not as the accumulation of past wisdom but rather as the very latest technique, and the very latest technique is often explained in terms of how it puts past ideas to rest. Very recent training has largely replaced, in the minds of many, the value of lifelong clinical experience. In this modern view, elders are people who require extra care, not people you turn to for an understanding of the world. And as far as a patient's right to evaluate his own treatment, the double-blind, placebo-controlled clinical trial has been developed. The patient's ability to know what really helps has been discredited as "merely subjective."

Up through the 1960s many believed that this social change in authority was irreversible and that technical knowledge would become the only kind of knowledge considered valid. But the 1960s brought deep change—ranging from the Hippie movement to the consumer movement, civil rights and women's liberation, even the Charismatic movement in Christian religion. All of these changes were rebellion against various kinds of authority and were a reassertion of the right of people to find, in their own experience, some valid basis for understanding and evaluating the world. The result has not been the complete overthrow of expert authority, but rather a process of trimming that authority back. In medicine, the idea of "informed consent," which requires doctors to tell patients what is proposed as treatment and why it is proposed, is an example of the reduction of medical authority and the return of some authority to the patient.

Folk medicine is made up of traditions in which the wisdom of past generations is gathered. Therefore, the idea that folk medicine contains important knowledge, some of which may have been forgotten in modern times, depends on a recognition of the value of life experience and the possibility that people really knew something—even before there were microscopes and X-ray machines. This idea is receiving renewed interest, thanks to the recent changes in cultural authority.

Ideally our society will find a balance on these issues. There is no need to decide between life experience and technical training, or between official medicine and folk medicine. Both seem to have great value. The greatest value will come from being able to understand what is appropriate to each. Herbal treatments clearly have some value, but they also have risks. The sense of closeness to nature and the avoidance of harsh side effects, which can come from the proper use of herbs, are best evaluated on the basis of life experience. Only the patient can answer: "How do these herbs make me feel?" and "How much did the side effects of the remedy bother me?" On the other hand, many serious illnesses require medical expertise for their successful management. Some patients believe they can increase the success of their medical treatment by also using folk remedies. This is a good idea, as long as there is an informed process in which both the doctor and the patient understand the treatments being used.

FOLK MEDICINE AND ALTERNATIVE MEDICINE

As the modern understanding of authority and life experience have improved in recent decades, we have also become aware that folk medicine has persisted, adapted, and grown. It has shared in the social processes by which alternative medicine has become so enormously popular.

The definition developed by the 1995 Complementary and Alternative Medicine Research Methodology Conference, sponsored by the NIH Office of Alternative Medicine, identifies alternative medicine as all health ideas and practices at any particular time in history or in any society that are different from those found in official medicine. Obviously, then, folk medicine is a kind of alternative medicine. But folk medicine and alternative medicine are not exactly the same thing. In the United States today there are important differences to bear in mind between folk medicine and the cosmopolitan alternative medicines. Folk medicine traditions are

- heavily dependent on oral transmission, although traditions sometimes can be influenced by print

- relatively informal in structure, although specialists may be trained through formal apprenticeships
- relatively uncommercial, although folk specialists (e.g., traditional herbalists) may receive some cash payments or barter

Based on these characteristics, it is reasonable to think of some traditions as being more or less "folk" than others. Still, Mexican-American curanderismo is obviously a folk medical tradition, and heart surgery and chiropractic are obviously not.

None of these characteristics disqualifies folk medicine as alternative medicine, however. In fact, by definition and by history, folk medicine is one of the basic—probably the most basic—aspects of alternative medicine. And yet most contemporary writing on alternative medicine makes no mention of folk medicine. At the same time, much of what is written about folk medicine ignores its place within alternative medicine. Unfortunately, it is really not possible to understand either one without knowing something about the other. The distinctive characteristics of folk medicine do set it apart from many other forms of health practices found in contemporary society—including many kinds of alternative medicine.

We can refer to the other forms of alternative medicine as "cosmopolitan," meaning that they are present in many different regions and are similar wherever they are found. All of conventional medicine and much of alternative medicine in the United States consists of cosmopolitan traditions. Homeopathy and chiropractic, two prominent alternative examples, each depends heavily on print—from professional journals to textbooks to popular works read by the public. Because of folk medicine's reliance on oral transmission, its traditions tend to change in ways that conform quickly to local conditions. The result is the development of many different regional traditions. Even though it contains similar practices and beliefs, Pennsylvania German folk medicine seems quite different from Mexican-American folk medicine in the Southwest. In contrast, while the ways in which chiropractic is used may vary in the two regions, chiropractic is recognizably the same in each place.

Cosmopolitan alternative systems tend to stay the same in very different places because print media has a conservative influence on the tradition. This influence is partly due to the formal institutions that maintain the use of print: chiropractic colleges, homeopathic institutes, certification, the development of a standard "canon" of published works. In turn, these formal institutions make it easier for cosmopolitan systems to generate a commercial base, from cash fees for service to insurance reimbursement. The resources that become available with a commercial base facilitate the use of print and electronic media, the development of formal institutions, and so forth.

Oral folk medicine traditions have retained many ideas for centuries, but other elements of folk medicine have changed very rapidly. This combination makes folk tradition very adaptable, and this is what accounts for its regional variation.

IN CLOSING

Most folk medicine traditions stress the underlying causes of disease as well as the immediate causes. The underlying causes are usually seen as some kind of imbalance or lack of harmony within the body. These causes range from sin to an improper balance of foods in the diet. A sick person may bear responsibility for the sickness, but it is also possible that the sickness is the result of someone else's wrongdoing. Folk medicine tends to have a strong moral tone, always trying to fix the blame for misfortune.

The moral element and the importance of harmony and balance are factors in folk medicine that lead to a sense of personal health's interconnectedness with the community, the physical environment, and the cosmos. This suggests a major function of all healing systems: the integration of the experience of sickness within a meaningful view of the world. Such an integration helps the sufferer to bring the maximum number of resources to bear on his illness and provides a rationale for efforts at prevention as well as treatment (such as protective amulets, blessings and pilgrimages, a good diet and exercise, and avoidance of poor social relations that could provoke witchcraft or the envy that leads to the evil eye). A rationale of this kind makes it possible to understand specific causes of disease on the basis of general principles, such as hot-cold balance or God's law. This complex, multicausal view of disease etiology and appropriate treatments has often been called the "holistic outlook" of folk medicine. This view is usually quite open to modern medical knowledge. It accepts medical ideas of etiology: It is believed a germ can cause a disease, for example. But, in folk medicine, a germ causes disease in a particular person (at a particular time) for any number of reasons, including sinfulness, evil eye, poor diet, or because of decreased vital energy.

An emphasis on a special kind of "energy" that is unique to living things is almost universal in folk medical systems, and it is crucial in mediating the concepts of harmony, balance, and integration. This energy element places folk medicine within the tradition that, in Western thought, has been called vitalism. Vitalism says that life is made possible by a non-physical kind of force, often called vital energy (from *vita*, the Latin word for life). This energy is often believed to be distinct from the physical body that it animates and to be capable of a separate existence. The idea of human souls can be an example of this kind of energy. This concept of vitalism provides links among a great variety of specific theories of healing and general physical and metaphysical theories. It is also one reason that folk medicine has such a strong affinity with religious belief.

In folk medicine, positive life energy is frequently contrasted with negative, life-destroying energies. Thus, disease may result from imbalances or the loss (or theft) of vital energy, but it may also be caused by the presence of negative energies. Both kinds of energy may be involved in natural and supernatural ideas of disease. For example, improper cooking of foods may destroy their vitality (or witchcraft may steal it), resulting in food that appears good but no longer can nourish, leading eventually to illness and death. Vital force may be taken directly, as in vampirism, or dislocated, as in soul loss. Negative thoughts may destroy the "will to live" or they may directly create disease. The powerful glance of someone with the evil eye may give a victim negative energy.

Many of the folk beliefs that involve "contagion" imply the exchange of such energies. Material objects may be endowed with negative energies and placed in the victims environment to cause illness (see "Rootwork," page 287). The residue of a victim's unique life force, which can be found in hair, nail parings, or an object long worn on the body, may serve to focus the transmission of negative force—as in black magical assault, which uses "poppets" or "voodoo dolls." The very widespread folk medical idea of the transference of disease (as to a tree or an animal) implies that disease is a form of negative energy. Positive energies, on the other hand, may be absorbed, as when fresh blood (the seat of life and vitality) is taken as a medicine.

Folk healers often view their activities as a transfer of good energy to a patient and, often, the removal of negative energy. When working on the material level, as opposed to the spiritual level, Mexican-American curanderos manipulate positive energies and expel negative vibrating energies (called *vibraciones)* with incantations and certain material "tools." This is done to correct the patient's field of vital energy. Similar ideas about energy were very popular among "magnetic healers" in the 19th century, as well as in modern alternative medical systems, such as chiropractic and homeopathy. These systems began in the 19th century, but their commitment to the idea of a special vital energy is part of what has kept them "alternative." Probably the most famous idea of vital energy in alternative medicine today is the Chinese concept of chi, also sometimes written qi (pronounced chee). This reference to the flow, transmission, and balance of life energies exists in folk medical traditions around the world and must certainly indicate the existence of some human universals in the perception of health, illness, and healing.

Another characteristic of folk medicine is that it provides meaning for disease and suffering at the same time that it seeks cause and cure. In addition to predicting and controlling suffering as much as possible, seriously sick people very often ask *why* they are sick in a moral or metaphysical sense. In religious terms, philosophers call this the question of theodicy—that is, a defense of God's goodness and omnipotence in view of the existence of evil. In the case of sickness, this evil is most often perceived as innocent suffering, as in "Why does God permit this?" The answers provided by folk medicine are extremely varied, ranging from the wickedness of others to a combined sense of the mystery of God's will and trust in God's ultimate goodness. These meanings of suffering are often very complex and serve several functions at the same time, including preventing disillusionment and alienation from religious belief; providing grounds for acceptance of suffering; and reinforcing believed methods for controlling sickness.

The complexity of these meanings illustrates another difference between folk and modern medicine: the variety of goals explicitly being served. The explicit goals of modern medicine can be briefly stated as the reducing of the harmful effects of disease. In most folk medical systems, this goal is found alongside a variety of non-medical goals; for example, assigning social responsibility for misfortune (as in witchcraft and the evil eye) and obtaining salvation in religious healing. There is also the goal of healing the environment. It is believed that preventing and healing disease in individuals can come about only in ways that also save and heal the individual's environment. So the same natural farming methods that produce foods free of toxins and high in essential nutrients also preserve the ecology and prevent the destruction of waterways by agricultural runoff. In this way, according to natural healing beliefs, the environment heals and is healed at the same time and in the same way. These broader views of healing found in folk medical beliefs generally offer sets of meaning that allow other kinds of misfortune (such as financial loss, family problems, natural

calamities) to be understood within the same framework as sickness itself.

Finally, the techniques of folk medicine are almost entirely ones that are broadly legal, require little or no technology, and are therefore available to practically everyone. Although the highly learned healer generally has a body of knowledge (plus a personal power) that requires time and special circumstances to acquire, the individual elements are nonetheless generally available to all. Thus, the materials of these systems can readily be organized into all levels of health behavior—from first aid and home treatment to the most specialized and authoritative forms. This makes it very easy for people to enter folk medical systems. Folk medicine lacks many of the official barriers found in scientific medicine, and it makes available to patients a wide range of options for varying levels of personal involvement and decision making. For many patients, this is an attractive feature of folk medicine.

In the pages to come you will find a great variety of folk medical practices. Some of these practices will seem simple, such as drinking cranberry juice to reduce the risk of urinary tract infections. Others will seem outlandish and bizarre, including those folk remedies that require animal sacrifice! The remedies described in this book come from many different communities and represent the accumulated ideas and observations of centuries of healers. Like scientific medicine, some folk medicine is obsolete, some is dangerous, and some is ahead of its time. But all of these ideas represent the struggles of human communities to make sense of disease, suffering, and death and to do something about the human condition.

—David Hufford, Ph.D.

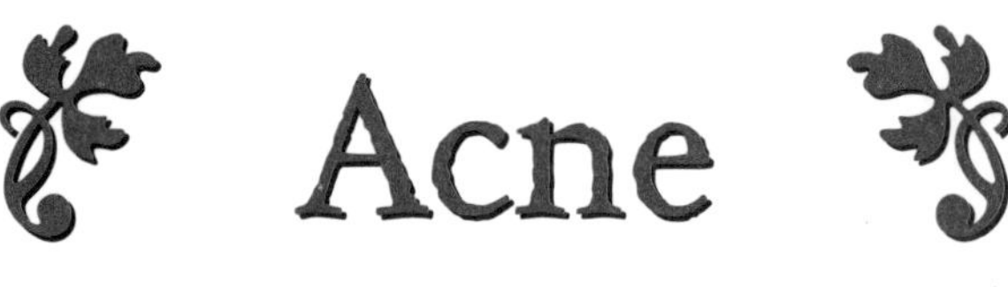

Acne

Although these folk remedies date back centuries, they have proven time and again that they have what it takes when it comes to treating acne

Acne often begins with the normal hormonal changes of puberty. The hormone testosterone increases at that time in both men and women and causes an increase in the size and secretions of the sebaceous glands in the skin that produce sebum (an oily secretion). Most excess oil produced by these glands leaves the skin through the hair follicles (the tubelike structures from which hairs develop). Sometimes, however, oil clogs these tubes and creates comedones (blocked hair follicles). Comedones are what form the initial bumps of acne.

If comedones are open to the surface of the skin, they are called blackheads. They contain sebum from the sebaceous glands, bacteria, and any skin tissue that accumulates near the surface. Comedones that are closed at the surface are called whiteheads.

Plugged hair follicles can rupture internally, resulting in a discharge of their contents into the surrounding tissues. Bacteria in the injured area can sometimes lead to more widespread inflammation and the formation of painful cysts. In severe cases, pitting and scarring result.

Acne normally resolves all by itself without specific medical treatment. For some individuals, however, acne can continue into the adult years. In women, acne may cycle with the menses, due to varying output of hormones. Oily cosmetics or moisturizers can sometimes cause acne or make an existing case worse. And although a link has not been medically proven, many people notice acne flare-ups when they're under stress. There is, however, no medical evidence to suggest that what you eat affects acne (see sidebar, "Dietary Myths and Acne," page 19).

Acne has no prevention or cure, but there are several treatments. The main treatment for mild acne is thorough cleansing with a mild soap two to three times a day. Some over-the-counter medications, particularly lotions or creams containing benzoyl peroxide, can help troubled skin as well. For persistent acne, a doctor might prescribe an antibiotic preparation that can be applied to the surface of the skin or an oral antibiotic, such as tetracycline. Antibiotics do not heal the pimples or prevent their formation, but they do prevent their infection or rupture, and subsequent inflammation of the surrounding tissues. Thus, antibiotics may also help to prevent scarring. Unfortunately, oral antibiotics can also kill the friendly bacteria

in the intestinal tract and cause unpleasant digestive side effects, such as gas, bloating, and indigestion. Antibiotics may also promote intestinal or vaginal yeast infections.

For severe acne, the drug isotretinoin may be prescribed. This drug works by temporarily suppressing the production of secretions by the sebaceous glands. This drug can have very serious side effects and should never be used without the supervision of a doctor. In fact, for patients taking isotretinoin, standard medical practice is to run routine blood and liver function tests each month to see if the drug is damaging the liver. In addition, isotretinoin should not be used by any woman who is—or who thinks she may be—pregnant. Use of this drug in any amount for even short periods during pregnancy is associated with an extremely high risk of birth defects.

Trying vitamin supplementation might make a prudent first course of action before trying prescription medications. Supplementation with zinc, for example, is one scientifically validated nutritional treatment of acne. (Some acne patients have lowered serum and tissue levels of zinc.) A 1989 double-blind clinical trial showed that zinc supplementation significantly improved the acne of the participants in the study.

Although the folk remedies that follow date back centuries, they have proven time and again that they have what it takes when it comes to treating acne.

Dietary Myths and Acne

It is commonly believed that two of the best ways to treat acne are to reduce fat and avoid chocolate. Scientific studies have not found any link between chocolate and acne (except in allergic-type reactions), but high-fat diets have been found to increase the flow of the skin's oily secretions. The advice to avoid fatty and greasy foods is consistent also with traditional Chinese medicine, which views acne as a "hot" condition and fatty foods as "heating." In Chinese medicine, "heating" foods or herbs may increase inflammation. Thus, symbolically, the fats add fuel to the fire. The herbs in this section, including burdock, canaigre, nettle, and red clover, are all considered cooling herbs in the Chinese system, and their folk use in North America is surprisingly consistent with the principles of traditional medicine in Asia. A number of scientific studies have shown that acne is a "Western disease"; that is, its incidence may be related to our modern diet because it does not appear in primitive societies that eat more traditional diets. Traditional diets lack refined foods such as sugar, white flour, and canned products. Further nutritional studies need to be carried out in the United States to verify these connections between acne and diet.

Remedies

CLAY PACKS: Many folk remedies call for the use of astringent washes and poultices. These remedies naturally absorb or "draw" the excess oily secretions out of the skin. Applying clay packs to the face is a popular acne remedy among today's Seventh Day Adventists, a religious movement that uses many natural remedies. (This remedy was also used by German immigrants at the turn of the century.) Today, you can purchase cosmetic grade clay for the same purpose.

☞ Directions: Using bentonite clay or other cosmetic clay, mix the clay into 1 cup of warm (not hot) water until it is the consistency of a thick pea soup. Apply it to the skin. Let it stay on for at least forty minutes—several hours if possible. Wipe off using water and a wash cloth. You may need to scrub with the cloth if the clay has dried completely—but don't scrub your skin too hard! Wipe the clay off over a bowl and discard the dry clay in your garden or on your lawn. (Clay can accumulate and stop up your plumbing pipes.) Repeat as often as desired.

MUNG BEANS: A Chinese folk remedy for acne is to apply a paste of mung beans to the face. The astringent properties of the beans draw the oil out of the skin.

☞ Directions: Use a coffee grinder to grind the dry mung beans to a powder. Mix with warm water and follow the instructions above for applying a clay mask.

CANAIGRE: Traditional Hispanic residents of the American Southwest use the herb canaigre *(Rumex hymenosepalus)* as a poultice to draw oil from the skin. Canaigre contains high amounts of tannin, which acts as an astringent.

☞ Directions: Chop or grind 1 ounce of the root, and simmer in 2 quarts of water for twenty minutes. Soak a cloth in the tea and apply it hot to the face for ten to fifteen minutes. Save the tea to reheat for future use. Apply the poultice once or twice a day until skin improves and complexion clears.

BURDOCK: Burdock tea has been used to treat acne throughout the eastern states and at least as far west as Indiana. Burdock *(Arctium lappa)* is slightly diaphoretic, which means it brings blood circulation to the surface of the skin to promote sweating. The increased local circulation of immune elements of the blood may help fight the infection and inflammation of acne. Burdock also contains a high amount of starch, and, applied locally, the starch may help absorb excess oils from the skin.

☞ Directions: To make a cup of burdock tea, take 1 ounce of the ground dried root and simmer it in 2 quarts of water for twenty minutes. Strain (saving the root) and drink 3 to 4 cups a day. You can also apply a poultice to the affected area. After making the tea, wrap up the leftover root in a

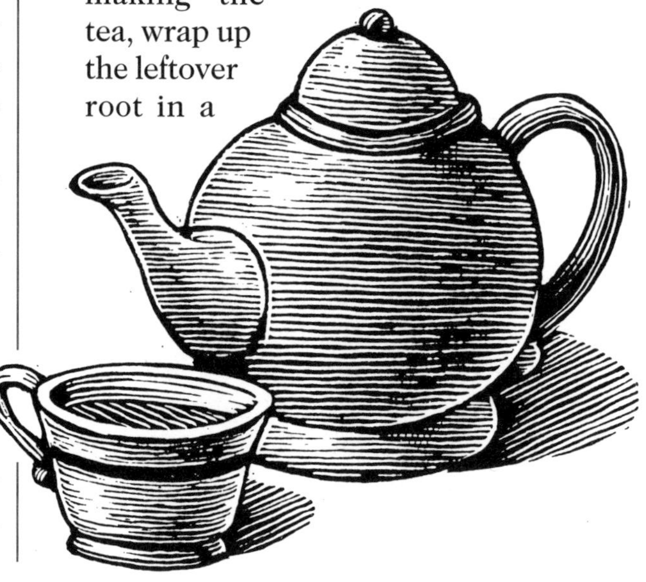

cloth. Moisten both the cloth and the root with a little of the hot tea. Apply for fifteen to twenty minutes. Do this as often as desired. Continue using until skin improves and complexion clears.

RED CLOVER: Indiana farmers today still utilize a poultice of red clover plants as a treatment for acne. Red clover *(Trifolium pratense)* contains several constituents that may thin the oily secretions of the face, making the oil easier to remove.

☞ Directions: Using just enough water to cover, simmer whole flowering red clover plants in a pot until tender. Strain, press the plants into a thick mass, and sprinkle with white flour. (The flour helps add consistency to the poultice and will help to draw the oils from the skin.) Place the poultice directly on the skin. Leave on for half an hour. You can use the red clover poultice several times a day. This poultice can last a few days if it's kept in the refrigerator between applications.

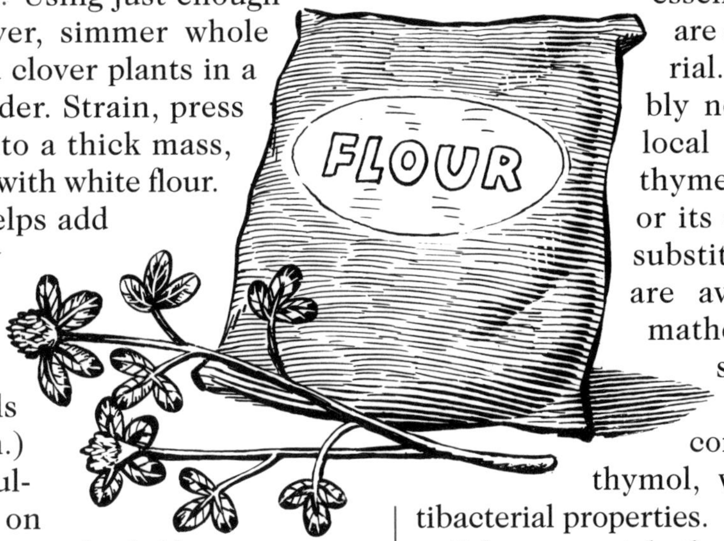

STINGING NETTLE: Drinking a tea of stinging nettle *(Urtica dioica)* is a Gypsy remedy for treating acne. You can also apply stinging nettle tea as a face wash. Nettle is astringent and drying and may help reduce the oily secretions of the skin.

☞ Directions: Place 1 ounce of dried stinging nettle leaf in a 1-quart canning jar. Fill the jar with boiling water. Cover and let sit overnight or until the water reaches room temperature. Drink 2 to 3 cups a day. You can also reheat a portion of the tea and apply it to the face as a warm wash once or twice a day. Handle carefully to avoid the plant's stinging hairs.

ESSENTIAL OILS: The Winnebago Indians of the last century treated acne by making a poultice of the boiled leaves of the wild bergamot plant *(Monarda fistulosa)*. Besides the oil-absorbing properties of the leaves, the essential oils of the plant are drying and antibacterial. This plant is probably not available in your local store, but common thyme *(Thymus vulgaris)* or its essential oil may be substituted. Essential oils are available where aromatherapy products are sold. Both wild bergamot and thyme contain the volatile oil thymol, which has mild antibacterial properties.

Other essential oils used as folk remedies for acne include the oils of juniper, thyme, and rose. If you decide to use essential oils, be sure to dilute them with alcohol or glycerin before applying them to the skin, however. Some pure concentrated oils can cause second- and third-degree skin burns if left in place for too long.

☞ Directions: Use a pleasant carrier oil or cream such as almond oil or cold cream. Use 6 to 8 drops of the concentrated oil for each ounce of the carrier. Mix well and apply to the face. Wipe off after twenty minutes. Apply once a day. Continue to use until skin improves. Avoid the eye area.

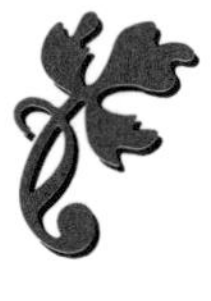

Allergies, Hives, and Hay Fever

For millions of Americans, each change of season brings its own brand of allergies and irritants—and a variety of folk remedies

Our bodies are constantly assaulted by substances from the environment, in the form of bacteria, viruses, molds, dust, pollen, and other potential invaders. Our immune system reacts to these substances through chemical and blood responses that attempt to neutralize the invaders or eliminate them from the body. One specialized immune response is the allergic reaction, in which specialized cells stimulated by an invading substance release the chemical histamine into the tissues. The histamine can cause swelling, increased circulation, and sneezing, actions designed to isolate the invader, eliminate it, or render it harmless. An allergic reaction can occur in the respiratory tract, digestive tract, skin, or eyes.

An allergic reaction is a healthy, protective response to an invader, but, in some individuals, the body overreacts, and the uncomfortable reactions are far in excess of what is necessary to neutralize the offending substance. The most noticeable allergic symptoms are sneezing, red swollen eyes, shortness of breath (in asthma), rashes, eczema, or the swelling that accompanies insect bites and stings. Food allergies can also cause symptoms in the digestive tract, but these are usually less noticeable to the sufferer than the external reactions above. The worst type of allergic reaction—called anaphylaxis—is an overwhelming allergic reaction that can lead to death. Any swelling of the airways or shortness of breath during an allergic reaction is a medical emergency.

Allergies tend to run in families, so some people may be genetically predisposed to having them. It has also been suggested that nutrient deficiencies common in the modern diet may also contribute to allergies. Dietary deficiencies of calcium and magnesium, which are common deficiencies in Americans, can also increase allergic symptoms. Studies have shown that the body's stores of vitamin C correlate inversely with the release of histamine during an allergy attack, so an abundant dietary intake of vitamin C may reduce allergy symptoms. Omega-3 essential fatty acids, such as occur naturally in cold-water fish and wild game, are also natural anti-inflammatory substances that can reduce the intensity of allergies.

Antihistamine drugs and avoidance of allergens are the most common conventional

treatments for symptoms of allergy. The drugs work by blocking the effects of histamine in the tissues, but they do not reduce its release. Desensitization involves medical treatments where small amounts of an allergen may also be injected into the body in the form of allergy shots in order to reduce the body's reaction to it.

The folk remedies listed here do not address the cause of allergies but may reduce allergy symptoms through their astringent or anti-inflammatory actions. Also, avoid herbal remedies that are made up of flower parts (such as chamomile and echinacea) because these contain allergic pollen.

Remedies

ALLERGIES AND HAY FEVER

HORSERADISH: Horseradish *(Armoracia rusticana)*, popular today as a sushi condiment, was an early American folk remedy for hay fever. If you've used it as a condiment, you're probably well aware that it causes watery eyes and a burning sensation in the sinus tissues. These effects are due to its constituent allyl-isothiocyanate, which is related chemically to the substances in watercress, red radish, and brown and yellow mustard. Scientific studies have shown that allyl-isothiocyanate has decongestant and antiasthmatic properties.

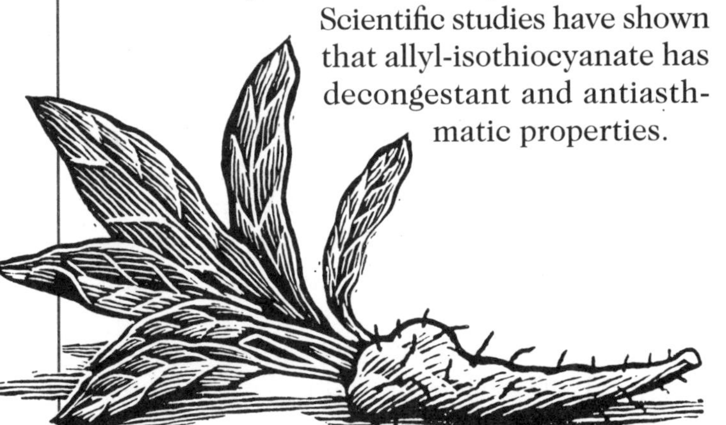

☞ Directions: Purchase grated horseradish as a condiment. Take a dose of ¼ teaspoon during a congestive hay fever attack. You can take horseradish as often as desired—or as much as you can stand!

An alternate method, if you have access to fresh horseradish root, comes from an old New England remedy. Take fresh horseradish roots, wash, and blend, skin and all, in your blender. Fill half of a 1-quart jar with the ground roots. Add enough vinegar to cover the roots, and close the jar tightly. Store the jar at room temperature. When suffering a hay fever attack, remove the cap, place your nose into the jar, and sniff or inhale. (Do this carefully at first to avoid irritating your nose and eyes.) Quickly replace the cap to keep the remaining aromatic substances from escaping. This treatment requires fresh-ground horseradish; most likely, it will lose its potency after four or five days.

HORSEMINT: In the folk medicine of southern Appalachia, horsemint *(Monarda punctata)* is a traditional treatment for hay fever. Horsemint may be inhaled, or you can drink it as a simple tea. Horsemint is not readily available in stores today, but its antiallergic constituent is probably the essential oil thymol. Scientific studies have shown that thymol reduces swelling in the bronchial tract, relaxes the trachea, and acts as an anti-inflammatory and mild antibacterial. The kitchen spice thyme also contains large amounts of this aromatic oil and can be substituted for horsemint.

☞ Directions: Place ½ ounce of ground thyme in a 1-pint jar and cover with boiling water. Close the jar tightly and let the mixture cool for half an hour. Remove the lid and inhale, taking a few deep breaths. Do this as needed throughout the day.

The Hair of the Dog That Bit You

In *Herbal Medicine Past and Present* (Volume I), by John K. Crellin and Jane Philpott, a traditional Appalachian herbalist named Tommie Bass, of northern Georgia, says: "You can make a tea from ragweed, or anything else you are allergic to, and drink 2 to 3 cupfuls while you have an allergy." According to Bass, who participated in a major study of folk medicine in the northern Georgia region during the 1980s, the method often works just "like an allergy shot."

Other folk remedies, originating in both Texas and the Ozark mountains, also call for the ingestion of substances to which you are allergic, such as locally grown bee pollen or honey. If you treat allergies in this manner, you may be taking a gamble, however. While the method undoubtedly works for some individuals, others may experience a worsening of allergies. And though rare, a life-threatening allergic reaction called anaphylaxis can occur from consuming pollen or teas from plants you are allergic to.

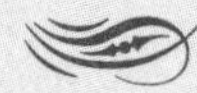

CHAMOMILE AND THYME OIL: German immigrants inhaled the fumes of chamomile tea *(Matricaria recutita)* to treat bouts of hay fever. In contemporary German naturopathic medicine, 3 to 5 drops of the essential oil of thyme is added to chamomile tea for the same purpose. (The action of thyme oil is described under the remedy Horsemint.) Chamomile contains the essential oil azulene and related oils that are anti-inflammatory and antiallergic, as well as the oil alpha-bisabolol, which is also an anti-inflammatory.

☞ Directions: Place ½ ounce of chamomile flowers in a 1-quart jar. Fill two thirds of the jar with boiling water. Add 3 to 5 drops of essential oil of thyme. Cover and let cool for half an hour. Open the lid and inhale the fumes, taking a few deep breaths. Repeat as desired throughout the day. (Be careful of inhaling chamomile flower dust, because the pollen causes allergy in some people.)

MINT TEAS: Inhaling, drinking, or washing affected skin areas with mint teas can be accredited in this country to the folk medicine of the Seneca Indians. The plants used to make the teas are peppermint *(Mentha piperita)* and spearmint *(Mentha spicata)*. In China, cornmint *(Mentha arvensis)*, which is similar in its chemical composition to peppermint, is used. (Mint teas have been used to treat allergies in China at least since the 7th century A.D.)

When consumed as a tea or inhaled, the essential oils in the mints act as a decongestant. When applied to the skin, the menthol

in peppermint and cornmint produces a cooling sensation and reduces itching. (Spearmint contains little menthol, however, so it does not have this effect on the skin.) All three of the mints contain other anti-inflammatory and mild antibacterial constituents.

☞ Directions: Place ½ ounce of dried mint leaves in a 1-quart jar. Fill two thirds of the jar with boiling water and cover the jar tightly. Let cool for half an hour. Strain and drink. The tea's fumes will also help relieve congestion.

EYEBRIGHT: The use of eyebright *(Euphrasia officinalis)* to treat allergies in the eastern United States dates back at least 150 years and may have had its roots among German immigrants. At the turn of the century, Eclectic physicians, a group of M.D.s who used mostly herbs as medicines, also used eyebright to treat allergy symptoms among their patients (see sidebar, "Eclectic Medicine," page 29). During the same period, the pharmaceutical companies Parke Davis and Eli Lilly sold eyebright allergy preparations to the public. Eyebright is still used today in Appalachia as a folk remedy for allergies.

Eyebright contains the constituents caffeic acid and ferulic acid, both of which have an anti-inflammatory effect. The caffeic acid also has specific antihistamine effects.

☞ Directions: You can purchase eyebright tincture in a health food store or herb shop. Take a dropperful every three to four hours during the height of allergy season.

Another option is to make your own tincture. Place 2 ounces of dried eyebright leaves in a 1-pint jar and fill the jar with grain alcohol or 100 proof gin or vodka. Cover the jar and let it stand in a cool, dark place for three weeks, shaking the jar each day. After three weeks, strain and store the solution in the refrigerator. Take as directed above.

HIVES AND ALLERGIC REACTIONS

BASIL TEA: A traditional Chinese folk remedy for treating hives is to bathe the skin in basil tea. Basil contains high amounts of caffeic acid, one of the key anti-allergic constituents also contained in eyebright.

☞ Directions: Place 1 ounce of dried basil leaves in a 1-quart jar and fill the jar with

continued on page 29

Bringing out Hives

In traditional African-American folk medicine, hives in a young baby are considered a good sign. It is believed that through hives, impurities in the body are released. In fact, some individuals believe that a fussy baby's mood can only improve if hives break out. Thus, catnip tea is sometimes given to relax a fussy baby and to help "bring out hives." Using catnip for this purpose is also a widespread practice among southern Appalachian whites, although it lacks any scientific verification.

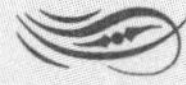

Animal Cures: Down on the Farm

Folk medicine has always made use of materials that are readily on hand, including common foods, such as honey and vinegar, and plants. Animals, numerous and easily accessible in rural life, have also figured prominently into the folk remedies of all cultures. But, while patients use them in the hopes of bringing about health benefits, the animals usually get the short end of the stick.

Some reported animal remedies appear so unreal that it's hard to believe they were ever really used. For example, one man in Illinois claimed that a woman could avoid headaches by binding a live toad to her forehead. Toads are commonly used in remedies, but, as a long term preventive, this seems more like a cruel joke, not a practical recommendation!

At the other end of the spectrum there are remedies that are very similar to the conventional treatments we use today. For instance, mutton tallow—the fat from sheep—was used in folk remedies to prevent and treat chapped hands and lips. In fact, all sorts of animal fats have long been used as emollients to soften and soothe skin. Today we use lanolin, an oil obtained from sheep wool, for the same purpose.

DOGS AND CATS: Cats and dogs evoke great loyalty from their human owners. Perhaps that is the reason these animals are not used in folk remedies as often as other domesticated animals. Nonetheless, there have been some uses reported. In the Southwest, it is said that if a Mexican Chihuahua sleeps on your bed, you will be cured of rheumatism. (The same has been said about guinea pigs, especially by the Slavic and German Americans.) For some, the belief is that the remedy works by transferring the rheumatism from the patient to the animal. Others believed that the remedy is advantageous to the health of the animal and the owner alike. Chihuahuas kept in the house are also said to prevent asthma. This belief probably originates from the fact that the dander from furry pets is a potent allergen, and Chihuahuas have very little fur.

The few reported remedies involving cats are less

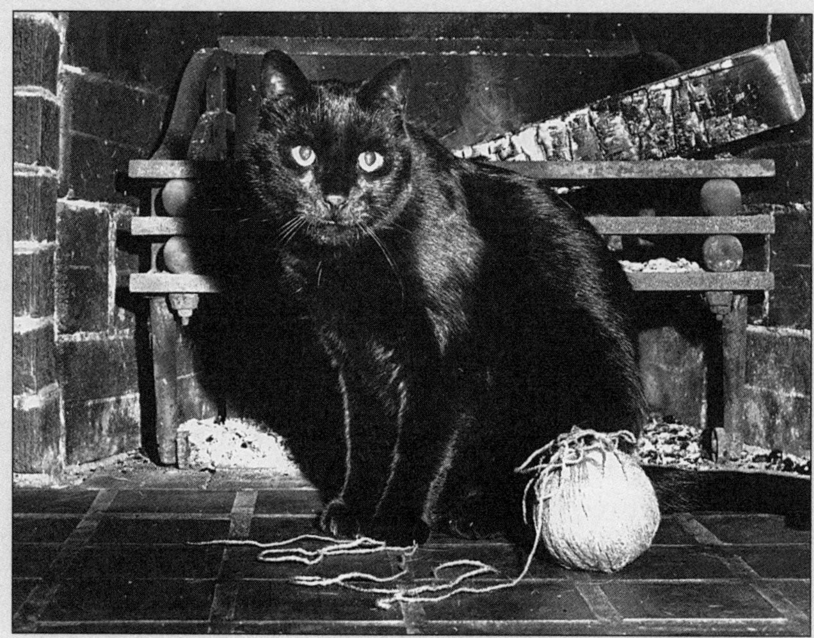

In folk medicine, some turn to the black cat as a cure-all.

favorable to the animals' well being. In Georgia, it has been said that to cure shingles (a painful infection by the herpes zoster virus that is accompanied by skin eruptions) a person should rub the blood of a black cat on the inflamed area. An even more gruesome treatment for shingles, found both in the Midwest and among Pennsylvania Germans, says to paint the shingles with the blood from the stump of a black cat's tail! An African-American remedy uses the black cat's blood on a lump of sugar to be taken internally.

In the United States and Europe, it is widely believed that cat's fur worn against the skin will absorb arthritic pain, and, as recently as the 1960s, cats' pelts were sold in French drugstores for this purpose. In Utah, wearing cat's fur against the skin is believed by some to cure tuberculosis and pneumonia.

CHICKENS: Farm animals figure more prominently into folk medicine, probably because butchering is inevitable for many of these animals. Chickens are used quite prominently in folk medicine—and we should remember that chicken soup is still widely reputed to have healing properties. Most medicinal uses of chickens have been much less savory and far from kosher, however! One treatment for colitis (inflammation of the large intestine) is a "tea" made by steeping a whole chicken—complete with feathers—in water. Some believe chicken blood, especially the blood of a black chicken, has healing qualities. A cure for shingles from Georgia involves pulling the head off a live black hen and holding the carcass so that the blood flows over the affected body part. A cloth is wrapped around the patient to catch the blood and the blood is then used as a dressing. The cloth is left in place until it falls off on its own accord—at which time the shingles will be gone. The same use of a black chicken's blood, for both shingles and hives, has been reported in remedies from the Midwest.

In some remedies it is the blood and meat that

Hog Magic

Hogs are famous for being completely consumable–right down to their squeal! So it is not surprising that even hogs' feet can be used in a tea (with pine buds and resin) for respiratory ailments. But some cures involving hogs were surprisingly magical. For example, a sore neck could be treated by rubbing it against a tree where a hog had rubbed; mumps were treated by rubbing the swollen areas with marrow from a hog jaw or by rubbing an ailing child's jaw on a pig trough. And, if the patient was too ill to get to the trough, the hog was brought to the sickroom so the child could rub his jaw directly on the hog's jowl!

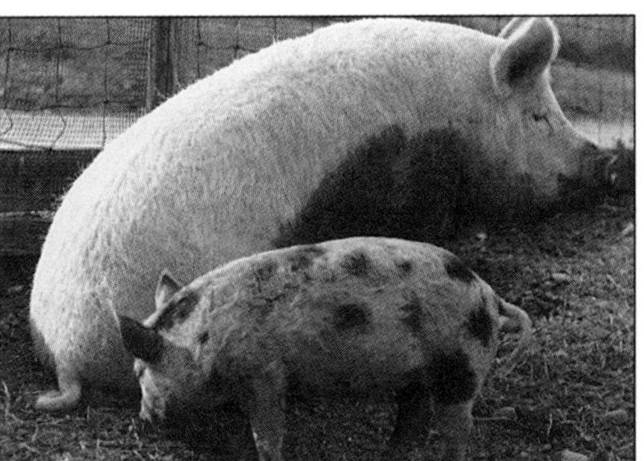

Hogs were used to remedy illnesses.

Animal Cures: Down on the Farm

affect the cure, as in the following treatment for snake bite, reported in Illinois. A chicken was split and one half of the raw carcass was tied over the bite area to draw out the poison. (While this practice may sound bizarre, realize that many people still believe that blood can be drawn from a bruise by holding a raw steak against it, especially in the case of a black eye.) A similar treatment from Maryland used additional magical elements: The raw split chicken (preferably black in color) was put on the feet of a feverish patient, while the chicken's feathers were burnt under the patient's bed. Finally, also from Maryland, a remedy that even the chicken could survive: Children with chicken pox were put in front of a chicken house so that chickens could fly over them. Like many animal remedies, this one probably has its origins in the belief that the disease can be transferred from the patient to the animal (see "Magical Transference," page 58).

HORSES AND MULES: At one time there were almost as many horses and mules as there were chickens, and the animals were equally valued in folk medicine. However, while chickens were expendable, horses and mules were not—most of the remedies left these larger animals completely intact! For example, in Georgia it has been said that sore eyes can be cured by washing them in a mule's watering trough, and, in both California and Utah, it has been reported that a toothache can be cured by kissing a mule. But most often it is the breath of horses and mules that seems to be the most powerful. In Illinois, it is said that kissing the nostrils of a mule will cure catarrh (inflammation of the nose and throat) and that tonsillitis is cured by having a horse blow in the patient's mouth. In California, if the horse is a full-bred stallion, his breath can be used to cure whooping cough (a serious scourge of childhood prior to pertussis vaccination). Other horse and mule remedies seem purely magical, such as the idea that sleeping in the hay with horses will relieve tuberculosis or that children's respiratory illnesses can be cured by simply being passed under the belly of a mule or horse.

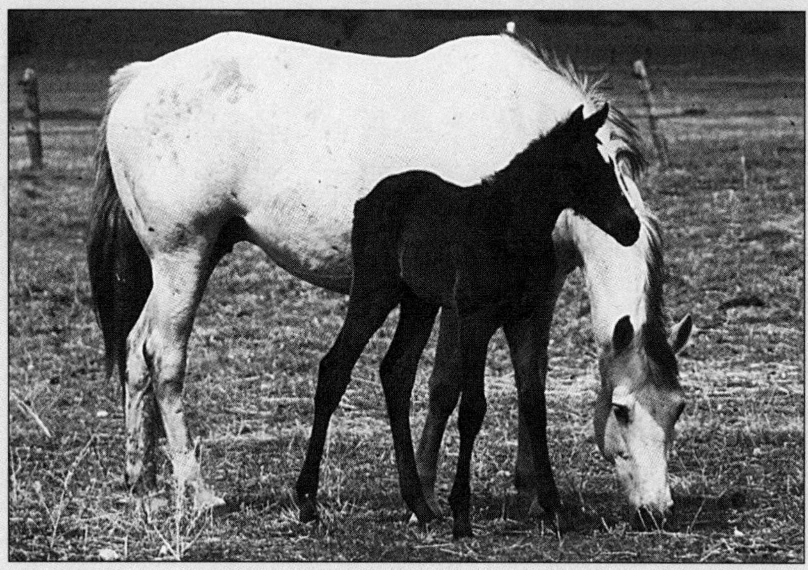

Remedies using horses usually left the animals completely intact.

Eclectic Medicine

The Eclectic movement was formed in the late 1820s and 1830s by medical doctors who were disgruntled with the medical methods used at the time, such as bloodletting and the administration of poisonous minerals like mercury. They sought knowledge of the "new" North American plants, ("new" compared to their knowledge of European plants) and turned to American Indian traditions and the folk medicine of the early states for inspiration. They formally named themselves "Eclectics" in the 1840s and began to experiment clinically with many herbal medicines. By 1900, the Eclectics had a number of medical schools throughout the country and produced sophisticated textbooks on clinical herbalism. During the first two decades of the 20th century, under pressure from the political organizations of more conventional doctors, the Eclectic schools lost their accreditation, and their graduates were denied licensing. The Eclectic Institute, the last Eclectic medical school, graduated the last group of Eclectic physicians in 1939.

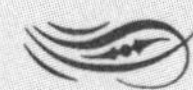

boiling water. Cover the jar tightly and let cool to room temperature. Use the solution as a wash for hives or itchy allergic skin rashes as often as needed.

ASAFOETIDA: Asafoetida *(Ferula assafoetida),* a relative of onions and garlic that is sometimes called "devil's dung," is a popular Alabama folk remedy for hives. Asafoetida contains the volatile constituents ferulic acid and umbelliferone, both of which have an anti-inflammatory effect. Umbelliferone also has an antiallergic effect.

☞ Directions: Add ¼ teaspoon of asafoetida powder (available in many supermarkets in the spice section) to 4 tablespoons of warm castor oil. Mix well. Apply the solution directly to hives. Be aware that this material has a strong, garlic-like odor.

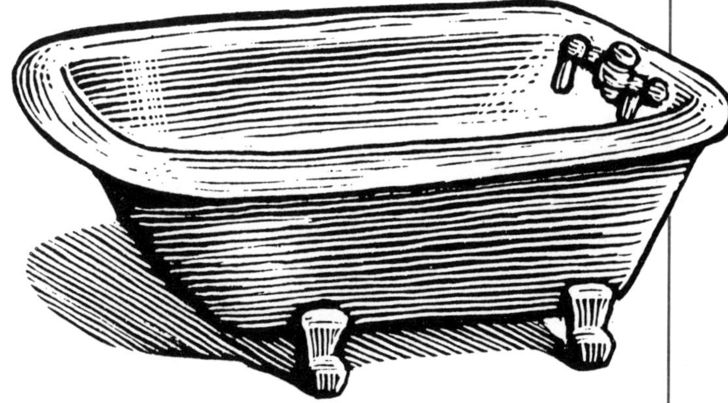

BAKING SODA BATHS: Taking a baking soda bath is an old New England folk remedy for soothing hives.

☞ Directions: Place a few handfuls of baking soda in warm bath water and soak for twenty to thirty minutes. You can enjoy baking soda baths as often as you like.

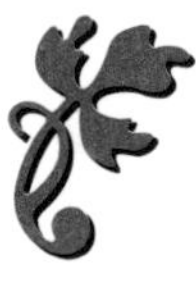

Anxiety and Nervousness

Probably no single situation or condition causes anxiety disorders. Rather, physical and environmental triggers may combine to create a particular anxiety illness

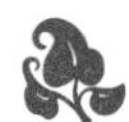

Everyone experiences some anxiety. Anxiety helps us stay alert and adapt to the ever-changing demands of our environment. Anxiety is really the body's "early warning system" against harm. When we feel danger, the alarm goes off to warn us and prevent injury. The body responds immediately to the alarm emotionally, physically, and behaviorally. Emotionally, we may feel fear, doom, or anger. Physically, our hearts race, muscles tense, breathing becomes rapid, and palms and feet start to sweat. We respond behaviorally by getting ready to fight or flee from danger.

The anxiety warning system works fine when there's clear and present danger, but anxiety can become a problem for people when they perceive harmless situations or people as threatening.

There is no single reason why some people experience episodes of chronic anxiety. Some of these individuals will benefit from visiting a psychotherapist, who can help them sort out internal conflicts or past conditioning that may be causing the emotional state. Any physical change, such as illness, can also cause anxiety. Anemia, diabetes, premenstrual syndrome, menopause, thyroid disorder, hypoglycemia, pulmonary disease, endocrine tumors, and other conditions can cause anxiety symptoms. Other individuals simply need to improve their nutrition and lifestyle—anxiety can be the symptom of several nutrient deficiencies or lifestyle habits that are common in modern society.

One of the most commonly overlooked causes of anxiety and nervousness in modern life is related to caffeine consumption. Even moderate amounts of caffeine can create nervous symptoms severe enough to earn a diagnosis of chronic anxiety—and a subsequent prescription of sedative drugs or referral to a therapist. The table on page 31 shows some symptoms of "caffeinism," taken from turn-of-the-century medical books, and compares them to symptoms of chronic anxiety found in contemporary medical literature.

You don't need to take a lot of caffeine in order to experience these symptoms. Some of us can get away with drinking a few cups

Symptoms of Caffeinism	Symptoms of Chronic Anxiety
anxiety	apprehension
tremors	trembling
insomnia	insomnia
nervous irritability	nervousness
hysteria	irrational thinking
heart palpitations	heart palpitations
mental confusion	difficult concentration
muscular weakness	motor weakness
physical exhaustion	chronic fatigue
headaches	headaches

of coffee every day, but others can develop the symptoms of caffeinism even from a small amount. In one scientific study, patients with anxiety disorder rated their symptoms on a standard test. Their levels of anxiety and depression correlated directly with the amount of caffeine they consumed. In another study, a group of six anxiety patients who consumed the caffeine equivalent of 1.5 to 3.5 cups of coffee—about the average daily intake for Americans—cut their intake to zero. Within 12 to 18 months, five of the six patients no longer experienced symptoms of anxiety.

One scientific theory suggests that anxiety is closely associated with the balance of the substances lactate and pyruvate in the body. These two substances are associated with energy production within the cells, and high lactate levels may cause anxiety. Alcohol, caffeine, and sugar all increase lactate levels, and the B-vitamins niacin and thiamine and the mineral magnesium all lower it. Deficiencies of the B-vitamins as well as omega-3 fatty acids, such as occur naturally in fish and wild game, may thus contribute to anxiety.

Conventional treatment of anxiety is primarily with drugs of the benzodiazepine class, such as Valium and Xanax. Anxiety patients are often treated by psychotherapists as well. Below are some natural remedies you can try to help ease feelings of stress and anxiety.

Remedies

VALERIAN: In folk medicine, valerian is considered a universal sedative. The Greeks used valerian as a relaxant and antispasmodic. The herb was also used in the folk medicine of India, Tibet, and Japan. Today, Mexicans and Mexican-Americans use varieties of the plant native to their regions. An African-American folk remedy from Louisiana is to put valerian root in a pillow and inhale its fragrance as you sleep. Valerian continues to be used as a sedative among today's Appalachians as well.

Valeriana officinalis, the European variety of the plant, was brought to the eastern colonies by immigrants for cultivation. It has

Driving Out Evil Spirits

Several of the sedative herbs in this section have been used traditionally to "drive out evil spirits" or to treat epilepsy, which in ancient times was considered to be a form of possession. Both valerian and rosemary are still used today in ritual purifications in southwestern and Mexican folk medicine.

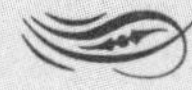

subsequently become native in the eastern United States. Valerian is recognized today as an official medicine for nervousness and anxiety by the German government. Its suspected active constituents are its essential oils. Valerian has proven to be as effective as the sedative Valium in some clinical trials, although it has no relationship chemically to that drug.

Valerian can cause stimulation rather than sedation in some individuals, however, especially those with "hot" constitutions, as might be indicated by feelings of warmth, by red flushed cheeks, and by desire for cool drinks. According to Chinese medicine, this strong "fire-type" personality should avoid alcohol and stimulating foods and, instead, balance their excess heat with cooling foods and calming herbs. Heating herbs such as valerian increase circulation, which is already excessive in those with a hot nature.

☞ Directions: Place 2 to 3 teaspoons of dried chopped valerian root in a cup and cover with boiling water. Cover the cup and let stand for fifteen minutes. Drink 2 to 3 cups a day for up to three weeks. Individuals who use valerian for longer than three weeks, or who use valerian to help them get to sleep, can ultimately develop lethargy and experience hangover-like effects.

Here is a recipe from gypsy folk medicine for valerian wine: Take 2 handfuls of chopped valerian root, 1 whole clove, 1 orange rind, 1 sprig of rosemary, and 1 quart of dry white wine. Place the dried herbs in a 1-quart jar and cover with the wine. Seal the container and allow to stand in a cool dark place for one cycle of the moon. Strain and store. Take 1 tablespoon of the mixture three times a day for up to three weeks. It should be noted that valerian has a disagreeable odor.

VALERIAN AND HOP: German immigrants of the late 18th century treated nervousness with a mixture of equal portions of valerian *(Valeriana officinalis)* and hop *(Humulus lupulus)*. Commercial combinations of these two herbs are still popular in Germany today. Hop has also been used as a sedative among British immigrants, Seventh Day Adventists, Indiana farmers, and residents of the American Southwest.

☞ Directions: Mix equal amounts by volume of dried and chopped valerian root and hop in a bowl. Place 1 tablespoon of the mixture in a cup and fill the cup

Hydrotherapy

The Seventh Day Adventist religion, which arose in the mid-1800s and advocates the use of natural remedies, remains an influential force in American folk medicine. The Seventh Day Adventists use a famous water treatment called a "neutral bath" to soothe nervousness or nervous exhaustion. In a neutral bath, the patient relaxes in water that is kept within a degree or two above body temperature for 20 to 40 minutes. Also, a cool compress placed on the head of a particularly agitated patient can prove to be very soothing.

with boiling water. Cover the cup and let stand for twenty minutes. Strain and drink 3 cups a day. Take nightly for up to three weeks.

CATNIP: Catnip tea has been used as a popular sleep aid in America since the arrival of European immigrants in New England. The popularity of the tea spread rapidly in the New World, and American Indians soon adopted its use. The Onondaga and Cayuga Indian tribes used it to calm restless children, and European New Englanders gave it to adults for nervous disorders, including nervous breakdown. Today, catnip remains a common folk remedy among residents of Appalachia.

☞ Directions: Place 1 to 3 teaspoons of the dried herb in a cup and cover with boiling water. Cover the cup and let stand for ten minutes. Strain and drink 3 cups a day. Use as needed.

An Endangered Sedative

Lady's slipper (*Cypripedium spp.*), an orchid native to swamps, bogs, and rocky places throughout the United States and Canada, was the universal medicine among American Indians residing in those types of areas. European colonists quickly adopted it as a valerian substitute. It was an official medicine, listed as a sedative in the *United States Pharmacopoeia* from 1863 to 1916. Due to loss of habitat and overharvesting, however, lady's slipper has practically disappeared from the marketplace in North America. Contemporary American herbalists consider it unethical to use this endangered species as a medicine.

SKULLCAP: More than a hundred species of skullcap *(Scutellaria spp.)* grow throughout the world. North American varieties of the herb were used by American Indian tribes such as the Penobscot, Iroquois, and Cherokee to treat diarrhea and heart disease and to promote menstruation and eliminate afterbirth. Skullcap received its common name, mad dog weed, in the 18th century, when the herb was widely prescribed as a cure for rabies. It is still used today in Appalachian folk medicine as a sedative. The suspected medicinal constituents are flavonoids and an essential oil.

☞ Directions: Put 2 or 3 teaspoonfuls of dried skullcap leaves in a cup and fill with boiling water. Cover and let steep for fifteen minutes. Strain and drink 3 to 4 cups a day as needed.

ROSEMARY: European and Spanish immigrants brought the herb rosemary *(Rosmarinus officinalis)* with them to cultivate in the New World. Rosemary was later used by early Californians to rid the body of "evil spirits" or to treat epilepsy, which in ancient times was considered to be a form of possession.

Rosemary has long been used in European and Chinese folk medicine to calm the nerves. Medical experts in the United States continue to recommend rosemary to treat ner-

continued on page 36

Measuring Health

Measurement is such a universal aspect of modern medicine that we often take its scientific nature for granted. Quantitative assessment plays a large role in modern medical practice and is used throughout life—from the time a new baby is weighed and measured until a senior citizen's potential bone loss is calculated. Measurement in diagnosis and treatment was a part of ancient medicine, too. In the first century, measurement was recorded in the works of the Roman naturalist Pliny the Elder. It has been a standard part of folk medicine ever since.

In folk medicine, just the act of measuring accords a great deal of power. In fact, in many parts of the United States, people believed that measuring a child under the age of one was very dangerous. It was said that doing so symbolized measuring the child for a coffin! Others believed that early measuring could stunt a child's growth.

In folk medicine, the most basic measuring technique uses a string or thread to measure—first from head to toe and then from fingertips to fingertips, with arms outstretched. According to early ideas of bodily proportion, these two measurements were supposed to be equal. If they were not, it was an indication that the patient was out of balance or had "lost his measure." A different kind of diagnostic measuring was reported from Kentucky, where it was said that if a "delicate" child was not three times as tall as his diameter, he had "decay." Although these kinds of diagnostic measurings are no longer common in American folk medicine, their use has been reported in Virginia, Pennsylvania, and Maryland.

The most common diagnostic measuring in American folk medicine compares the length of the foot to the child's height. Popular belief generally holds that the height should be seven times the length of the foot, from the heel to the tips of the toes. If the measurement is not in this proportion, it is a sign of wasting sickness. Once referred to as a "nonthrifty" child, today the condition would be called "failure to thrive."

Measuring for the treatment of disease involves using strings or threads of specific colors. In Illinois, for example, erysipelas (an acute infectious disease of the skin; also called "St. Anthony's Fire") was treated by using three different strings—one red, one white, and one blue. Sometimes, disposal of the measuring strings suggested that magical transference was at work.

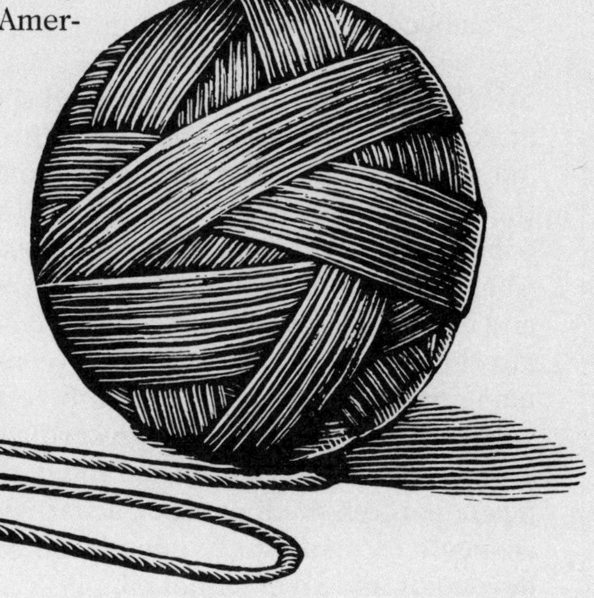

In Pennsylvania, erysipelas was treated by measurement with a red string that then had to be burned in the fireplace. In Virginia, the string was made into a loop through which the child was passed nine times. It was crucial the loop did not touch the floor. Then the string was placed somewhere where it would wear out quickly. As the string wore away, it was believed that the child would recover. In Indiana, a similar ritual was used for children of abnormally short stature. After measuring the child, a loop was made, the child stepped through, and the loop was brought up over his head. This was done three times while the practitioner said "In the name of the Father, Son, and Holy Ghost, Amen." A variety of folk healers might use such practices. In some parts of the country, in Illinois for example, these healers are called "string doctors."

Other uses of measurement in healing deal with asthma and croup, two airway illnesses that can cause frightening respiratory distress. Asthma is a chronic airway disease characterized by wheezing when the patient exhales. Croup is brought on by upper respiratory infection and causes wheezing when the patient breathes in. These distinctions are not consistently made in folk medical terminology, however, so the cures for asthma and croup are often interchangeable and can also apply to other respiratory illnesses such as bronchitis.

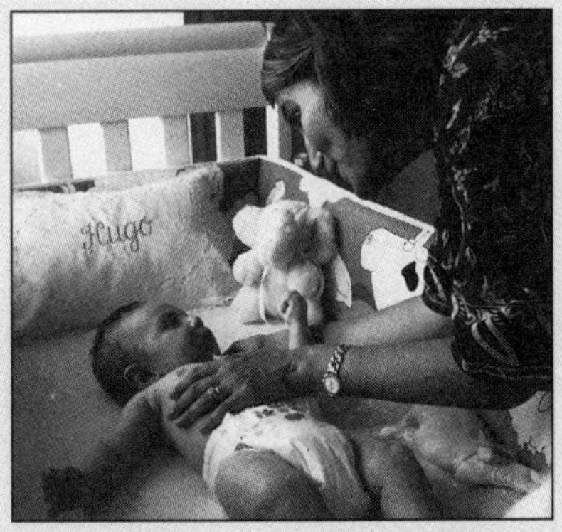

Abnormal growth of a child is always a parent's concern.

One cure for croup that is found in Maryland has counterparts all over America and Europe. A healer (or parent) must drill a hole in a door frame at the height of the sick child's head. The healer then places a lock of the child's hair in the hole. The hair plug is cut even with the frame. When the child has grown past the plug, it is believed the croup will be gone for good.

In California, exactly the same practice has been reported to cure asthma, along with another asthma cure that calls for plugging a lock of the child's hair in a window sill. The Maryland cure, however, brings in an additional magical element: The cure specifies that the measurement be done at sunrise.

In addition to strings, asthma cures often used sticks during measurement treatments. For example, in Tennessee in the 1930s, it was reportedly popular to treat asthma by measuring the child with a sourwood stick. The stick was then left in a dry place where the child couldn't see it. When the child grew taller than the stick, the asthma was expected to go away.

Airway diseases are often worse in young children because, compared to adults, their small airways have more difficulty coping with mucus. Thus, it may be that these remedies that require measuring and the growth of the child are simply "marking time"—and waiting for maturation of the airways.

Although ritual measurement is not limited to the diagnosis and treatment of children in American folk medicine, that is by far its most common use. Perhaps this is to be expected since childhood is a time when growth is normal—and abnormal growth is always a cause of serious concern.

American Ginseng

American ginseng (*Panax quinquefolius*) grows in the Appalachian mountains and has long been used as a sedative and tonic by the people who live there. A related species of ginseng, *Panax ginseng*, is perhaps the most famous tonic herb in China, although Chinese herbalists use that plant as a stimulant rather than a sedative.

In the early 1700s, Jesuit priests noticed American ginseng growing in the Canadian woods and initiated export of the plant to China. Some 100,000 tons have been shipped there in the last 250 years. Ginseng harvesting and export became an important economic force in the early American colonies, among American Indians and traders alike. Wild ginseng is now almost extinct in North America, but large quantities are grown commercially in Michigan and Wisconsin, mostly for export to China, where demand for it remains high.

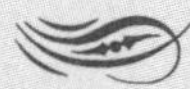

vous conditions. Rosemary's analgesic and antispasmodic properties are also recognized by the German government; the herb is used there as an official medical treatment for spastic conditions, including epilepsy.

☞ Directions: Add 1 or 2 teaspoons of the dried herb to a cup and fill the cup with boiling water. Cover the cup and let stand ten minutes. Strain and drink 2 to 3 cups a day as needed.

VERVAIN: Vervain *(Verbena spp.)* has long been used in folk medicine as a sedative among residents of the Southwest and Appalachia. It has been used in European medicine since antiquity for the same purposes. Its constituent verbenalin promotes relaxation. Vervain is claimed to be especially useful for recovery from the exhaustion of long-term stress.

☞ Directions: Add 1 or 2 teaspoons of the dried herb to a cup and fill with boiling water. Cover the cup and let stand ten minutes. Strain and drink 2 to 3 cups a day as needed.

PASSION FLOWER: Of 19 passion flower species worldwide, eight have been used as sedatives by various cultures. Passion flower *(Passiflora incarnata)* is native from Florida to Texas and may also be found as far north as Missouri. The herb is abundant in South America; it's long-time use as a sedative there is recorded in Brazilian folk medicine.

The passion flower species *P. incarnata* was introduced into American professional medicine in 1840 after medical doctors in Mississippi experimented with it and demonstrated its sedative effects. Thereafter the herb was mainly used by doctors of the Eclectic school (see "Eclectic Medicine," page 29). Passion flower is still popularly used as a sedative among residents of southern Appalachia and among the Amish. The herb is also widely cultivated in Europe for medicinal purposes; it is approved by the German government as a sedative medicine.

Passion flower is a gentle sedative and is often combined with other plants. Most likely, its active constituent is an alkaloid, called passiflorine (or harmane).

☞ Directions: Place 1 heaping teaspoon of dried passion flower in a cup, fill the cup with boiling water, cover, and steep ten minutes. Strain and drink as needed.

MOTHERWORT: Motherwort is a mild relaxing agent often recommended by herbalists to reduce anxiety and depression and treat nervousness, insomnia, heart palpitations, and rapid heart rate. Motherwort *(Leonurus cardiaca)* has been used in Europe since antiquity as a sedative and to treat menstrual irregularities. It probably came to North America with physicians among the British colonists. American Indian tribes later adopted the herb's medicinal uses.

Today, in Germany, motherwort is an approved medicine for treating anxiety. It is also used in contemporary Chinese medicine for the same purpose. The herb contains a chemical called leonurine, which may encourage uterine contractions, however. Thus, you will want to avoid motherwort if you are pregnant or trying to conceive.

☞ Directions: Place 1 to 2 teaspoons of motherwort herb in a cup and fill the cup with boiling water. Cover the cup and let stand for ten to fifteen minutes. Strain and drink. The tea's taste is bitter, so you may wish to mix it with other herbs. Don't drink more than 2 to 3 cups a day.

CELERY AND ONIONS: Some contemporary Indiana residents, according to a survey of folk remedies in the state, suggested eating celery and onions to overcome nervousness. Both celery and onions contain large amounts of potassium and folic acid. Studies have shown that deficiencies of each of these nutrients can cause fatigue, insomnia, and nervousness.

☞ Directions: Eat 2 cups of either celery or onions, or a combination of the two, raw or cooked, with each meal for a week or two.

Gypsy Wisdom

According to Wanja von Hausen's *Gypsy Folk Medicine*, when asked about anxiety, a gypsy folk healer in Spain replied, "Fear is part of life. But you are ashamed when you experience fear, as if it were a sin. So, the result of fear is depression, insomnia, and hopelessness. You cannot escape these unless you face the fear."

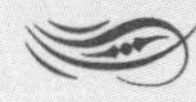

ASAFOETIDA: Asafoetida *(Ferula assafoetida)*, a relative of garlic and onions, is a traditional medicine from Asia. Its usage as a calming agent probably

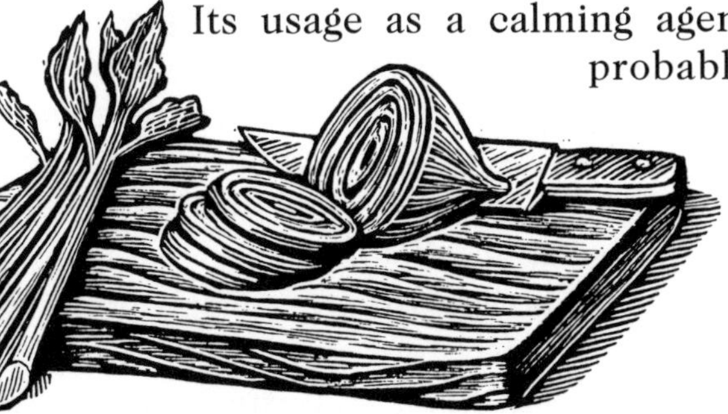

arrived in North America by way of immigrating European physicians. The Eclectic physicians of the 1920s used asafoetida as a sedative. The herb is still used today in Appalachian folk herbalism to treat nervousness.

Asafoetida has at least two sedative constituents, including ferulic acid, which is analgesic, antispasmodic, and acts as a muscle relaxant, and valeric acid, which induces sleep, relaxes muscle, and acts as a sedative.

☞ Directions: Stir 1/4 teaspoon of asafoetida powder into a little warm water and drink. Do this two or three times a day. If asafoetida begins to cause heartburn, reduce the dose or try another sedative. Asafoetida has a strong, disagreeable garlic-like odor.

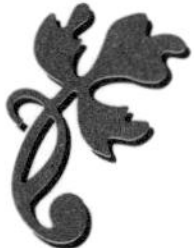

Arthritis

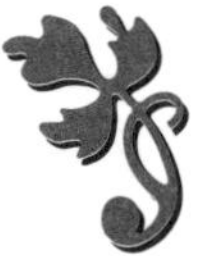

Millions of Americans are caught in the grip of some form of arthritis or rheumatic disease. While there are no cures, there are folk remedies you can try to help ease your discomfort

In a nutshell, arthritis means "inflammation of the joints." Rheumatism is an old medical term that was used to describe inflammation of either joints or muscles. Rheum was thought to be a watery mucus-like secretion, sometimes brought on by cold weather. Joint or muscle pain was thought to be caused by such secretions trapped in the tissues. Although the concept is not far from the truth—inflammation is usually accompanied by swelling and a build-up of fluid—the modern explanation of arthritis is much more precise.

Today's medical experts suggest there are at least 23 varieties of arthritis, including rheumatoid arthritis and osteoarthritis, the two most common types. With osteoarthritis—sometimes called degenerative joint disease, or DJD—there is a gradual wearing away of cartilage in the joints. Healthy cartilage is the elastic tissue that lines and cushions the joints and allows bones to move smoothly against one another. When this cartilage deteriorates, the bones rub together, causing pain and swelling. Permanent damage and stiffness of the joints is possible.

Rheumatoid arthritis can attack at any age. This form of arthritis affects all the connective tissues, as well as other organs. The precise cause of rheumatoid arthritis is unknown. Some researchers believe that a virus triggers the disease, causing an autoimmune response whereby the body attacks it own tissues. However, evidence for this theory is inconclusive. What is confirmed is the progression of the condition. First, the synovium (the thin membrane that lines and lubricates the joint) becomes inflamed. The inflammation eventually destroys the cartilage. As scar tissue gradually replaces the damaged cartilage, the joint becomes misshaped and rigid. Rheumatoid arthritis may damage the heart, lungs, nerves, and eyes.

A medical examination and diagnosis is required to identify the cause and nature of any chronic joint or muscular pain. Other "rheumatic" diseases include arthralgia (pain in a joint), fibrositis ("muscular rheumatism"), and synovitis (inflammation of the joint membrane).

There is no simple cure for arthritis. Conventional treatment for chronic joint pain is to use drugs to suppress the inflammation in order to reduce pain and also prevent tissue destruction. Usually, simple aspirin-related pain medications, called nonsteroidal anti-inflammatory drugs (NSAIDs), are first prescribed. Corticosteroids may be prescribed for more serious illness, especially when tissue destruction is evident. In about 15 percent of rheumatoid arthritis cases, these measures are ineffective, and stronger substances are used. Oral or injectable gold may prove helpful in treating rheumatoid arthritis. Some drugs usually used for cancer treatment may also be helpful.

Alternative physicians usually treat arthritis by recommending short fasts, screening for food allergies, recommending avoidance of processed foods, introducing fish and fish oils to the diet as well as anti-inflammatory herbal and nutritional supplements, and using natural methods to improve digestion. Alternative physicians may also recommend the substance glucosamine sulfate, which provides natural building blocks for cartilage, as a dietary supplement for those suffering from osteoarthritis. Scientific studies have suggested that supplementation with B vitamins, vitamin E, and some multiminerals (including the trace elements copper and selenium) may also improve the disease. On the other hand, studies have shown that nightshade vegetables—potatoes, tomatoes, bell peppers, and chili peppers—may provoke joint pain.

Very few of the herbs or foods recommended in folk literature for treating arthritis have been tested clinically for anti-inflammatory effects. Many of these herbs and foods contain plant constituents for which such effects are known, however.

Remedies

CELERY: The remedy of eating raw or cooked celery seeds *(Apium graveolens)* or large amounts of the celery plant to treat rheumatism arrived in North America with the British and German immigrants. Using celery to treat rheumatism persists today in North American professional herbalism. Various parts of the celery plant contain more than 25 different anti-inflammatory compounds. And, taken as a food, celery is rich in minerals: A cup of celery contains more than 340 milligrams of potassium.

(A potassium deficiency may contribute to some symptoms of arthritis.)

☞ Directions: Place 1 teaspoon of celery seeds in a cup. Fill the cup with boiling water. Cover and let stand for fifteen minutes. Strain and drink. Drink 3 cups a day during an acute arthritis attack.

ANGELICA: Angelica *(Angelica archangelica)*, an herb that has been used in European folk medicine since antiquity, can be used to treat arthritis. The Western variety of angelica has 12 anti-inflammatory constituents, ten antispasmodic (muscle relaxant) constituents, and five anodyne (pain-relieving) ones. The Chinese sometimes use their native variety of the plant *(Angelica sinensis)* for the same purpose. The Chinese species is sold in North America under the names *dang gui* or *dong quai.*

☞ Directions: Place 1 tablespoon of the cut roots of either species of angelica in 1 pint of water and bring to a boil. Cover and boil for two minutes. Remove from heat and let stand, covered, until the water cools to room temperature. Strain and drink the tea in 3 doses during the day for two to three weeks at a time. Then, take a break for seven to ten days and start the treatment again if desired.

ROSEMARY: A collection of remedies by folklorist Clarence Meyer called *American Folk Medicine* suggests drinking rosemary

Aspirin-like Compounds in Plants

Over the past hundred years, aspirin has been one of the most common treatments for inflammatory arthritis. Today we have a wide variety of aspirin-like drugs, such as ibuprofen and naproxen, which are collectively called nonsteroidal anti-inflammatory drugs, or NSAIDs. (You can also think of them as New-Sorts-of-Aspirin-In-Disguise, because, like aspirin, these drugs all work in pretty much the same way.)

Aspirin was developed as a less toxic substitute for methyl-salicylate, which comes from the wintergreen plant *(Gaulteria procumbens).* Wintergreen was used as a traditional American Indian treatment for rheumatism and headache. Aspirin-like compounds are also contained in the herbs black cohosh *(Cimicifuga racemosa),* black haw *(Viburnum prunifolium),* pipsissewa *(Chimaphila umbellata),* and white willow bark *(Salix alba).* Therapeutically, these herbs are not as powerful as aspirin or today's NSAIDs, but they are less likely to cause gastrointestinal bleeding, a side effect that afflicts from two to four percent of regular NSAID users and causes 2,000 to 3,000 deaths a year.

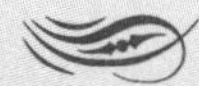

tea to treat arthritis. The same remedy is used in the contemporary folk medicine of the Coahuila Indians in Mexico. Rosemary has not been tested in clinical trials, but it was used to relieve pain and spasm by doctors of the Physiomedicalist school, a group of M.D.s in the second half of the 19th century who used only herbs when treating patients. The plant's leaves contain four anti-inflammatory substances—carnosol, oleanolic acid, rosmarinic acid, and ursolic acid. Carnosol acts on the same anti-inflammatory pathways as both steroids and aspirin, oleanolic acid has been marketed as an antioxidant in China, rosmarinic acid acts as an anti-inflammatory, and ursolic acid, which makes up about four percent of the plant by weight, has been shown to have antiarthritic effects in animal trials.

☞ Directions: Put ½ ounce of rosemary leaves in a 1-quart canning jar and fill the jar with boiling water. Cover tightly and let stand for thirty minutes. Drink a cup of the hot tea before going to bed and have another cupful in the morning before breakfast. Do this for two to three weeks, and then take a break for seven to ten days before starting the treatment again.

Potato Magic

A magical arthritis remedy from the Appalachians, and also from rural Louisiana, is to carry a potato around with you. In fact, some say, in order for the remedy to work, the potato must be carried in the right-hand pants pocket; others insist that you must carry an Irish potato.

WINTERGREEN: Wintergreen *(Gaulteria procumbens)* was used to treat arthritis by the Delaware, Menominee, Ojibwa, Potawatomi, and Iroquois Indian tribes. The plant was accepted in the United States as an official medicine for arthritis in 1820; it is still included—in the form of wintergreen oil—in the *United States Pharmacopoeia* today. The chief active pain-relieving constituent in wintergreen is methyl-salicylate. This compound can be toxic when consumed in concentrated wintergreen oil, even when applied to the skin, so, if you want to use this plant, stick with using the dried herb. (Aspirin was developed as a safer alternative to methyl-salicylate.)

☞ Directions: Place 1 or 2 teaspoons of dried wintergreen leaves in a cup and cover with boiling water. Cover the cup and let steep for fifteen minutes. Strain and drink 3 cups a day. Do this for two to three weeks, and then take a break for seven to ten days before starting again.

BLACK COHOSH: An American Indian treatment for arthritis, in both the Seneca and Cherokee tribes, involved using the root of black cohosh *(Cimicifuga racemosa)*. White settlers in the eastern states eventually adopted the plant's use, as did the Eclectic physicians of the last century (see sidebar, "Eclectic Medicine," page 29). There are five species in the *Cimicifuga* genus worldwide that have been used to treat rheumatism. Black cohosh contains aspirin-

continued on page 44

The Power of Amulets

In folk medicine there is a constant interaction between the spiritual and the material as well as the mental and the physical. This is what makes folk medicine holistic. A good example of material–spiritual holism can be seen in the use of amulets. Amulets are material objects said to have spiritual power. They are used either to protect against harm or to help obtain something good. Amulets are used to ward off fire, violence, witchcraft, lightning, disease, evil spirits, or anything dangerous and undesirable. On the positive side, amulets may be used to draw good luck, health, love, success, or supernatural powers.

Amulets come in many forms. The rabbit's foot and the horseshoe—both of which have a reputation for bringing good luck—are probably the most familiar to Americans. And good luck, of course, always includes good health. In fact, some folk practices regarding amulets are very health specific. For example, the foot of a mole, worn around the neck on a string, has been a popular way to prevent illness and promote long life in the southern United States. The horseshoe, another amulet of good fortune and health, is generally hung above a doorway, illustrating that amulets can be placed on houses as well as on people. Amulets can also be placed on valued animals to protect them.

PLANT AMULETS: Throughout the world, plants and plant parts are among the most common items used as amulets. Sometimes these plant amulets are quite elaborate. In India, one of the most powerful amulets is made by gluing together bits of wood from ten different types of sacred trees and then wrapping the wooden mass with gold wire. Other plant amulets are simple and use just a seed or other plant part. A clove of garlic, widely reputed to repel evil forces, is perhaps the best known of these simple amulets. Garlic is also believed to have healing powers. Spruce needles, carried in powdered form, have been used as a medicinal amulet by the Shoshone Indians. Since spruce needles are a source of vitamin C, the connection between biological and spiritual methods may be similar to that of garlic. Buckeyes, the shiny brown nuts of the horsechestnut tree, are used as a general purpose amulet as well as a specific one to prevent or treat rheumatism, that is, aches and pains of all sorts. Although not as well known in popular culture as garlic, the use of buckeyes as medicinal amulets is found throughout the United States.

METAL AMULETS: Metal amulets are found throughout the world, and some scholars have suggested that the wearing of jewelry—both metals and stones—originated in the wearing of amulets. Sometimes it is difficult to decide whether an object worn on the body to treat or prevent illness is functioning in a natural or a supernatural way. For example, many people insist that wearing copper, usually worn as a bracelet but occasionally placed in the shoes or elsewhere on the body, has a magical curative effect on arthritis.

Is the copper bracelet an amulet? Most skeptics would say that the bracelets are not magical. Instead, the bracelets are believed to work by providing a source of subtle electrical energy that offers the curative effects. As with garlic and spruce needles, copper amulets remind us that in folk medicine the distinction between natural and supernatural varies from one person to another and is often very uncertain and difficult to prove.

WRITTEN AMULETS: Amulets can also be written materials. These materials range from entire books to magical charms written on pieces of paper and then sealed inside a small bag. The Pennsylvania German Powwow book, *The Long Lost Friend*, states on its title page, "Whosoever carries this book with him, is safe from all his enemies, visible and invisible . . . [and cannot be] drowned in any water, nor burn up in any fire, nor can any unjust sentence be passed upon him." John George Hohman, compiler of *The Long Lost Friend*, was the first to publish a Himmelsbrief, or "Letter from Heaven." These letters, reputed to be Divine in origin, have been used as amulets in Christian countries for centuries. In Italian-American tradition they are called "Santa Letter di Gesú Cristo." Similar use of written materials is also found in Jewish and Islamic traditions.

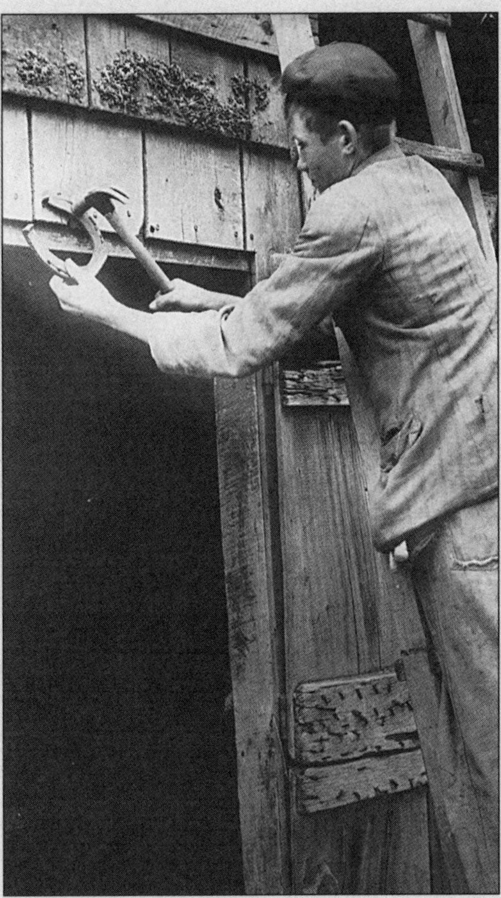

The horseshoe is believed to bring about good luck.

EVIL AMULETS: Amulets are sometimes used as a kind of sorcery to cause illness. In Louisiana, for example, hoodoo bags, also called "sachets," often contain dried snake skin or lizard skin, graveyard dust, dead flies, rusty nails, bits of bone, and other materials traditionally associated with malevolent magic. If these amulets are hidden in the victim's vicinity, those who follow the hoodoo tradition believe these evil amulets can cause sickness and even death. Hoodoo is a blend of Haitian vodun, Cuban Santeria, and other New World religious systems that combine Christian, African, and American Indian elements.

Among the most common amulets found in American folk medicine are those that protect against the "evil eye," the spiritually powerful glance that can cause illnesses ranging from headache to potentially fatal "wasting away." A common evil eye amulet is the cornu, a small horn-shaped object. The cornu is sometimes worn as jewelry or it can be seen dangling from a car's rearview mirror. Today it is usually made of red plastic. It is likely that many who use the cornu are unaware of their most basic purpose, however.

like substances as well as other anti-inflammatory and antispasmodic constituents.

☞ Directions: Simmer 1 teaspoon of black cohosh root in 1 cup of boiling water for twenty minutes. Strain and drink the tea in 2 divided doses during the day. Do this for two to three weeks, and then take a break for seven to ten days before starting the treatment again.

SESAME SEEDS: A remedy for arthritis from Chinese folk medicine is to eat sesame seeds. One-half ounce of the seeds contains about 4 grams of essential fatty acids, 175 milligrams of calcium, 64 milligrams of magnesium, and, notably, .73 milligrams of copper. Increased copper intake may be important during arthritis attacks because the body's requirements go up during inflammation. (See the remedy in this section, "Copper Bracelets," page 47.)

☞ Directions: Grind up ½ ounce of sesame seeds in a coffee grinder and sprinkle on your food at mealtime. You can use this treatment for as long as you like.

Counterirritants and Arthritis

A universal approach to relieving arthritis pain in all cultures is the application of a counterirritant, or substance that irritates and inflames the skin over the painful area. Cayenne pepper, pine pitch, bee and scorpion stings, and modern over-the-counter remedies such as Ben Gay ointment are all used for this purpose. Physiological tests show that such treatments increase blood flow to the area by as much as four times and also increase blood flow and temperature in the muscles beneath the skin.

Any relief from such treatments is due to this increase of circulation to the area. Counterirritation may also increase local or systemic levels of endorphins, natural pain-killing substances that can be more potent than opiates.

ALFALFA: Alfalfa *(Medicago sativa)* is often promoted in health food stores as an arthritis remedy—in the form of capsulated alfalfa powder. Alfalfa contains l-canavanine, however, an amino acid that can cause symptoms that are similar to those of systemic lupus, an autoimmune disease that can also cause joint pain. Some scientific studies show that these symptoms can occur in both animals and humans as a result of eating alfalfa. Thus, the remedy below is best taken in the form of a tea rather than powder; the amino acid is not present to any significant amount in alfalfa tea. Alfalfa tea is rich with nutritive minerals. It is a recommended folk remedy for arthritis in southern Appalachia.

☞ Directions: Place 1 ounce of alfalfa tea in a pot. Cover with 1 quart of water and boil for thirty minutes. Strain and drink the quart throughout the day. Do this for two to three weeks, and then take a break for seven to ten days before starting again.

PINE PITCH AND TURPENTINE: American Indians of the Six Nations tribes of the northeastern United States and southeastern Canada used pine pitch (congealed pine sap) applied externally as a counterirritant treatment for arthritis (see sidebar, "Counterirritants and Arthritis," page 44). The practice was later adopted by residents of Appalachia. Today, turpentine, which is made from pine pitch, is used there for the same purpose.

☞ Directions: Mix a small amount of turpentine with lard or vegetable oil to keep it from burning the skin. Apply over the area of the arthritis pain. Leave it on for ten to twenty minutes. Wipe off.

MUSTARD PLASTER: Perhaps the most famous of the counterirritant treatments for arthritis is the mustard plaster. This treatment is used throughout Europe and also in Appalachia and China. The irritating substance in mustard is allylisothyocyanate, which is related to the acrid substances in garlic and onions. This constituent is not activated, however, until the seeds are crushed and mixed with some liquid. Only then does the mustard produce the irritation necessary for the counterirritant effect.

☞ Directions: Crush the seeds of white or brown mustard *(Brassica alba, Brassica juncea)* or grind them in a seed grinder. Moisten the mixture with vinegar, then sprinkle with flour. Spread the mixture on a cloth. Place the cloth, poultice side down, on the skin. Leave on for no more than twenty minutes. Remove if the poultice becomes uncomfortable. After removing the poultice, wash the affected area.

HOT PEPPERS: Cayenne pepper *(Capsicum spp.)* appears in counterirritant potions in China, the American Southwest, and throughout Ohio, Indiana, and Illinois. External and internal use of cayenne pepper was a key element of Thomsonian herbalism, which was popular throughout rural New England and the Midwest in the early 1800s. Cayenne works by reducing substance P, a chemical that carries pain messages from the skin's nerve endings, so it reduces pain when applied topically. Try this simple cayenne liniment.

☞ Directions: Place 1 ounce of cayenne pepper in 1 quart of rubbing alcohol (a poison not for internal use). Let stand for three weeks, shaking the bottle each day. Then, using a cloth, apply to the affected

Medicinal Marijuana

The United States is currently embroiled in a debate over the medicinal use of marijuana, with some states wanting to legalize it for medical purposes, and the federal government opposing such use. A Hispanic remedy, widespread in Mexico and the American Southwest, uses marijuana to treat rheumatism. (Scientists have recently discovered that cannabinoids, constituents of marijuana, are effective against arthritis pain.) The marijuana is not smoked, however, but soaked in alcohol. Once the alcohol turns green from the marijuana, it is rubbed onto the afflicted areas.

Blood Purifiers

Traditional "blood purifiers" mentioned in Appalachian folk literature as being treatments for arthritis include sassafras (*Sassafras albidum*), sarsaparilla (*Smilax officinalis*), and burdock (*Arctium lappa, Arctium minus*). Residents in the American Southwest insist red clover (*Trifolium pratense*) and yerba mansa (*Anemopsis californicum*) do the trick. Practitioners of folk medicine in New York recommend dandelion root (*Taraxacum officinale*) as the best treatment for arthritis.

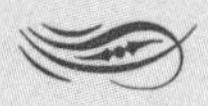

area during acute attacks of pain. Leave the solution in place for ten to twenty minutes, then wipe clean.

GINSENG LIQUOR: The Iroquois Indians used American ginseng *(Panax quinquefolius)* as a treatment for rheumatism. Today, the Chinese use the herb for the same purpose. Be sure to use American ginseng, however, not Asian ginseng *(Panax ginseng);* Asian ginseng can actually aggravate the pain of arthritis. Ginseng contains constituents called ginsenosides, which have a variety of pharmacological actions. Both the American and Asian varieties of the plant are classified as adaptogens, meaning that they increase the body's ability to handle a wide variety of stresses. The Iroquois Indians made a tea of the plant's roots and added whiskey. You might prefer the traditional Chinese formula below.

☞ Directions: Chop 3½ ounces of ginseng and place in 1 quart of liquor like vodka. Let the mixture stand for five to six weeks in a cool dark place, turning the container frequently. Strain and take 1 ounce of the liquid after dinner or before bedtime every night for up to three months. Then, take a break for two weeks before starting the treatment again.

HOP TEA: Hop is native to Europe and can be found in vacant fields and along rivers there. The Pilgrims brought hop *(Humulus lupulus)* to Massachusetts, and it quickly spread south to Virginia. The hop plant contains at least 22 constituents that have anti-inflammatory activities, including several that act through the same cellular mechanisms as steroid drugs. Four constituents have antispasmodic properties, and ten may act as sedatives. The fresher the plant, the better. Today, a popular remedy for rheumatism in Mexico and the American Southwest is hop tea.

☞ Directions: Place 2 or 3 teaspoons of hop leaves in a cup and fill with boiling water. Cover the cup and let stand for

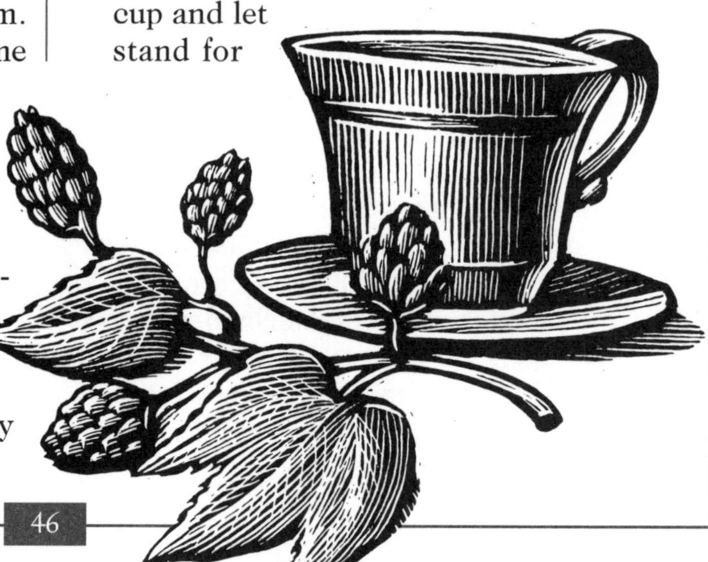

Chaparral

Chaparral (*Larrea tridentata*) is widely promoted in health food stores as a treatment for arthritis. In the early 1990s, reports of liver toxicity for chaparral appeared in scientific documents, and 18 cases of adverse effects to chaparral have since been reported to the Food and Drug Administration (FDA). Two of those patients required liver transplants. The individuals who were poisoned took powdered chaparral in the form of capsules, ingesting toxic constituents that are not present in the traditional teas.

Chaparral was widely used by the American Indians of the Southwest. These Indian groups used chaparral either externally as a wash or internally as a tea, however; they did not take it in the form of powdered capsules. Pima Indians recommended using only the new growing green parts of the plant for the tea, a consideration not always followed in today's herb commerce where old dire leaves are just as likely to be used.

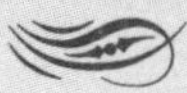

fifteen minutes. Drink the tea while it's warm. The tea is bitter. Drink 1 to 3 cups between dinner and bedtime as needed.

WILD YAM: Wild yam *(Dioscorea villosa)* was used by physicians of the last century to treat spasms of smooth muscle that often accompany gallbladder attacks or painful menstruation. Wild yam contains diosgenin, a steroid constituent with anti-inflammatory properties. Wild yam root itself has not been tested for such activity. Some southern African-Americans drink a tea of wild yam to treat muscular rheumatism. (Some eat the root of the wild yam instead.) This remedy was learned from the American Indians and is also recorded in the folk literature of contemporary whites in the Appalachian mountains of northern Georgia.

☞ Directions: Place 1 ounce of wild yam root in a 1-quart canning jar. Add a few slices of fresh ginger root. Fill the jar with boiling water, put the lid on tightly, and let the mixture stand until it reaches room temperature. Drink 2 to 3 cups of the tea each day for three to six weeks, then take a break for seven to ten days.

COPPER BRACELETS: The recommendation for arthritis patients to wear copper bracelets is common throughout European and American folk literature. Copper is a nutrient that may play a role in modifying arthritis. The nutrient takes part in key antioxidant systems that help prevent inflammation and is also necessary for the formation of connective tissue. The normal daily requirement of copper for an adult is

continued on page 50

Counterirritants: Like Cures Like

A counterirritant is anything that produces one irritation with the intention of relieving another. For example, you have used a counterirritant if you have ever applied a "balm" that produces a sensation of heat when rubbed onto sore muscles. The idea behind these remedies is that the medicinal irritation will produce, or enhance, a bodily reaction that will help overcome the initial problem. The balms operate by increasing local blood flow. In addition to such direct activity, counterirritants follow an ancient healing idea that sometimes "like cures like," as in the system of medicine known as homeopathy.

The most common counterirritants in folk medicine are "rubefacients." (The name is derived from the Latin word meaning "to make red.") These irritating medicines, when they are applied to the surface of the body, can cause the skin to become red by bringing more blood to the surface. Powdered mustard is the most frequently used rubefacient; it is usually used in the form of a mustard plaster. Mustard plasters are a kind of poultice in which mustard, flour, and water (or vinegar) are mixed and smeared on a cloth and then applied to the body. (It's important to note that, while the mustard plaster does create a sensation of heat, if it is left on too long it can actually cause burns.) These plasters are used to soothe sore muscles and joints and are applied to the chest to treat respiratory infections. Mustard foot baths have also been traditionally recommended for treating respiratory infections, although, in this case, the logic of how the plaster works is less obvious.

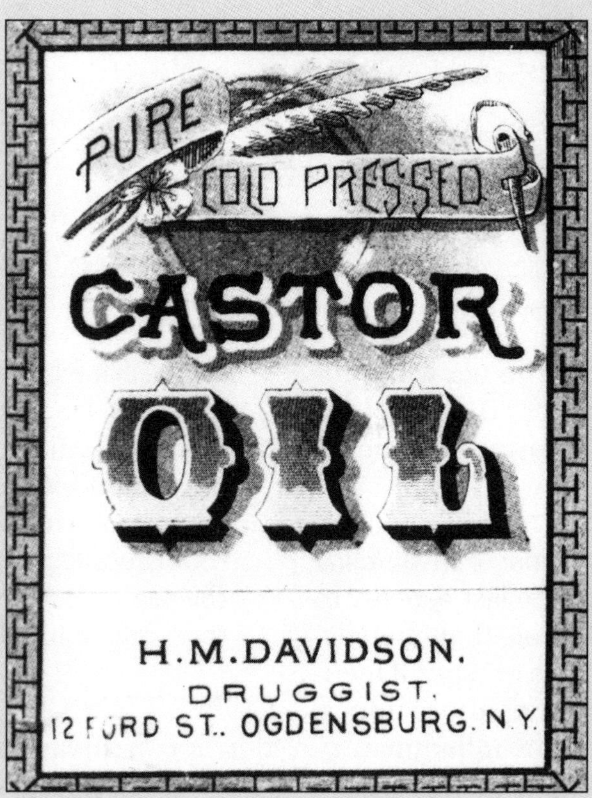

One of many treatments used in healing.

Pepper, another rubefacient, is also known for its irritating properties. In Connecticut, for example, a winter remedy for tonsillitis uses slices of salt pork, warmed in a pan. The pork slices are placed on a soft cloth and sprinkled with pepper. The cloth is wrapped around the patient's throat and left in place until the sore throat is gone.

Like these mustard and pepper cures, many counterirritants sound more like recipes for meals than medicines. Some recipes are decidedly inedible, however! For example, alum, which can refer to a variety of metal compounds but usually refers to aluminum potassium sulfate, is used in folk medicine as an astringent or styptic. Astringents and styptics are substances that constrict tissue, especially blood vessels. For this reason, although they are irritants, they also help stop bleeding. In Indiana, "burnt alum" is made by heating alum until it boils and a white residue forms. The residue is then applied directly to canker sores.

A remedy from Georgia for hemorrhoids combines three irritants—snuff, alum, and camphor. Snuff, made from tobacco and originally sniffed into the nose to receive nicotine or produce sneezing, has the rare distinction of being both a medicinal and a recreational irritant! (Forms of tobacco other than snuff have also been used medicinally. For example, it remains a widespread belief that an earache can be cured by blowing smoke into the affected ear.)

Also from Georgia comes the recommendation that a mixture of mothballs (of which camphor is usually a main ingredient), table salt, and gasoline can relieve inflammation. Although this remedy did not mention the exact manner in which this mixture was to be used, hopefully users did keep it away from open flames! Other volatile fluids, especially turpentine and kerosene, have often been combined with animals fats (such as tallow) or vegetable oils (such as castor oil) to make poultices that are applied with flannel cloths. These mixtures have been especially popular for the treatment of chest infections and respiratory ills, with the intention, presumably, of bringing more circulation to the vicinity of the lungs. In Georgia, a mixture of kerosene and castor oil is sometimes used as a treatment for corns.

Dangerous Practices

Perhaps because they are popular as topically applied counterirritants, volatile fluids, such as kerosene and turpentine, have also been used as inhalants and gargles, and, in some cases, they have been taken internally. In Maryland, it was believed that the labored breathing of croup could be relieved if the infant wore a piece of flannel soaked in kerosene and inhaled the fumes. Actually, it is very unhealthy to breathe the fumes of any petroleum product.

Even more drastic is a remedy reported from many states that recommends gargling with coal oil or kerosene for a sore throat. However, the unhealthiest of these practices for sore throat are the recipes in which kerosene or turpentine was mixed with sugar and swallowed. All of these remedies are very dangerous. If even a small amount of kerosene or turpentine is inhaled into the lungs—easily done with these substances—a serious, potentially fatal, chemical pneumonia could result.

Diuretic Herbs

Taking diuretic herbs as a treatment for arthritis has been recommended in various customs throughout the world; in North America, it was prescribed by physicians of the last century. The European colonists introduced the use of celery seed *(Apium graveolens)* to the eastern colonies as a diuretic and antirheumatic. The Seneca Indians used horsetail *(Equisetum arvense)* as a diuretic to treat arthritis, the Aztec Indians of Mexico used corn silk *(Zea mays)*, and the Allegheny tribe used parsley *(Petroselenium sativum)*. The Seneca and Pacific Northwest Indian tribes recommended pipsissewa *(Chimaphila umbellata)*. Various eastern Indian groups took cramp bark *(Viburnum opulus)* and black haw *(Viburnum prunifolium)*.

The rationale for this diuretic prescription is not clear, but its use remains widespread. Contemporary Appalachians use pipsissewa as well as Joe-Pye weed *(Eupatorium purpureum)*. Pipsissewa, cramp bark, and black haw, in addition to their diuretic properties, also contain aspirin-like anti-inflammatory compounds.

1.5 to 3 milligrams, but that requirement may be higher in patients with rheumatoid arthritis (but not osteoarthritis). A 1976 clinical trial demonstrated that copper bracelets could be an effective treatment for arthritis. Patients in the trial who wore copper bracelets had fewer symptoms than those who wore colored aluminum look-alikes. The researchers also found that the bracelets lost as much as 1.7 milligrams of copper a day, some of which may have dissolved in the individual's sweat and been absorbed through the skin.

☞ Directions: Wear a copper bracelet around your wrist or ankle—the more surface area the bracelet covers, the better. (It is unlikely to absorb too much copper. Copper toxicity occurs after ingesting about 60 milligrams of copper, an amount that is many times more than what is found in copper jewelry.)

EPSOM SALTS: In the town of Epsom, England, in 1618, a substance called magnesium sulfate was found in abundance in spring water. The colonists brought the substance, named Epsom salts, to this country. Magnesium has both anti-inflammatory and antiarthritic properties and it can be absorbed through the skin. Magnesium is one of the most important of the essential minerals in the body, and it is commonly deficient in the American diet. A New England remedy for arthritis is a hot bath of Epsom salts. The heat of the bath can increase circulation and reduce the swelling of arthritis.

☞ Directions: Fill a bathtub with water as hot as you can stand. Add 2 cups of

Dog Nap

A widespread folk practice to cure rheumatism is to sleep with a dog, with the animal resting against the affected area. In Mexico and the American Southwest, the dog is sometimes shaved. Physiologically, this may be an alternative to a hot water bottle or a heating pad, because the heat from the dog's body keeps the area warm. The practice has a darker side, however. Some cultures believe that the disease will go into the dog, the patient will be cured, and the dog will die. This use and superstition is also recorded in the medical practices of some southern African Americans as well as in the folk medicine of residents of North Carolina, Kentucky, Indiana, Illinois, Texas, Kansas, and Nebraska.

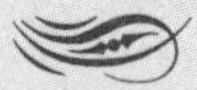

Epsom salts. Bathe for thirty minutes, adding hot water as necessary to keep the temperature warm. Do this daily as often as you'd like. (If you are pregnant or have cardiovascular disease, however, consult your doctor before taking very hot baths.)

HYDROTHERAPY: Water treatments for arthritis, which have become popular throughout the United States in the last century, invariably involve heat. Hot water or steam increases the circulation, which in turn can reduce local inflammation and swelling. These techniques are used today in parts of Appalachia and among the Seventh Day Adventists.

☞ Directions: Try one of the following treatments: Take a steam bath in a sauna. Soak in a hot tub, or, if there is one in your area, a hot spring. You can also try placing hot towels on the afflicted area.

STINGING NETTLE: A gypsy folk remedy for arthritis is to drink the juice of nettle leaves. Stinging nettle is an official remedy for rheumatism in Germany. In botanical medicine classes at the National College of

Bee Stings

A counterirritant method you may rightly recoil from is to allow yourself to be stung by a bee. The origins of the treatment are unclear, but it was used in the eastern United States in the early 1800s. Later, the medical profession made alcohol tinctures of either whole bees or of bee venom for patients' external and internal use. Internal use proved to be potentially toxic, however. Eventually the homeopathic physicians created a diluted form of the same tincture, which is still available in health food stores under the name *Apis mellifica*, or simply Apis.

Wild Cucumber Bark

The best plant for treating arthritis, says traditional Georgian Appalachian herbalist Tommie Bass, is wild cucumber bark according to *Herbal Medicine Past and Present* (Volume II) by John K. Crellin and Jane Philpott. This herb is generally not available in the herb trade, but it may be worth your while to track it down. Says Bass: "More people call for the wild cucumber bark to treat rheumatism and arthritis than any other bark or herb I know of. It can be put in drinking alcohol or made as a tea. Take a teaspoon of it three times a day and one tablespoon at night if it's not too much of a laxative. We've had people that had to walk on canes or crutches that's laid them down after using the cucumber bark."

Wild cucumber was prescribed by physicians of the last century as a laxative. When taking wild cucumber bark, the dose should be kept below that which loosens the bowels.

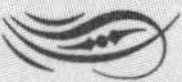

Naturopathic Medicine in the United States, it is taught that stinging nettle is the most important herb to consider for treating early-onset arthritis. A 1996 laboratory analysis of nettle juice showed an anti-inflammatory effect similar to that of steroid drugs.

☞ Directions: Purchase nettle leaf juice in a health food store and take as directed on the package. If you know how to identify and harvest nettles, collect your own (they must be harvested before they flower), and juice them in a juicer. Take 1 tablespoon of nettle juice three times a day. You can freeze the juice for later use.

Also, you can make a tea of the dried leaves. Place 1 ounce of dried nettle in 1 quart of water. Bring to a boil and then simmer for thirty minutes. Drink 3 cups a day for as long as you'd like.

FASTING: Fasting on water or vegetable juices to cure an acute arthritis attack is a treatment recommended in many folk systems. It is used today in European spa therapy and among Seventh Day Adventists in North America. Several scientific trials have shown the benefits of a four-day water fast in reducing the symptoms of an acute arthritis attack. A possible benefit of fasting is that it relieves the body of the burden of producing digestive enzymes, thus freeing up resources for the process of healing arthritis damage. Fasting may also reduce the load of allergenic foods in the system. Vegetable juices of celery, carrot, or beet are also mineral-rich and can help replenish the body's mineral stores.

☞ Directions: Fast for thirteen days. Drink juice from raw potatoes and or carrots—mixed in with a total of 1 tablespoon of cosmetic-grade facial clay—every day. During the fast, also drink 1 tablespoon of nettle juice three times a day. Don't practice this fast more than once every three months. Consult your physician before starting any fast.

Asthma

The suffocating symptoms of asthma are much more frequent in our society today than in the times of our ancestors. In fact, just since 1980, the incidence of asthma has risen more than 60 percent in the United States

Asthma now affects some fourteen million Americans and claims about five thousand lives a year. Asthma is the most common chronic disease among children, affecting one in five. Because it may be a life-threatening condition, any individual with asthma should be under the care of a physician.

Asthma is a respiratory disorder marked by unpredictable periods of acute breathlessness and wheezing. Asthma attacks can last from less than an hour to a week or more and can strike frequently or only every few years. Attacks may be mild or severe and can occur at any time, even during sleep.

The difficult breathing occurs when the small respiratory tubes called bronchioles constrict or become clogged with mucus or when the membranes lining the bronchioles become swollen. When this happens, stale air cannot be fully exhaled but stays trapped in the lungs, so that less fresh air can be inhaled.

Asthma attacks can result from oversensitivity of the bronchial system to a variety of outside substances or conditions. About half of all asthma attacks are triggered by allergies to such substances as dust, smoke, pollen, feathers, pet hair, insects, mold spores, and a variety of foods and drugs. The allergic trigger cannot always be identified, and sometimes food allergens complicate the picture. An individual who is allergic to a specific food may experience "allergic overload" when consuming it and then overreact to a simple pollen or other airborne allergen that normally would not cause a serious problem. Attacks not related to allergies can be set off by strenuous exercise, breathing cold air, stress, and infections of the respiratory tract.

Modern physicians treat asthma with drugs delivered by inhalers, including, in serious cases, steroid drugs. Recent research has demonstrated that prolonged use of inhaled steroids can cause severe side effects similar to those experienced by users of oral steroids, however. Inhaled steroids nevertheless remain an essential and sometimes lifesaving part of treatment for severe asthma.

Why does the body overreact to a simple allergen? One possible explanation is a deficiency of the body's natural anti-inflammatory prostaglandins, substances naturally derived from the fats of cold water fish and wild game. The decline of these foods in the modern diet may be contributing to the increased incidence of asthma. The body can make these substances from certain vegetable oils, but the process is much more complex and can be inhibited by deficiencies of magnesium, zinc, vitamin B_6 or vitamin C—all common deficiencies in the modern American diet. Science has linked each of these deficiencies—as well as the reduced consumption of cold water fish—to asthma, but the evidence is not strong enough to implicate a single deficiency in all cases. Modern science has also demonstrated that increased salt consumption worsens (and reduced salt consumption improves) the severity of asthma. Although controversial, the industrialization of agriculture and food processing over the last few decades may have contributed to the increased incidence of asthma by exacerbating these deficiencies or excesses. Charles Cropley, a naturopathic physician in Colorado, recently described his dietary regimen for patients with asthma: "Nothing out of a can, nothing out of a box."

If you suffer from asthma, you might want to consider the folk remedies below. After all, these remedies have helped the many generations before us breathe a little easier.

Remedies

LICORICE: Licorice root has long been used to treat coughs and bronchial problems in many cultures throughout the world. It has expectorant properties and also contains anti-inflammatory constituents similar to steroids, although much weaker. Licorice is not so effective in treating an acute asthma attack, but daily use over a long period of time may reduce the body's tendency to overreact to allergens.

☞ Directions: Cut 1 ounce of licorice root into slices, cover with 1 quart of boiling water, and steep for 24 hours. Strain and drink 1 or 2 cups a day. Licorice can cause high blood pressure and salt imbalances if taken for long periods. Don't take the above doses if you already have high blood pressure, and don't continue to take the herb in any case for longer than six weeks. (Note that real licorice is not a common ingredient in United States candy. Instead, anise oil is substituted, which has a similar taste.)

Amish Wisdom

The basic Amish treatment program for asthma includes eliminating all refined foods—such as sugar, flour, soft drinks, homogenized milk, coffee, black tea, and chocolate—from the diet. Prudent avoidance of airborne allergens is also a customary treatment of asthma among the Amish.

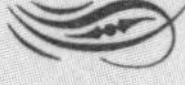

MORMON TEA: Mormon tea, the common name for a variety of plants in the *Ephedra* genus, was used as a decongestant for allergies in western American folk medicine among American Indians, Hispanics, and settlers from the eastern states. A more potent Asian relative called *ma huang* is used in the same way in traditional Chinese medicine.

The medicinal constituents involved are ephedrine and pseudoephedrine, which also appear in over-the-counter allergy medicines. The American ephedra species do not contain reliable amounts of these constituents. Ma huang and ephedrine-containing drug combinations have been responsible for a number of deaths in the United States in recent years, but generally not when taken as allergy medications. Weight-loss formulas and pep pills sometimes contain ma huang or ephedrine. In this form they are consumed in much larger amounts than in allergy medications and present a greater risk of side effects. Ephedra is contraindicated in heart disease, hypertension, thyroid conditions, prostate disease, anxiety, pregnancy, and concurrent use of pharmaceutical drugs, except with approval of your physician. Mormon tea itself is not usually available in herb or health food stores, but ma huang often is.

☞ Directions: Cover 1 teaspoon of Chinese ephedra with 1 cup of boiling water. Let steep ten minutes. Drink the full cup when suffering an acute asthma attack. Prepare the tea ahead of time and keep it in a sealed container in the refrigerator.

Emetic Therapy and Asthma

A popular treatment for asthma from the last century was to use an emetic—a substance that induces vomiting. Some herbs were used for this purpose. More often, smaller doses were taken to simply produce expectoration of mucus. The principle of "emetic in large dose but expectorant in small dose" applied to dozens of herbs, including ipecac, bloodroot, and mustard seed. There is no scientific evidence supporting the effectiveness of these herbs in treating asthma, however, possibly due to the difficulty in accurately measuring expectoration.

GARLIC: Garlic *(Allium sativum)* has long been used to treat bronchial problems in many cultures. Like many of the other herbs used to treat asthma, garlic acts as an expectorant in low doses and an emetic in higher doses, especially if taken on an empty stomach. The Seventh Day Adventists use garlic in the following way to treat an acute asthma attack.

☞ Directions: Take 2 cloves of garlic and crush well or blend in a blender. Mix in 2 cups of hot water (105°F). Add a pinch of salt. Drink 1 cup rapidly. (Though this remedy may induce vomiting, it may also abort the asthma attack.) Then drink a second cup, which will usually stay down.

Also, you can try simmering the garlic in water for twenty minutes. (This destroys some of the irritating substances that cause nausea.) This treatment came from the 12th century German mystic Hildegarde von Bingen.

MUSTARD SEED: An old New England remedy calls for 1 teaspoon of mustard seed *(Brassica spp.)*, taken morning and evening, in the form of a tea or soup. Mustard contains irritating and expectorant sulfur-containing compounds. Like garlic, it can induce vomiting in larger doses and was used for this purpose by the Eclectic physicians of the late 19th and early 20th centuries in cases of narcotic poisoning.

☞ Directions: Crush and moisten the seeds well in order to release the constituents. Let the freshly crushed mustard seeds sit in a warm soup or tea for ten to fifteen minutes before drinking. Take two to three times a day.

DAISY BLOSSOMS: White daisy blossoms *(Chrysanthemum leucanthemum)* were an early traditional asthma remedy in the eastern United States. By the turn of the 20th century, this plant had become a standard medical treatment of the Eclectic physicians.

☞ Directions: Take 4 ounces of white daisy blossoms and crush them well. Pour 1 pint of boiling water over them. Steep for one hour and strain. You can take 2 to 3 tablespoons two to three times a day.

HONEY: Honey has been used in traditional Chinese medicine for more than two thousand years. It is used to treat conditions ranging from asthma, cough, and chronic bronchitis to stomachache, constipation, chronic sinus congestion, canker sores, and burns. To cure a cough, a simple folk remedy from China recommends drinking a tea consisting of hot water and a tablespoon of honey. (This treatment probably isn't strong enough to treat an asthma attack, but it might help thin mucus and prevent congestion.) Expectorant syrups made from honey or sugar are widespread throughout the folk traditions of the world. In the United States, honey syrups appear in the folk medicine of New England, Appalachia, and the Southwest.

GARLIC AND HONEY: Some syrups combine the healthy benefits of both garlic and honey. Such syrups appear in the folk traditions of both New England and the Southwest.

☞ Directions: Place 8 ounces of peeled and sliced garlic in 1 pint of boiling water. Let soak for 10 to 12 hours, keeping the water warm, but not boiling. Strain and add 2 pounds of honey. Bottle the mixture. Take 1 teaspoon of the mixture when you're congested.

MULLEIN AND HONEY: You can use the mullein plant to make an asthma syrup, too. Mullein *(Verbascum thapsus)* came from Europe to North America with the European colonists and is now naturalized throughout the United States and Canada. Its use as a cough medicine was quickly adopted by various Indian tribes, including the Mohegan, Delaware, Cherokee, Creek, and Navaho. The Penobscot, Potawatomi, and Iroquois used mullein specifically to treat asthma. It was an official medicine in the *United States Pharmacopoeia* from 1888 to 1936. Today, it is an approved medicine for treating coughs in Germany.

Jimsonweed

Here's a folk remedy to avoid. Jimsonweed (*Datura stramonium*) was used to treat acute asthma attacks by many groups throughout the United States, including American Indians, New Englanders, Indiana farmers, and settlers in the American Southwest. Jimsonweed seeds were smoked in a pipe or cigarette to calm an acute attack.

Hyoscyamine and scopolamine, two alkaloid constituents of the plant, are proven bronchodilators, and they also dry the secretions of the mucous membranes. The plant is so powerful that some individuals can receive a medicinal dose by simply touching the leaves or inhaling its fragrance, however. High doses can cause temporary psychosis and nightmarish, fearful hallucinations—hence its common names "Devil-weed" and "Loco-weed." The plant or seeds may be fatally poisonous if eaten and should never be kept within reach of children.

☞ Directions: Place ½ pound of mullein leaves in a 1-quart jar. Fill the jar with boiling water and let cool to room temperature. Strain. Add honey to the tea until it is the consistency of syrup. Take 1 tablespoon of the syrup when suffering an asthma attack.

NETTLE AND HONEY: This home remedy comes from German immigrants who settled in the New York area. Nettle juice *(Urtica dioica, Urtica urens)* and nettle syrups may still be purchased in Germany today. American physicians of the 19th and early 20th centuries also used nettle to treat some types of allergic conditions. Nettle is an unusually mineral-rich plant. An ounce of the dried herb contains more than two-thirds of the minimum daily requirement of magnesium, which is a frequently deficient mineral in asthma patients.

☞ Directions: Take ½ pint of nettle juice, boil it, remove the scum from the pot, and mix the remaining juice with an equal part of honey. Take 1 tablespoonful in the morning and evening.

ELDER FLOWER PILLOW: Another remedy from the eastern states of the last century is to sleep on a pillow stuffed with dried elder leaves or flowers *(Sambucus spp.)*. As you sleep, you'll inhale the plant's aromatic oils and breathe a little easier.

☞ Directions: Take 4 ounces of dried elder leaves or flowers and place inside a pillow. (Be careful of allergic reactions to the flower's pollen.)

EGG SHELLS AND MOLASSES: An early 18th century asthma treatment in the eastern United States was to mix roasted egg shells with blackstrap molasses. This mix-

continued on page 60

Magical Transference

Around the world, one of the most widely observed ideas in folk medicine is the belief that disease can be magically transferred from a sick person to another person, animal, or object. The desired result? The sick person becomes well. The idea of transference is rooted in a fundamental concept that scholars call "sympathetic magic." Sympathy refers to a relationship between people or things in which each is affected by whatever affects the other. When we feel another's sorrow we say that we are sympathetic; what we mean is we feel the effects of what the other person is experiencing. In sympathetic magic this connection can exist between things that have been in contact (such as a foot stepping on a nail) or things that are very similar (such as a person and a photo of that person).

Magical transference may take place either directly or symbolically. For example, when a nail that has pierced your foot is then cleaned and carefully bandaged, the magic transfer is direct. When a picture of the patient is used for diagnosis or treatment, the picture serves as a symbol of the patient. In some cases it is difficult to distinguish between direct and symbolic transfer. For example, there was a healer in Maryland who had been very effective at curing warts by gazing at them. A patient who had been successfully treated by the healer returned when he developed a new wart on his hand. The healer looked at the wart, then rolled up his sleeve to reveal an arm covered with warts. After commenting that he had room for another one, he began to stare at the patient's new wart.

The idea of healers at least temporarily taking a patient's symptoms onto themselves—and feeling weakened or experiencing the patient's specific aches and pains after a healing session—is common in folk medicine. One religious healer in Philadelphia—a man who worked by placing his hands on a sick person's head and praying—said that some people drained him so much that he was forced to lie down for hours afterward. (The healer likened this to a transfer of energy that he experienced in mental hospitals. There, he said, simply walking through the halls could drain him of his energy.) Other healers have specific ways of making certain the negative energies of an illness pass through them instead of settling within them. One Pennsylvania German powwow (see page 102) always made a vigorous shaking movement with the arm he was not laying on the patient. He used this movement to ensure that if something passed into his healing hand it would go out of him through the other.

Many cures involve transferring disease to an inanimate object or sometimes a plant. For example, the following remedy was collected in Illinois: To relieve a "stitch" (a pain in the side), pick up a rock, and spit on the ground under it. Those who have reported this practice specifically say that "the pain will be transferred to the rock," although it is hard to understand exactly how that would work! From Utah comes the belief that jaundice can be cured by hanging a carrot in the patient's basement. It is believed that as the carrot dries up it will absorb the jaundice. (In this case the "sympathy" transfer includes the coloring of the carrot and the characteristically yellow color of jaundice.)

Another very common method of transferring disease is called "plugging," in which hair from a sick person is placed in a hole that has been bored in a tree. Once the hole is plugged, the disease is thought to be trapped in the hole. Sometimes the hole has to be plugged while the hair is still attached to the head, and then the hair is cut off. Asthma is the disease most often treated with this cure. And, depending on the area, certain trees are thought to be more effective than others. For example, in New York, apple trees are popular; in Pennsylvania, sugar maples are used in this remedy.

According to other remedies, in order for one person to be cured, another person or animal must actually develop the disease. Often this belief has led to the keeping of pets specifically to prevent or treat disease. Among German Americans, guinea pigs are used this way. In Nebraska it is said that keeping cats in the house will cure asthma—when nine cats have contracted asthma from you, you will be cured! Another report told of a child sick with "dumb ague" who was treated by placing a puppy in his crib. The puppy became sick and broke out in sores, and the child soon recovered. The most common remedy of this kind reported in the United States is sleeping with dogs to cure rheumatism. Invariably the dog is said to contract the rheumatism, eventually becoming crippled or even dying.

And if sacrificing "man's best friend" is not bad enough, there are many beliefs about the transfer of disease to another person. This transfer is often specific and intentional. Some wart cures call for rubbing a wart with a coin and leaving the coin in the road so an unsuspecting passerby will pick it up and carry it off—along with the wart. Another widely reported belief says that when a sick and well person sleep together, the sick one improves at the healthy one's expense. Similarly, in a sort of vampire fashion, many have insisted that if a young and an old person sleep together, the older one drains away some of the younger one's youth!

A Dangerous Practice

It is a potentially dangerous belief that people can be cured by transmitting their disease to another. Fortunately, in most cases, the method of transmission is unlikely to be effective. But one very widespread belief has been the source of a great deal of suffering—the belief that sexually transmitted diseases can be cured through sexual intercourse with an uninfected partner. Frequently this belief specifies that the partner is to be a virgin or even a sexually immature child. This tragic belief is ancient and widespread. In some locations the belief is less dangerous because it specifies intercourse with an animal. For example, in some parts of the Middle East it is said that intercourse with a mare will cure syphilis.

ture makes an effective mineral supplement. The egg shells are almost pure calcium carbonate, and molasses is one of the most mineral-rich foods on earth. The dose of molasses below contains a significant portion of the recommended dietary allowance of magnesium, and this amount has been found in some scientific studies to be an effective treatment for asthma. (The treatment is remarkably similar to a traditional Mongolian remedy for leg cramps due to calcium deficiency, where black pepper berries are mixed with egg shells, which are roasted until brown and then crushed into powder.)

☞ Directions: Roast 3 egg shells until brown. Crush into a powder. Mix with half of a pint of molasses. The dose is 1 tablespoonful three times a day for as long as desired.

Sweating

A common folk medical treatment of the 19th century was to induce sweating. In *Home Remedies: Hydrotherapy, Massage, Charcoal, and Other Simple Treatments*, co-author Calvin Thrash, M.D., a contemporary teacher and advocate of the Seventh Day Adventist school of natural medicine, writes, "Anything that increases perspiration of the skin will encourage increased activity of the mucous membranes."

Mucous secretions become thick in asthma. When an individual sweats, however, the belief is that the flow of mucus will increase. The increased flow thins the secretions and makes them flow more easily, helping to relieve difficult breathing. Sweating practices are contraindicated in patients who are thirsty or dehydrated, a caution probably overlooked in the 19th century traditions to the detriment of the patient. On this topic, Thomsonian herbalist George Letsum made a play on his name: "First I pukes 'em, then I sweats 'em, and if they dies, then I lets 'em."

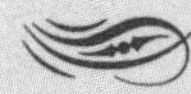

FOOT BATH AND TEA: A Seventh Day Adventist treatment for asthma is to induce sweating by putting the feet in warm water and drinking a tea made of catnip *(Napeta cataria)* or pennyroyal *(Hedeoma pulegioides)*. Catnip and pennyroyal are both diaphoretics—they bring circulation to the skin and produce sweating. Don't use this treatment during pregnancy, however; both these herbs promote menstruation. (See "Sweating," this page, for other contraindications.)

☞ Directions: Fill a bathtub or a smaller tub with hot water. Put the feet in the water while drinking the hot tea. (This treatment is contraindicated in diabetics, however, because the feet might be burned.)

To make the tea, place 1 ounce of catnip or pennyroyal leaves in a 1-quart jar and cover with boiling water. Cover the jar tightly and let steep for ten to fifteen minutes. Strain and drink.

HERBAL FORMULA: A tea formula from the last century combines licorice root *(Gly-*

cyrrhiza glabra), mullein leaves *(Verbascum thapsus),* horehound leaves *(Marrubium vulgare),* lungwort *(Pulmonaria officinalis),* and sage *(Salvia officinalis).* All these herbs have subsequently been used in North American, British, and German herbal medicine, and licorice, mullein, horehound, and sage have all been listed as official medicines in the *United States Pharmacopoeia.*

☞ Directions: Place ½ ounce of each of the herbs in 1½ quarts of water. Boil for 20 minutes. Strain when cool. Drink 5 ounces (the amount that would fill a wine glass) at bedtime.

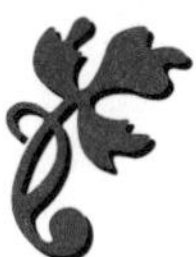

Bites and Stings

Humans, insects, and reptiles all strive to live comfortably in the same space. Unfortunately, humans inevitably get bitten and stung as a result

When bees, wasps, scorpions, and snakes attack humans, it's usually because we threatened them or their living space. On the other hand, insects such as mosquitoes, biting flies, ticks, chiggers, and fleas are predatory pests that view humans as good opportunities for a bite to eat. Their bites are more likely to be itchy than painful. With any bite or sting, the species' venom, or sometimes the tiny insect itself, penetrates the barriers of the body. The combination of the effects of the poison and the body's attempt to eliminate it can cause pain, swelling, or itching near the bite site.

Most bites and stings are not a serious medical concern, but there are a few exceptions. In some people, the stings of bees, wasps, and hornets can cause a potentially fatal allergic reaction called anaphylactic shock. Any shortness of breath, difficulty breathing, or swelling in the airway after a sting is a medical emergency requiring immediate attention. Tick bites can cause Lyme disease or Rocky Mountain spotted fever. Bites of the black widow spider and brown recluse spider can also cause serious medical symptoms; any reaction following a spider bite requires medical attention.

The bites of the poisonous snakes in North America are not usually life threatening to healthy adults. Of about 8,000 such bites in the United States each year, fewer than 15 cause fatalities; the deaths occur mostly in children and the elderly. The illness from a poisonous snake bite can be quite severe, however, and should be treated as a medical emergency. Any snake bite can cause an infected puncture wound, which requires careful cleaning and medical attention. The *Centruroides exilicauda* scorpion, native to Arizona, New Mexico, and the California side of the Colorado River, is the only North American scorpion that can cause serious illness or death. The folk remedies here are for normal itches and pains associated with bites and stings, not for the more exotic complications caused by Lyme disease, anaphylactic shock, or snake bites.

Remedies

MINTS: American Indian tribes have used various species of mint for the relief and prevention of insect bites. For example, peppermint *(Mentha piperita)* contains camphor, which is cooling to the skin and helps to relieve itching.

☞ Directions: Place 1 ounce of peppermint leaf in a 1-quart canning jar and cover with boiling water. Seal the jar tightly and let stand until the water cools to room temperature. Apply to mosquito bites or other itchy areas with a cloth. Reapply as desired.

PENNYROYAL: Early American colonists introduced European pennyroyal to North America, but found the Indians were already using American pennyroyal *(Hedeoma pulegioides)*. The herb was used by American Indians to prevent deer tick bites. In the *Frank C. Brown Collection of North Carolina Folklore,* a North Carolina source says: "Pennyroyal beaten on the legs will keep insects away." Pennyroyal contains eleven separate constituents with identified insect-repellent properties.

☞ Directions: Purchase the essential oil of pennyroyal. Put 8 to 10 drops in some almond oil, mix, and apply—especially around the ankles, neck, and scalp—to repel ticks and other insects.

My Scorpion Bite

Once in Arizona, I was bitten by a *Centruroides exilicauda* scorpion, the only potentially lethal poisonous scorpion in North America. I didn't know I'd been bitten, but thought I'd been stabbed by a cactus thorn. Soon my arm was numb, an itchy rash crept up my legs to the knees, and my pulse rate rose to more than 100 beats per minute. I went to bed but didn't figure out what had happened until I woke the next morning and my pulse rate was still over 100. Realizing it was a scorpion bite, I began taking large hourly doses of *Echinacea angustifolia*—a folk remedy of the Plains Indians for rattlesnake bites. Nothing much happened for the first five hours, but then I fell asleep and woke as if nothing had happened, and the rash was gone. I have only a small scar from the bite—and a fondness for American Indian herbalism—to show for it today. —*Paul Bergner*

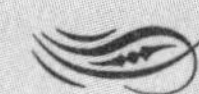

TOBACCO: The Mayan Indians moistened the leaves of wild tobacco *(Nicotiana rustica, N. glauca)* with saliva and applied the leaves to a bite or sting. The Six Nations, a league of Indians that extended from the Hudson River to Lake Erie, also used tobacco to treat insect bites. Using tobacco in this manner later passed into Appalachian folk medicine, where tobacco poultices are still used today to treat bee, hornet, yellow jacket, and wasp stings as well as spider bites. In the folk medicine of the Southwest, a strong tobacco tea is applied to tick bites to help draw the tick out. Physicians of the last century also supported tobacco's antiseptic qualities: They used tobacco ointments and tobacco poultices to treat skin conditions.

☞ Directions: Mix tobacco from cigarettes, cigars, chewing tobacco, or snuff with water and apply directly to a bite or sting. Leave the mixture on as long as you like.

Snakeroots

What's in a name? Everything when it comes to treating a snakebite. According to University of Michigan ethnobotanist Daniel Moerman, Ph.D., at least three unrelated plant species have been called black snakeroot and two have been called Sampson's snakeroot. There's also a broom snakeroot, Seneca snakeroot, white snakeroot, and Canada snakeroot. There are three rattlesnake roots and one rattlesnake weed, plus Kansas, Missouri, and Virginia snakeroots. Virginia snakeroot (*Aristolochia serpentaria*) was used for treating snakebites by the Mohegan Indians and by Mexican Indians. Kansas snakeroot, or *Echinacea angustifolia*, was widely used by the Plains Indians to treat rattlesnake bites.

The other plants, as far as we know, were called snakeroot because they looked like snakes. These plants all proved to have high success rates, of course, when it came to curing snakebites. The benefits attributed to any of them, however, are in a large part due to the fact that most snakebites in North America are nonfatal, and most patients will get better without treating the wound at all.

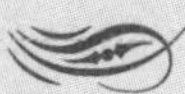

ECHINACEA: Echinacea *(Echinacea angustifolia, E. purpurea)*, also known as Kansas snakeroot, was a snakebite remedy of the Plains Indians introduced into medical practice in the United States in the mid-1880s. Dr. H.F.C. Meyer, M.D., a Nebraska doctor, learned how to use echinacea to treat snakebites from an American Indian woman. He experimented with the plant for about fifteen years; he even injected himself with rattlesnake poison and used the plant as an antidote. Echinacea was later identified by science as an immune stimulant. Today, it is one of the most popular herbal remedies in North America and in Europe, especially in Germany, where it is prescribed by physicians for colds, flu, and infections.

☞ Directions: Take a tincture of echinacea root with you when hiking in rat-

continued on page 67

Odors That Heal

Throughout history, people have associated certain odors with death and disease. Calamities such as floods, earthquakes, and war left the landscape littered with odorous decaying bodies—both human and animal. In the wake of these catastrophes, epidemic outbreaks of disease were common. And, during times of plague and other virulent diseases, it was sometimes impossible to bury the dead fast enough to prevent the stench of decaying corpses from pervading the town.

These experiences supported the belief that disease could be caused by bad odors. Such odors were called *miasmas*, from the Latin word meaning "to pollute." Miasmas were also believed to be given off by swamps and other damp environments that were thought to be unhealthy. Foul smells have even been associated with spiritual evil, as in the relationship between Hell and Satan and the smell of brimstone—an old word for sulfur. The connection between odors and spirits is a natural one, since both are invisible and each can be accompanied by powerful effects. (The word spirit comes from the Latin word for breath, which is another potent but invisible substance.)

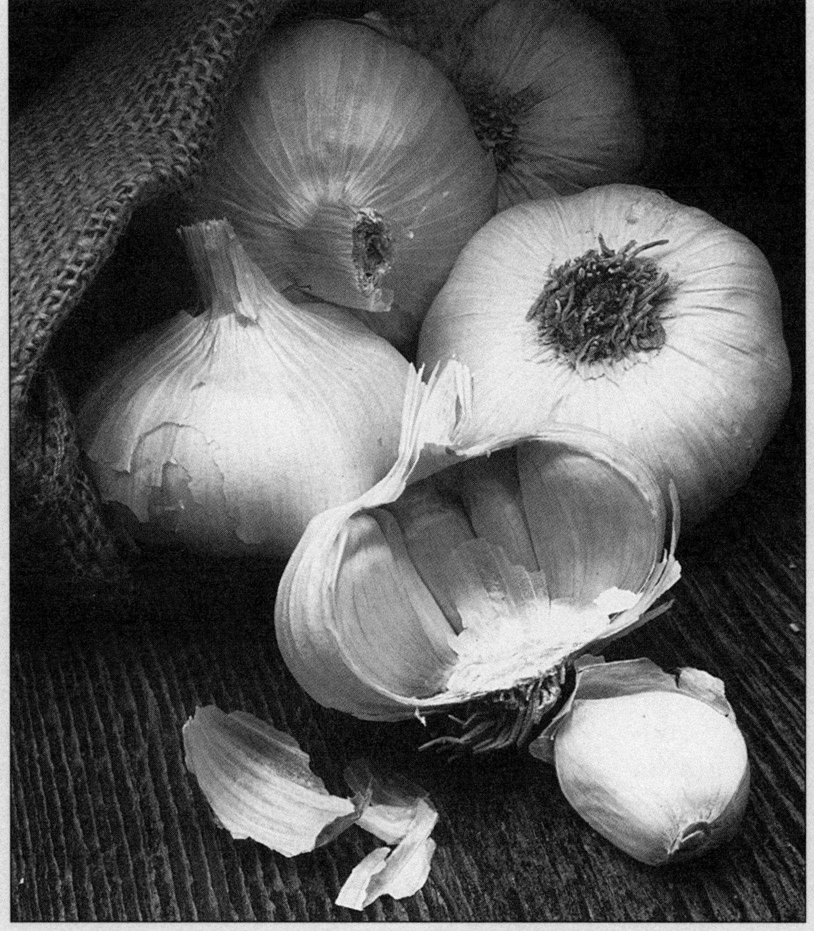

Garlic has a long history in folklore—as medicine and protection.

Since bad smells were thought to have the ability to cause disease or produce other evil influences, it was natural that strong counter-odors would be considered a protection against them. The idea of evil odors and powerful counter-smells is illustrated in a medieval European-Jewish tradition. On the Sabbath, according to the belief, the spirits of the wicked were allowed to roam free and did not return to Gehinnom (Hell) until after Sabbath prayers were finished. The Habdalah ritual, conducted at the conclusion of the Sabbath, customarily included the smelling of strong spices. One purpose of this was to protect the faithful from smelling the foul odor of Hell until the fires of Gehinnom were rekindled after the Sabbath.

In addition to its association with brimstone, sulfur is one of the most notable odors in folk medicine. The smell of rotten eggs, for example, is primarily the odor of hydrogen sulfide. Allicin, the substance that gives garlic its odor as well as its antibacterial properties, is another sulfur compound. Garlic has a long history in folklore as a potent protector from disease and evil spirits (such as vampires). For these reasons, garlic is not only consumed as a healthy food and medicine but it is also worn to fight the odors that bring about disease. A remedy from Maryland recommends wearing a ball of garlic around the neck and praying to get rid of worms. It is believed that the garlic smell will suffocate the worms. The prayer illustrates garlic's spiritual connection.

While garlic combats evil odors with a sort of "like cures like" approach using sulfur, other remedies have focused on using opposite kinds of smells. One of the most popular has been the smell of camphor. Camphor, usually in the form of a white crystalline substance, is obtained from the oil of a tree (*Laurus camphora*) native to China and Japan. Marco Polo, returning from his 13th century voyage to China, reported that camphor was highly favored by the Chinese as both a medicine and an embalming agent. Camphor later became popular in Europe and America; it is still commonly used in liniments as a counterirritant for aches and pains, rubbed on the chest for respiratory infections, and applied to the skin to repel insects. (Camphor was once the main ingredient in moth balls!) One of the most popular folk uses of camphor was to wear it in a bag tied around the neck as either a preventive or a treatment for respiratory infections. Although ancient Chinese medicine and Western folk remedies have sometimes included

The Excrement Pharmacy

Considering the use of foul odors in folk medicine, including stable odors, it is not surprising that tradition has also made use of excrement and urine. In fact, the practice of using these substances was so common that, in German tradition, the practice had a name: Dreck-Apothec, or excrement pharmacy.

A tea made from sheep dung was once used throughout North America as a treatment for measles. Human excrement was also believed to have healing virtue. In both England and America, children with respiratory illnesses were placed in the privy to get the benefit of the odor!

Human urine has been used for medicinal purposes in many traditions, including Ayurvedic medicine in India. In Utah and California, the urine of a faithful wife has been reported as a treatment for sore eyes. In Georgia, putting olive oil, warm milk, or hot urine in the ear was a remedy for earache.

the internal use of camphor, this is not considered safe today.

Unpleasant animal and human smells are also believed to cure sickness. Folklorists in England and the United States have found that the air of a stable can be used as a treatment for a variety of childhood sore throats and respiratory ailments, including whooping cough. If the child is well enough, spending the day playing in a stable is thought to be healthful. And some cures even specify holding the sick child over a "steaming manure pile"!

It was also common to treat a sore throat by wrapping it with a dirty sock, a remedy once found all over the United States. Similarly, running your fingers between your toes and then smelling your fingers was said to relieve coughs and sore throats. From Maryland comes a remedy for whooping cough in which garlic is worn in the shoes to produce a powerful odor. In Georgia a similar treatment advises putting sulfur in the shoes!

The most important foul-smelling remedies, however, have involved the use of asafoetida, whose common name is "Devil's Dung." Native to Iran, Pakistan, and Afghanistan, the root of this plant yields a gum that has a powerful odor produced by a sulfur compound. Used in Hindu medical tradition for over a thousand years, the plant, despite its odor, was also the most popular spice in ancient Rome. Today it is a component of Worcestershire sauce. In American folk medicine it has been used internally as a medicine and worn externally for its odor-producing protection. Asafoetida was commonly put on cotton and placed in a cloth bag, preferably red flannel, and worn around the neck. As with camphor, it fills the nostrils with an overpowering counter-smell! One recipe from Georgia leaves nothing to chance. It combines asafoetida with onions, camphor gum, sulfur, cinchona bark (from which quinine comes), poke berry roots, myrrh, and sassafras. The ingredients are to be worn in a bag around the neck.

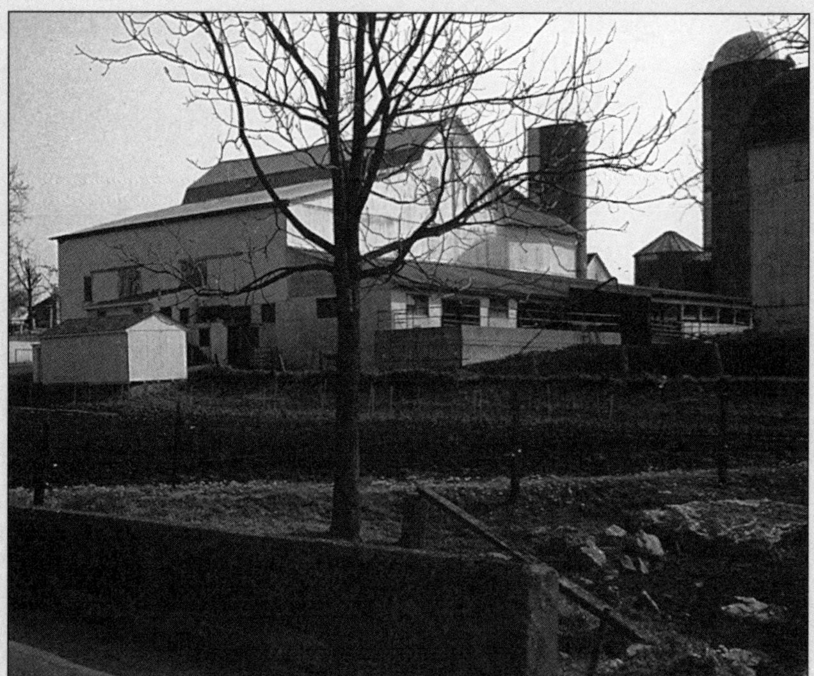

Playing in a stable is considered a remedy for whooping cough.

Louisiana Snake Magic

Louisiana folklore recalls the magical traditions of Africa and the voudon. A book of Louisiana folk remedies suggests that, if bitten by a snake near water, you need to beat the snake back to the water. Then, you must dip the bitten area of your body into the water. If you do this, the snake will die instead of you. Another folk remedy for treating snakebites suggests cutting open a black hen, and while she is still jumping, holding her over the bite. When the hen has stopped fluttering, the poison will be gone. Specialized "snake doctors" in rural Louisiana would also suck on snakebites, attempting to remove the poison. As mentioned above, all these remedies seemed to work—because most people recover from a snakebite with nothing more than a little bed rest.

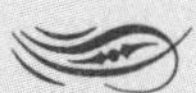

tlesnake country. If bitten by a snake, take a 1-teaspoon dose every half an hour and drink plenty of liquids. Snakebites are considered a medical emergency, however, so you should go to a medical facility as soon as possible.

PLANTAIN LEAVES: Plantain *(Plantago spp.)*, the common four-leafed weed that grows in lawns and around sidewalks throughout the country, was once called "White Man's Footprint" by the eastern American Indians because it came to this country with the European immigrants and spread wherever they went. Various tribes quickly adopted the plant as a medicine for treating bites, stings, and minor wounds. The Six Nations (see remedy, Tobacco) used the plant specifically to treat spider bites. Plantain leaves are still used today in the folk medicine of Indiana, North Carolina, and the Southwest. Plantain's chemical constituents may explain its ability to soothe pain and promote wound healing: It contains at least fifteen constituents with identified anti-inflammatory properties, seventeen with bactericidal properties, six analgesics, and five antiseptics. It also contains the constituent allantoin, which promotes cell proliferation and tissue healing.

☞ Directions: Crush a small handful of fresh plantain leaves and apply locally to bites and stings. Applied externally, the plant stimulates and cleanses the skin and encourages wounds to heal faster. You can apply fresh leaves every fifteen to twenty minutes. Leave on as long as desired.

GARLIC AND ONIONS: Cultivated garlic *(Allium sativum)*, onions *(Allium cepa)*, and their wild relatives have appeared in the medical records of all major civilizations since ancient times. Both garlic and onion have been used as antidotes to the poisons of bites and stings, taken internally or applied externally to the bite area. In North American folk medicine, the Amish and residents of Indiana apply crushed garlic or raw onions directly to snake, scorpion, or insect bites. Garlic and onion have also been used for this purpose in New England,

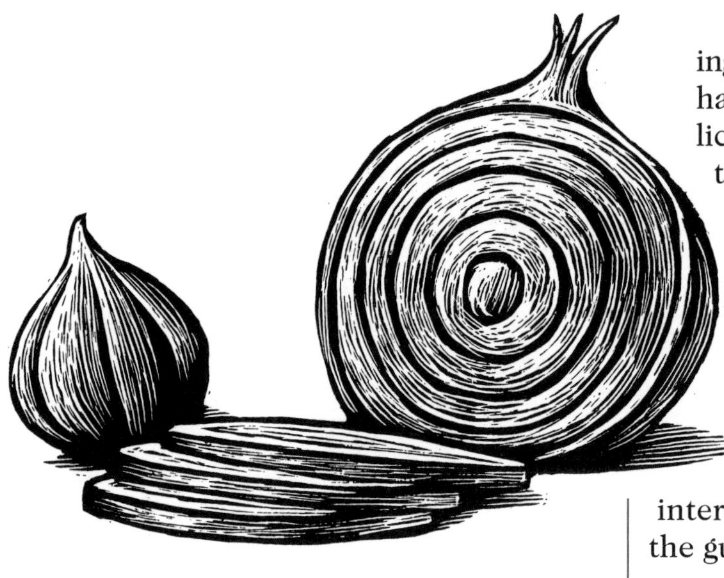

in the Southwest, and in Chinatowns of the West Coast.

Both garlic and onions contain broad spectrum antibiotic and anti-inflammatory substances that can disinfect and soothe a bite or sting.

☞ Directions: Crush a clove of garlic and mix it with a little water or saliva. Apply directly to the bite area. Also, you can blend up 3 cloves of garlic in 1 cup of wine, and let the mixture sit overnight. Wash any infected bites or stings hourly with the wine mixture the next day.

Place a thick slice of onion over the bite area. Leave on as often as you like.

VINEGAR: In the folklore of New England, rural Indiana, the American Southwest, and among Gypsies and the Amish, a vinegar wash is recommended for treating bites and stings.

☞ Directions: Use undiluted vinegar as a wash to stop itching or to relieve the pain of stings. Also, you can try this Gypsy recipe: Take a handful of thyme *(Thymus vulgaris)* and seal it in a bottle of vinegar for one cycle of the moon, in the sun if possible. Shake the bottle every morning and evening. Then, after an additional half cycle of the moon, crush seven garlic cloves and add them to the bottle. At the end of the second lunar cycle, strain and bottle the liquid. Use as a wash for itchy or infected bites.

CHARCOAL: A charcoal poultice is a medical treatment of the Seventh Day Adventists for insect and snake bites. Charcoal has strong drawing properties and is sometimes taken internally to neutralize ingested poisons in the gut.

☞ Directions: Wet as much crushed charcoal as you need to cover the injured area. Place the charcoal directly over the area and cover with a clean cloth. Replace the poultice every ten to fifteen minutes until relief is obtained.

BAKING SODA: Applying baking soda paste to spider bites and bee stings to relieve pain or itching is a folk remedy still used today in North Carolina, New England, the Southwest, and among the Amish. This remedy reportedly reduces swelling and pain if applied to the skin immediately after the bite has occurred.

☞ Directions: Moisten baking soda with water and apply the mixture directly to the affected area. You can also use vinegar to moisten the baking soda, or mix the baking soda with equal parts of salt and add water to form a paste. Leave on for as long as desired.

CLAY: Using clay or mudpacks to treat bee and wasp stings seems to be a universal folk remedy. In North America, it appears in the folk literature of southern blacks, Canadians, New Englanders, New Yorkers, North Carolinians, the Aztec Indians of Mexico, and contemporary Hispanics in Texas and New Mexico. Some people believe it works by literally drawing the toxins out.

☞ Directions: Apply mud or cold clay (any kind of clay soil or cosmetic clay will do) to the sting area to relieve pain and reduce swelling. When the clay dries, apply new clay. Repeat this as long as necessary.

KEROSENE: A remedy from contemporary southern Appalachians is to apply kerosene to bee stings to relieve pain and swelling.

☞ Directions: Wash the sting area with kerosene, or soak a cloth in kerosene and apply it to the area as a poultice. Kerosene itself can be irritating, so don't keep the poultice in place for more than twenty to thirty minutes.

Bladder and Kidney Infections

Be aware that changes in urine and urinary habits that do not seem to have an obvious cause may be a sign of disease

The urinary system includes those organs of the body that produce or eliminate urine. By controlling urine flow, the system maintains proper water balance in the body. Changes in urine and urinary habits that do not seem to have an obvious cause may be symptoms of disease. An accurate diagnosis by a physician is the first step to proper treatment.

Most pathological conditions of the kidney and bladder are not appropriate for self-treatment with folk or home remedies. Even bladder infections, the least serious of common urinary tract conditions, require a diagnosis to rule out sexually transmitted diseases or more serious kidney involvement. Most of the folk remedies below for treating urinary tract infections work in the same way as conventional treatment recommendations, however. For example, drinking adequate water to wash out bacteria is a standard procedure in both folk and conventional medicine for treating urinary tract infections.

Most of the folk remedies in this section use herbs with mild diuretic properties. These herbs increase the flow of urine through the urinary tract, helping to wash out irritating substances. In Germany, the use of such mild diuretics is called "flushing out therapy"; in that country, the therapy is a routine conventional treatment for bladder infections and stone prevention. Research has shown that mild diuretics increase urination and reduce joint swelling. Thus, mild natural diuretics are also used in Germany for treating the swollen joints of arthritis.

An important restriction on the use of herbal diuretics, however, is in cases of edema resulting from heart, kidney, or liver disease. (The condition was once known as "dropsy.") Edema requires careful medical attention—and properly monitored doses of diuretics. Although some folk remedies were once used to treat edema, during the 20th century, modern medical science has discovered much safer and more effective treatments for the condition.

The remedies in this section are found in many cultures throughout the world. In fact, most of these remedies would be included in classes on urinary tract herbs in medical schools in Germany, where doctors and pharmacists are required by law to receive training in medical herbalism.

A topic not included in this section is urinary difficulties due to prostate problems. Any obstructive problems of the urinary tract due to enlargement of the prostate require conventional medical attention to determine the cause.

Remedies

BEARBERRY: The herb bearberry *(Arctostaphylos uva ursi)*, sometimes called uva ursi (*bearberry* in Latin), was first recorded as a medicinal herb in the 13th century Welsh herbal *The Physicians of Myddfai.* The berries of the plant are a favorite food of bears—thus its name. Its use as a diuretic and lower urinary tract disinfectant is recorded in subsequent centuries throughout the British Isles and northern Europe. American Indians, including the Cheyenne and Thompson tribes, have used the plant for the same purposes. Today, bearberry is used as a diuretic in the folk medicine of Indiana and also by Spanish Gypsies from Spain.

Bearberry is still one of the most often prescribed urinary tract herbs by professional medical herbalists in North America and Europe, and it is approved in Germany for use by medical doctors in the treatment of bladder infections. Arbutin, a constituent in bearberry, is broken down in the body and transformed into an antimicrobial substance that is excreted in the urine, thus delivering an antibiotic directly to the site of the bladder infection. What's more, animal research in Spain in 1994 demonstrated that bearberry teas could lower the risk factors for kidney stones and kidney infections, although the effect was mild. Avoid using bearberry during pregnancy or lactation.

☞ Directions: Simmer ½ ounce of bearberry leaves in 1 pint of water for five minutes. Let steep until the water reaches room temperature. For a bladder infection, strain and drink 1 ounce three times a day for up to five days.

STINGING NETTLE: The Chippewa and Sioux Indian tribes used the leaves of the stinging nettle plant *(Urtica spp.)* as a mild diuretic for flushing out the urinary tract. It is used the same way today by Gypsies in Europe. Stinging nettle is also used as a diuretic by contemporary professional medical herbalists in North America and Europe and is an approved medical treatment for bladder infections in Germany. Besides having a mild diuretic effect, nettle is highly nutritious. An ounce of the leaves contains a large

Kidney Stones

A myth perpetuated in many modern herbals and collections of folk remedies is that certain herbs or foods will "dissolve stones." Kidney stones are formed when certain salts become too concentrated in the urine. Once formed, they do not readily dissolve back into the urine, however, and must either pass down the urinary tract or be broken up or dissolved by conventional medical means. Certain individuals, sometimes referred to in conventional medicine as "stone formers," tend to suffer repeat attacks of kidney stones. For them, the best treatment for kidney stones is prevention, which involves drinking plenty of water to dilute the urine. Drinking large amounts of fluids, particularly at night, reduces urine concentration so that stones cannot form.

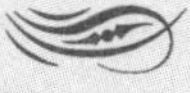

portion of the daily requirement for several minerals.

☞ Directions: Simmer 1 ounce of stinging nettle leaf in 1 quart of water for twenty minutes. Strain and drink 3 to 4 cups a day for a week or two.

CORN SILK: Corn silk *(Zea mays),* the hairy projections from the end of an ear of corn, was introduced as a medicine to the Western world after the European conquest of Mexico, Central America, and South America. Corn, native to those areas, is now cultivated not only in the Americas, but as far away as Africa, India, and China. Corn silk tea was used as a diuretic by American Indians in the conquered regions and is now used in the same way in folk traditions throughout North America and Europe. It has even entered into formal Chinese medical traditions, where it is called "yu mi shu." It is often prescribed as a diuretic by professional medical herbalists of Europe, North America, and Australia.

☞ Directions: Fill a 1-quart jar one-third full of fresh corn silk. Pour enough boiling water to fill the jar, cover, and let cool to room temperature. Strain and drink the quart in 4 doses during the day for seven to ten days.

GOLDENROD: If you're not allergic to this common cause of hay fever, goldenrod *(Solidago spp.)* may be as useful to you as a mild diuretic that helps to flush out the urinary tract. It was used for this purpose by the Chippewa Indians; it is used in the same way today in the folk medicine of Indiana. (Goldenrod was also used in Europe as a treatment for wounds—the flowers would be packed into a wound to stop the bleeding.) Goldenrod is approved for medical use in Germany as a mild diuretic and treatment for bladder infections.

☞ Directions: Place a handful of goldenrod flowers in a 1-pint jar and fill with boiling water. Cover and let cool to room temperature. To treat a bladder infection, strain and drink the pint in 3 doses during the day for seven to ten days.

"JOE-PYE" WEED: Queen of the meadow *(Eupatorium purpureum, Eupatorium maculatum)* was used medicinally by eastern American Indians, including the Cherokee and Mohawk tribes, before the arrival of European colonists. An Indian healer named Joe Pye reportedly used it to treat a group of colonists suffering from typhoid fever, and the survivors of the epidemic named the plant in honor of him—thus, Joe-Pye weed. It is also called "gravel root" because of its prominent use as a treatment for kidney stones.

Queen of the meadow was used by Eclectic physicians from about 1848 until the group's demise in the 1940s. The Eclectics preferred Queen of the meadow over some other diuretic plants because of its mild, non-irritating effects. One of the Eclectic physicians, Harvey Felter, M.D., stated in a turn-of-the-century medical book, *King's American Dispensatory*, that the herb was effective in treating kidney stones for two reasons—first, because it increased the flow of urine, preventing stone formation or washing out existing stones, and second, it reduced inflammation and pain in the urinary tract. Felter disputed the common myth that the plant could dissolve kidney stones that had already formed, however.

Queen of the meadow is recommended in the folklore of North Carolina residents for treating or preventing painful urinary tract conditions. The plant is still prescribed as a diuretic for bladder infections and kidney stones by professional medical herbalists in North America, although it has not been used in North American or European conventional medicine since the time of the Eclectics (see "Eclectic Medicine," page 29).

☞ Directions: Add ½ ounce of queen of the meadow to a pint of water. (Queen of the meadow may be sold in your herb shop under the name "gravel root.") Cover and simmer for twenty minutes. Let cool to room temperature. Drink 2 to 3 cups a day, while also drinking plenty of water.

WATERMELON: Watermelon seed tea *(Citrullus vulgaris)* is a folk diuretic mentioned in the literature of Indiana and North Carolina. It is also recommended by the Amish and the Seventh Day Adventists, the latter being a religious movement that advocates natural remedies and alternative medicine. Watermelon seed was also used as a diuretic by Eclectic physicians during the last century. Today, it is not commonly found in medical herbalism, probably because it is not always available in herb stores.

☞ Directions: Place a handful of fresh watermelon seeds in the bottom of a 1-pint jar and fill with boiling water. Let cool to room temperature. Strain and drink a pint of the tea each day for seven to ten days.

PUMPKIN SEEDS: Another diuretic often mentioned in folk literature is pumpkin seeds *(Cucurbita pepo)*. The folk traditions of New England, Indiana, and Louisiana all suggest taking a few pumpkin seeds to promote urination. The Eclectic physicians of the last century followed the practice until the group's demise in the 1940s.

Contemporary German physicians use pumpkin seed preparations to treat difficult urination that accompanies enlarged prostate

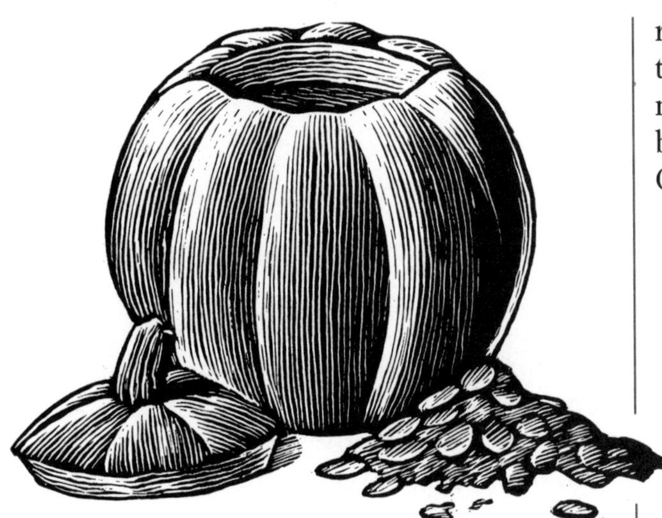

(when prostate cancer as a cause has been ruled out). Two constituents in pumpkin seeds, adenosine and cucurbitacin, both have diuretic properties.

☞ Directions: Crush a handful of fresh pumpkin seeds and place in the bottom of a 1-pint jar. Fill with boiling water. Let cool to room temperature. Strain and drink a pint of the tea each day.

Also, you can eat pumpkin seeds according to taste. It is best to remove the shells and eat them with little or no salt.

JUNIPER BERRIES: The ancient Egyptians used juniper berries as a diuretic. Juniper berries have been used for the same purpose by American Indians of the Tewa, Paiute, Shoshone, Cree-Hudson Bay, and Iroquois tribes. Today, juniper berries are recommended as a diuretic in the folk medicine of New England and the southern Appalachians. Contemporary medical herbalists warn that the aromatic oils in juniper berries can increase kidney irritation, and that it should not be used if kidney infection accompanies bladder infection. (The studies showing the resulting kidney irritation used concentrated oils in animals, not berries in humans, but due caution is in order.) Juniper berries are approved for use as a diuretic in Germany.

☞ Directions: Place 1 to 2 tablespoons of juniper berries in the bottom of a 1-pint jar. Fill with boiling water and cover tightly to prevent the escape of aromatic oils. Strain and drink the pint during the day. Do not try this remedy if you have kidney disease. The tea should not be consumed for more than three weeks. Take a break for two to three weeks between courses of treatment. This remedy should not be used by persons who have an existing renal disease.

WATER: The most obvious diuretic to increase the flow of urine is water. Simply drinking plenty of water—6 to 8 glasses a day—can increase urine flow, dilute the urine to prevent stone formation, and wash out bacteria that may cause infections. Some of the benefits of the mild diuretic teas used by physicians in Germany and by professional herbalists in North America come from the tea's increased volume of water. German physician R.F. Weiss, M.D., suggested that individuals who are prone to forming stones should, one day a week, consume a quart and a half of water rapidly (within fifteen minutes) to wash out any tiny stones that may be forming.

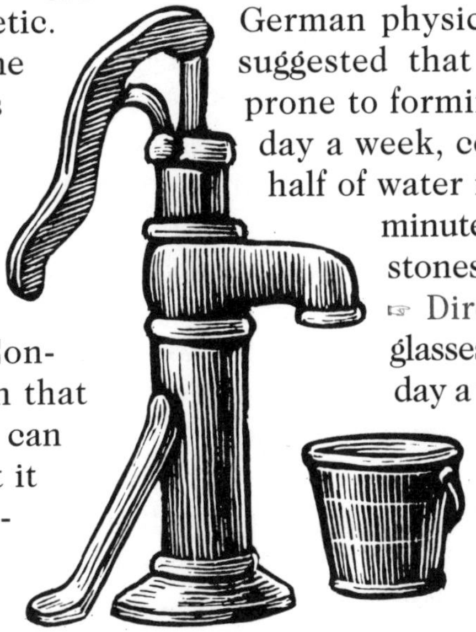

☞ Directions: Drink 6 to 8 glasses of water a day. Or, one day a week, drink 6 glasses of water in rapid succession, within fifteen minutes, to flush out the urinary tract.

continued on page 76

Magic in Folk Medicine: Control and Illusion

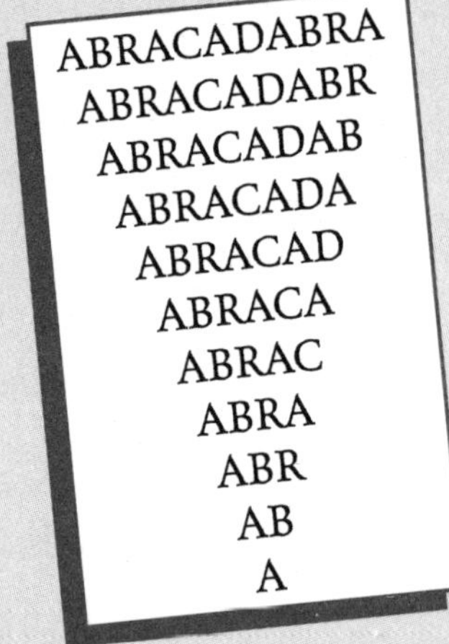

As early as the second century, physicians described abracadabra as a magical word effective against inflammations or fevers. Written on a piece of parchment or paper and worn as an amulet, it continues to be used in many different folk medicine traditions in the United States and Europe. Such words, written in blocks so that they can be read in more than one way, have long been popular for magical use. In the form of abracadabra shown above the idea seems to be that as the word itself disappears, so will the problem against which it is used.

This idea that two things can be supernaturally linked, so that what happens to one will happen to the other, is very prevalent in magic and applies both to healing and harming. In one of the most common folk medicine rituals, a wart is rubbed with a piece of potato, and the potato is buried under the eaves of a house or barn; as the potato rots, the wart disappears. In an act of sorcery made famous by Hollywood, bits of a person's nails or hair are placed on a crude doll that is injured with pins or fire; the victim experiences the pain of these actions and falls sick.

Sir James Frazer, an early anthropologist who systematically studied magical ideas from all over the world, called such a connection between two things that were once in contact—such as the wart and the potato or the hair and the victim—"contagious magic."

The similarity in the effects—the way in which the wart rots away like the potato or the victim experiences the injury to the doll—Frazer called "homeopathic magic," from the Latin *homeo-*, meaning "like" or "similar." (This is the same word history that, in alternative medicine, gives us the word *homeopathy,* although the ideas are quite different.) Frazer coined the term "sympathetic magic" to refer to the thinking in homeopathic and contagious magic. Sympathy refers to a relationship between persons or things in which each is affected by whatever affects the other.

What Frazer called sympathetic magic is common in folk medicine all over the world, but so are many other forms of magic. Another very common form of magic is called "spirit magic," in which the effects are brought about by spirits cooperating with the practitioner to heal or harm—whatever the practitioner seeks to accomplish. Although most cultures throughout history have assumed that real magic exists, skepticism on that subject began to emerge in western civilization in the late Middle Ages. Both religious reformers and Enlightenment philosophers saw magic as a form of trickery used by religious officials to create awe and, therefore, belief in the populace. Although jugglers and other entertainers used illusions to entertain, modern stage magic dates from the late 1700s when Joseph Pinetti, who called himself a "Professor of Natural Magic," performed tricks in Paris that would become the staples of modern magicians. In his act he included such tricks as escaping from chains and having his wife describe—while blindfolded—objects shown to him by audience members. Over a century later, Ehrich Weiss, whose stage name was Harry Houdini, became famous with similar—if not more difficult—tricks. Houdini also showed his audiences that some magical feats were nothing more than trickery and illusions. He did this on stage by recreating the effects being reported from the seances of local spiritists and mediums. The tradition of stage magicians as debunkers of magical or other extraordinary claims continues today. For example, "psychic surgeons" have frequently been accused of sleight of hand by stage magicians who can recreate similar effects.

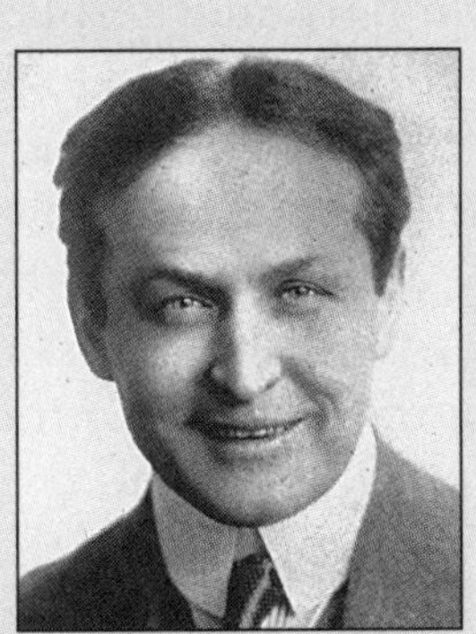

Harry Houdini

"Psychic surgery" is a kind of folk medicine found in the Philippines, South America, and in the United States among groups from these areas. The healers usually operate in a trance, and they describe themselves as under the control of the spirit of a deceased physician, often a surgeon. They appear to remove objects of various kinds from the bodies of their patients either through unbroken skin or through incisions made with their bare hands. These healing rituals are very impressive and have often been filmed by investigators. The patient lies on a table on his back, belly exposed. The healer then presses on the belly, blood suddenly appears, and after probing a moment longer the healer holds up an object apparently removed from the patient's body. The blood is wiped off the patient's belly. There is no wound or scar, and the patient reports no pain. The object removed varies from what looks like a blood clot to bits of metal or other odds and ends. Skeptics, with the help of stage magicians, have shown that similar acts can be reproduced by skilled magicians.

The psychic surgery healers come from spiritualist religious traditions, and their healing practices are often part of a larger and more complex religious system involving belief in communication with spirits. Some healers insist that the objects they remove "materialize" in their hands. Others have said that using illusions occasionally aids in the healing process. In any case, film documentaries of such healings show that these events can be very impressive indeed!

There have, no doubt, been people skillful at creating illusions throughout history, and many of them used their skills for personal profit by pretending that their illusions were real—fraud of all kinds is ancient. But it is equally true that many who use magic for practical purposes like healing are quite sincere in their efforts. Also, many "magical" elements in folk medicine actually involve self-care, as in the wart cures mentioned above, so no sleight of hand could be involved.

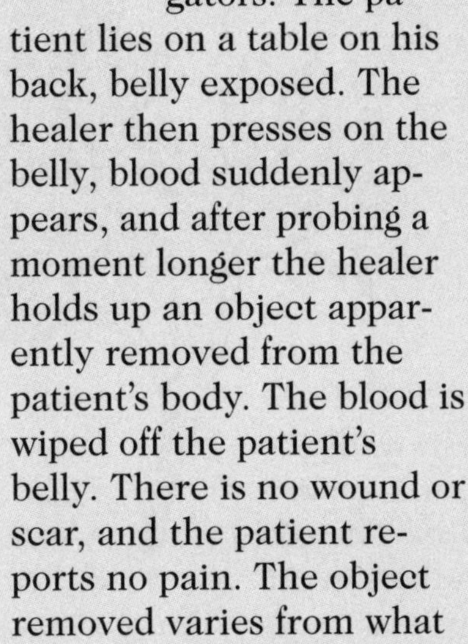

CRANBERRY JUICE: One of the most famous folk remedies for bladder infections—widely followed today throughout North America—is to drink cranberry juice. This remedy is especially well known in the folk medicine of New England.

This remedy, which has been studied in modern clinical trials, has been found to be effective in preventing, but not treating, bladder infections. A study conducted at the Brigham and Women's Hospital in Boston, and published in the prestigious *Journal of the American Medical Association* in 1994, found that consumption of about 12 ounces of commercial cranberry juice each day for a month reduced bacterial counts in the lower urinary tracts of elderly women. Several other trials have shown similar results. (Using cranberry juice as a preventive may be very useful to bedridden elders, who are at higher risk for bladder infections.)

Constituents in the cranberry juice help to prevent bacteria from sticking to the walls of the urinary tract, making the bacteria easier to flush out. Once the infection is underway, however, and the bacteria have set up shop, the cranberry juice is not of much use.

☞ Directions: Obtain a sugar-free cranberry juice or juice concentrate from a health food store. (The brands in supermarkets contain enough sugar to depress the activity of the immune system.) Drink 8 to 12 ounces of the juice a day to prevent recurring infections.

PLANTS CONTAINING BERBERINE: A New England folk tradition suggests using the plant goldthread *(Coptis trifolia)* to treat urinary tract infections. Drs. Agatha Thrash, M.D., and Calvin Thrash, M.D., authors in the tradition of the Seventh Day Adventists, suggest using goldenseal *(Hydrastis canadensis)* for the same purpose. Nineteenth century physicians of the homeopathic school of medicine used tinctures of Oregon grape root *(Mahonia aquifolium, Berberis aquifolium)* for urinary tract infections.

The three plants have a constituent in common, called berberine. Berberine has strong antibacterial properties. Berberine is not very well absorbed across the intestinal wall, though the most prominent use of these plants is for intestinal infections. The small amounts that are absorbed, however, are excreted through the kidneys and concentrated in the urine. This could explain the therapeutic effect, if any, on urinary tract infections. Goldthread is usually not available in the herb marketplace, and goldenseal is now an endangered species, facing extinction in North America. Oregon grape root is readily available at low cost, however.

☞ Directions: To treat urinary tract infections, simmer 1 tablespoon of Oregon grape root in a pint of water for twenty minutes. Cool to room temperature. Strain and drink the pint during the day for seven to ten days.

PARSLEY: The ancient Egyptians, Greeks, and Romans all used parsley *(Petroselinum crispum)* as a diuretic. The practice continues today both by Gypsies and in the folk tradition of New England. Parsley, which originated in the eastern Mediterranean region, was introduced to England in the year 1548, and, within a hundred years, it was recommended in British medical herbals for use as a diuretic in cases of severe edema (dropsy).

Sugar

The Spanish Gypsy folk healer Pilar, the source of the remedies in a book called *Gypsy Folk Medicine* by Wanja von Hausen, recommends against adding sugar or honey to diuretic teas used for treating urinary tract infections. This is sound advice, from a medical point of view, for any infection, actually. Clinical studies have shown that about 2 ounces of sugar—the amount in the average soft drink—depresses the activity of the immune system's white blood cells by about 40 percent. Cranberry juices sweetened with sugar should be avoided for this reason. Although a clinical trial showed that sugar-sweetened cranberry juice does help prevent bladder infections, it is likely that the juice may be more effective without the sugar.

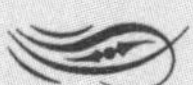

Although edema is now treated with conventional medicine, parsley can still be used to remedy other conditions. Parsley is approved by the German government for use as a mild diuretic and for treatment of bladder infections. For safety's sake, use parsley root rather than parsley seeds, parsley juice, or parsley leaves. (Parsley seeds can stimulate uterine contractions or irritate the kidneys. Parsley juice can also stimulate uterine contractions and should thus be avoided during pregnancy. And, although parsley leaves are nutritious, they do not contain much of the diuretic constituents of the plant.) The following formula is a modification of a Gypsy diuretic formula used for urinary tract infections and kidney stones.

☞ Directions: Take a handful of parsley roots and cut them into small pieces. Place them in 1 quart of water, bring to a boil, and simmer for ten to fifteen minutes. Remove from the heat and stir in a handful of rose blossoms. Steep, covered, for ten minutes. Strain and drink 5 to 7 cups of the tea during the course of a day for seven to ten days. Do not use in excessive amounts. Do not use during pregnancy and lactation.

ANISE: The Amish use anise seed *(Pimpinella anisum)* as a diuretic. Hispanics in the Southwest use it the same way—as did the ancient Egyptians and Greeks. The Greek herbalist Dioscorides, whose book of herbal medicine was used by doctors in Europe for at least 1600 years, stated that anise seed "provokes urine." Anise, better known in medical herbalism as a digestive stimulant, is probably one of the mildest diuretics in this section.

☞ Directions: Crush 1 teaspoon of anise seeds in a grinder or with a mortar and pestle. Place in a cup and fill with boiling water. Cover well, and let steep for ten minutes. Strain and drink 2 to 3 cups a day. Don't take anise except as a simple food spice in pregnancy, however, because anise can stimulate uterine contractions when taken in the above dose.

HORSETAIL: Horsetail *(Equisetum arvense)* was used as a medicine by the ancient Greeks. It has been used specifically as a diuretic in Western traditional medicine since the 1500s. The Iroquois Indians used a North American species of the plant *(Equisetum hymenale)* for the same purpose. Today, horsetail is used as a diuretic in the Hispanic folk medicine of the Southwest.

Horsetail is approved by the German government for use as a diuretic and for treatment of bladder infections. In 1994, animal research in Spain demonstrated that horsetail teas also lowered the risk factors for kidney stones and kidney infections, although the effect was mild. Note: Do not confuse this plant with marsh horsetail *(Equisetum palustre)*, a larger plant that contains toxic alkaloids.

☞ Directions: Place 1 tablespoon of horsetail herb in a 1-pint jar and cover with boiling water. Cover and let stand for ten to fifteen minutes. Strain and drink the pint in 3 doses throughout the day. Do not take horsetail for longer than three weeks on a daily basis, because it can irritate the digestive tract when taken for long periods.

BURDOCK: Burdock *(Arctium spp.)* has been used since ancient times as a mild diuretic. The Iroquois Indians used the root for this purpose. In 17th century Great Britain, the plant's seeds were used specifically for treating the bladder and kidney stones.

In Germany, burdock is commonly used in contemporary medical practice, even though a review by the German government failed to find adequate clinical research to justify its use. However, in 1994, animal research in Spain demonstrated that, while burdock root teas did lower the risk factors for kidney stones and kidney infections, the effect was mild. And, although burdock is widely used in contemporary North American professional herbalism, its most common use in this country is as a "blood cleanser," not a diuretic.

☞ Directions: Place 1 ounce of burdock root in 1 quart of water in a pot and simmer, covered, for twenty minutes. Let cool to room temperature. Strain and drink the quart of tea throughout the day. Do this for up to three weeks.

BUCHU: The Hottentot tribe of southern Africa first acquainted Europeans with the use of buchu *(Barosma betulina)*. In 1821, it was imported to England. By 1840, it appeared in the *United States Pharmacopoeia* as an official medicine; it remained listed in following editions until 1940. It was used for treating urinary tract infections by all schools of medicine during that period. (The Eclectic physicians cautioned that the plant's oils could further irritate those urinary tract infections that are accompanied by burning or stinging pain, however.) The plant's constituents are probably its aromatic peppermint-like oils. Buchu is used by conventional doctors in Germany as a mild diuretic and for treatment of bladder infections.

☞ Directions: Place ½ ounce of buchu leaves and ½ ounce of marshmallow root *(Althea officinalis)* in 1 quart of water. Cover the pot and simmer on the lowest heat for thirty to forty minutes. Allow to cool to room temperature. Strain and drink 1-ounce doses three to four times a day for seven to ten days.

FORMULA: A diuretic herbal formula combining several of the herbs in this section appeared in an anonymous personal letter in 1931 and is listed in a collection of remedies called *American Folk Medicine* by folklorist Clarence Meyer. Here is the formula slightly modified for more modern times.

Demulcent Herbs

Demulcents are a class of herbs that soothe irritated mucous membranes. They have a slimy mucous-like texture when mixed with water. The demulcents marshmallow (*Althea officinalis*), slippery elm (*Ulmus fulva*), and mullein leaf (*Verbascum thapsus*) all have been used in North American folk traditions to soothe urinary tract inflammation. The demulcents are often combined with diuretic herbs and taken as teas.

In the traditional herbalism of many cultures, demulcents are also used to treat sores in the mouth, sore throats, digestive tract ulcers, and irritations of the bronchial tract and lungs. The slimy substances can obviously soothe tissues they come in direct contact with, such as a sore throat or stomach ulcer. How they affect the lungs or urinary tract is a mystery, though, because the demulcents are completely digested and eliminated through the digestive tract. Even contemporary science has no explanation for the widely observed soothing action of these herbs on the urinary tract.

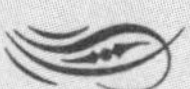

☞ Directions: Mix 2 ounces of buchu leaves, 2 ounces of uva ursi leaves, and 1 ounce of juniper berries. Grind them with a mortar and pestle and mix well. Place a teaspoon of the mixture in a cup, fill with boiling water, and let steep four to five minutes. Strain and drink 2 to 3 cups a day. Don't take this formula if you have active kidney disease.

CLEAVERS: Cleavers *(Galium aparine)* is most commonly used in contemporary medical herbalism as a "blood cleanser" (see section, Blood Purifiers) for skin conditions. But a tea made of cleavers—also known as goose grass or bed straw (it was also used to stuff mattresses)—has been used as a diuretic as well. The Ojibwa Indians used it for this purpose, as did the physicians of the Physiomedicalist and Eclectic schools—groups of doctors from the 19th and early 20th centuries who primarily used herbs as medicines.

☞ Directions: Place 1 ounce of cleavers in a quart of water and simmer for ten to fifteen minutes. Let cool to room temperature. Drink the quart of tea in 3 to 4 divided doses throughout the day.

WATER IMMERSION: The Seventh Day Adventists recommend sitting in a hot tub to promote urination. According to clinical research over the last ten years, full water immersion (up to the neck) can indeed produce this effect. (Apparently, the increased water pressure on the body promotes increased excretion of urine.) Research shows the same effect regardless of whether hot, cold, or neutral-temperature water is used.

☞ Directions: After drinking 2 to 3 glasses of water, immerse yourself for thirty to forty minutes in a hot tub, swimming pool, or other body of water.

Patent Medicines

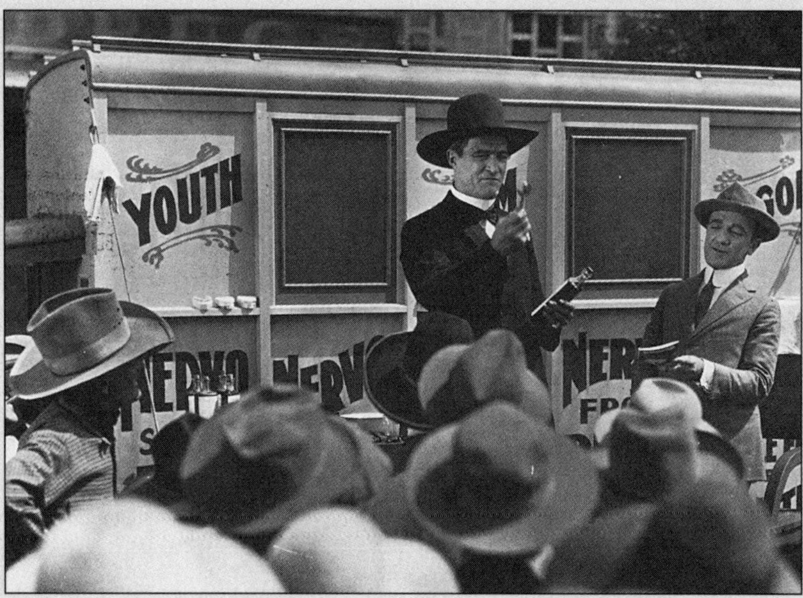

The medicine vendors and customers of days gone by.

From colonial times until the early 20th century the drug industry was a free-for-all. Effective drugs that were available competed with all sorts of panaceas that ranged from useless to dangerous. In this wild marketplace, patent medicine vendors were advertising pioneers.

At first, prepackaged remedies were imported, but after the Revolution, American entrepreneurs made and marketed their own medicines. Hundreds of hopeful medicine-makers took out patents for their compounds but couldn't compete with the advertising budgets of those who were successful. The heavy trend in promotion accelerated through the century and was boosted by the Civil War—from which many soldiers returned addicted to bottled medicines. The war also expanded the audience for newspapers, which soon became heavily subsidized by medicine accounts. When the price of newsprint rose, marketers turned to almanacs, handbills, and, above all, the outdoors—where buildings, boulders, and whole hillsides were emblazoned with their products' names.

Salesmanship reached fever pitch in the "medicine shows" of the 1880s. There the product was secondary to entertainment. The Kickapoo Indian Medicine Company, for instance, might have 75 shows touring the country at one time. Founded by three white men, it employed American Indians to enact dire scenarios from which they were saved by a medicine called Kickapoo Indian Saqwa. The sales team for Hamlin's Wizard Oil included a singing quartet. William Rockefeller (John D. Rockefeller's father) used his talents as marksman, ventriloquist, and hypnotist to attract

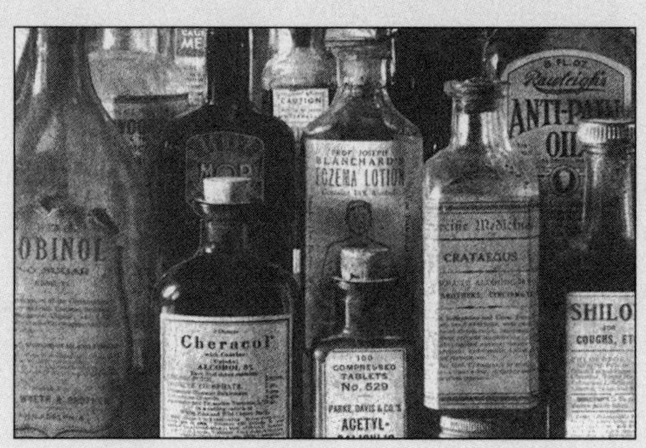

A remedy existed for practically every illness.

Midwest crowds to his medicinal products. Other salesmen posed as Quakers, Shakers, and Oriental mystics—whatever it took to move the goods. Many "doctors" and "professors" were addicted to their own wares, which sometimes contained alcohol, opium, chloroform, or cocaine. (Other products were not so dangerous. They contained colored water or candy, like Princess Lotus Blossom's Vital Sparks.)

Snake oil, which was actually fat rendered from a snake, was among the top-selling medicines of the time. The product was used to treat a variety of ills, from arthritis to earache. Ingredients in a bottle of snake oil usually included the oil, but it could also include anything but the oil. Thus, throughout the history of the U.S. patent medicine industry, the terms "snake oil" and "snake oil salesman" have been used to describe any dubious product and its seller.

Snake oil really was among the nostrums flooding the land. But why was it singled out to represent all the bogus products? Classic associations, like the serpent in the garden, probably helped. Contemporary emblems were likely the key, however. The perennially popular Swaim's Panacea bore a label depicting Hercules battling the many-headed snake-like Hydra. On the label for Dr. Hostetter's Celebrated Stomachic Bitters Tonic, a naked St. George slays the fabled dragon. In 1905, writer Samuel Hopkins Adams published two series of articles in *Collier's* magazine—one on patent medicines and the other on medical quacks. In his expose, he attacked 264 companies and individuals by name, exposing their involvement in drug sales that were dangerous and addictive. The American Medical Association then distributed 150,000 copies of Adams' "The Great American Fraud." This action marked the beginning of the end for unregulated drug sales. In 1906, Congress passed the Pure Food and Drug Act, which was the beginning of federal regulation. Ironically, consumption of patent medicines increased after the Pure Food and Drug Act of 1906, because with the worst products off the market, those remaining were believed to be safe.

Medicine from Around the World

Snake oil has indeed been used in homemade medicines, along with goose grease, rabbit lard, polecat grease, and skunk oil. Patent medicines generally strove for a more exotic appeal. Besides alleged American Indian sources, far-flung locales were evoked. Dr. Lin's Celestial Balm of China, Bragg's Arctic Liniment, Hayne's Arabian Ointment, Jayne's Spanish Alternative, and Druid Ointment ("handed down from mystic days when Stonehenge was a busy temple") were just a few choices. Household remedies tend to be specific ("For rheumatism, apply oil from a cooked snake on the sore area") but commercial ones were notorious cure-alls. Helmbold's Extract of Buchu claimed to help at least 21 separate ailments from "confused ideas" to "paralysis of the organs of generation."

Blood Purifiers and Blood Builders

The concept of blood purification remains alive and well in contemporary professional medical herbalism in North America, Great Britain, and Australia

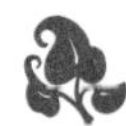

European and North American folk remedy books from the 18th and 19th centuries make frequent references to foods and herbs that "purify the blood." This concept was also important in conventional and alternative medicine in these centuries and survives today among practitioners of folk medicine. The "blood" in the traditional concept of bad blood did not really refer to the blood at all, but actually to the extracellular fluid that bathes the cells. The blood itself comprises only about five percent of the fluids in the body, while the extracellular fluid makes up about twenty percent. The rest of the body's water lies within the cells.

The composition of the blood is tightly controlled by the physiological mechanisms of the body, so it does not become "bad" in any sense. The extracellular fluid, on the other hand, accumulates the metabolic wastes of all the cells, the waste byproducts of infection and inflammation, and toxic byproducts of poor digestion. An overload of such materials in the extracellular spaces is probably what physicians of the last century referred to as "bad blood." These doctors included such medical conditions as abscesses, arthritis, boils, chronic infection, chronic inflammation, eczema, gangrene, psoriasis, septicemia, skin ulcers, and chronically swollen glands in their list of illnesses arising from "bad blood" and used "blood purifying" herbal medicines and diets to treat them. In folk medicine, the term "spring tonic" is equivalent to "blood purifier" in 19th century medicine. People felt the need to use such tonics in the Spring—after months of reduced activity and a lack of fresh fruits and vegetables during the winter.

The concept of bad blood has been abandoned completely in modern medicine, due to advances in the science of physiology and to a lack of clinical trials of most of the herbs formerly used. If you see references to such terms in books of folk or herbal medicine, know that they do not apply to true blood diseases in the modern sense. But the concept of blood purification is alive and well in contemporary professional medical herbalism in North America, Great Britain, and

Australia, even if the term itself is not accurate. Five of the ten most often prescribed herbs by professional herbalists in these countries, recorded in a 1994 poll, were traditional blood purifiers.

The actions of the herbs are varied. They include immune stimulants such as echinacea and garlic; circulatory stimulants such as cayenne; bitter liver-stimulating herbs such as dandelion, yellow dock, and goldenseal; diuretics like nettle; and sweat-inducing herbs such as burdock and boneset.

Remedies

BURDOCK: Burdock root *(Arctium lappa, Arctium minus)* has long been a universal "blood purifier" among North American peoples. Its medicinal value was noted by the ancient Greeks; it arrived in North America via the European colonists. Burdock's medicinal use was rapidly adopted by the Mohegan, Delaware, Chippewa, Omaha, Potawatomi, and Cherokee Indian tribes. It is used today in the folk medicine of Pennsylvania Germans, the Amish, Indiana farmers, and residents throughout Appalachia. Burdock has become naturalized throughout North America except in Texas and Alaska and parts of Canada.

Burdock was an official medicine in the *United States Pharmacopoeia* from 1831 to 1842, and again from 1851 to 1916. It was recommended as a diuretic, mild laxative, and treatment for skin ailments. Modern scientific studies show that burdock root has anti-inflammatory properties, slightly opposes the tendency of the blood to clot, and scavenges destructive free radicals from the blood.

☞ Directions: Simmer 1 ounce of burdock root in 1 pint of water for twenty minutes. Strain when cool. Add 3 or 4 tablespoons of molasses. Drink the entire contents over the course of a day. Repeat daily for one to two weeks.

ECHINACEA: Echinacea *(Echinacea angustifolia, Echinacea purpurea)* was used extensively by the Northern Plains Indians to treat burns and wounds as well as the bites of snakes and poisonous insects. Echinacea was adopted by the Eclectic medical profession in the mid 1800s, and became their most-often prescribed medicine by about 1920. The Eclectics, a group of M.D.s who primarily used herbs as medicines, classified the plant as a blood purifier and used it to treat life-threatening blood infections. German physicians began using the plant by the 1830s, and, in that country, it remains a frequently-prescribed medicine today. Folklorists have also discovered the use of echinacea in the folk medicine of the Appalachians in northern Georgia, but its use undoubtedly arrived there in the last century from outside the area.

Echinacea root is used primarily to boost the immune system and help the body fight disease. Besides bolstering several chemical substances that direct immune response, echinacea increases the number and activity of white blood cells, raises the level of interferon (a substance that enhances immune function), increases production of substances the body produces to fight cancer, and helps remove pollutants from the lungs. Many studies support echinacea's ability to fend off disease. It is perhaps the best known remedy of the modern folk herbal.

Echinacea is not effective as a tea for immune-building properties, but must be taken as a tincture, or, as in the case of the Plains Indians, the whole root can be chewed.

☞ Directions: Purchase an alcohol tincture of echinacea at a health food store or herb store. To prevent illness, take 1 dropperful three times a day. If you are sick with a cold or flu or feel a cold coming on, take a dropperful mixed with a little warm water every 2 hours.

To make your own tincture, purchase 1 pound of echinacea root. In a jar, cover the root with grain alcohol or 100 proof liquor. Close the jar tightly. Store in a cool dark place for three weeks, turning or shaking the jar daily. Then strain and store in the refrigerator. Use as directed above.

GARLIC: Garlic *(Allium sativum)* has been prized for millennia, used by the Egyptians, Hebrews, Romans, Greeks, and Chinese. It has appeared in the ancient medical texts of every traditional form of medicine. Garlic is one of the most extensively researched and widely used of plants. Its actions are diverse and affect nearly every body system. The herb boasts antibiotic, antifungal, and antiviral properties and is reported to be effective against many influenza strains. Garlic inhibits blood clotting and keeps platelets from clumping, which improves blood flow and reduces the risk of stroke. Its widest known folk use is as a tonic to "ward off" disease or evil.

Because garlic was not native to this country (it may have originated in southern Siberia), Indian tribes in the eastern United States used garlic's native botanical cousin, the onion, as a spring tonic. European immigrants brought their native folk uses of garlic with them, and the garlic plant was ultimately naturalized here. A single clove (not the whole bulb) of garlic a day has shown to have preventive effects against disease.

☞ Directions: One of the best ways to consume garlic is to eat it raw. You can eat up to 3 cloves a day. When cooked, the stronger the flavor is, the more medicinal value it has. Alternately, try blending 1 to 3 cloves of garlic in a cup of your favorite juice, warm water, or wine, and let stand covered overnight. Strain and drink the next day, in 3 divided doses, with meals.

CAYENNE PEPPERS: Cayenne peppers *(Capsicum spp.)* were used by the Aztec Indians as a remedy for "bad blood." The practice continues in the folk medicine of the American Southwest, although the usual form of administration is as a seasoning in food. Cayenne peppers are a strong circulatory stimulant and were one of the main remedies of the Thomsonian movement of folk herbalism during the first half of the 19th century. The stimulation of blood circulation to the periphery of the body is presumably how the peppers "purify" those areas where circulation is believed to have stagnated. Because chiles are so heating, they are probably best suited to those individuals with "cold" constitutions—those with cold hands and feet and a tendency to chill easily. Says Dr. William Cook, author of a mid-19th century medical herbal called *The Physio-Medicalist Dispensatory*: "Cayenne is as out of place in a hot constitution as a bonfire on the Fourth of July."

☞ Directions: Use chiles freely as a food condiment. Alternately, sprinkle ¼ teaspoon of cayenne powder into 1 cup of warm water and add a little lemon juice. Drink the mixture twenty minutes before meals. Do this three times a day for up to two weeks. Adjust the quantity of the pepper to your taste.

DANDELION: Through their writings, the Arabs were the first to introduce dandelion's *(Taraxacum officinale)* healing and nutritive abilities to the Europeans. By the 16th century, dandelion was considered an important culinary and blood-purifying herb in Europe. The root was recommended to treat liver diseases, such as jaundice and cirrhosis. The remedies requiring the use of dandelion traveled to North American with European immigrants; some eastern American Indian groups also used dandelion for healing purposes. The dandelion has become naturalized in this country throughout temperate regions.

Dandelion was an official medicine in the *United States Pharmacopoeia* from 1831 to 1926, recommended as a diuretic, tonic, and mild laxative. Modern scientific trials show that dandelion acts as a mild diuretic and increases the flow of bile from the liver, and, in one animal trial, it helped to restore depleted immune function.

Dandelion roots contain inulin and levulin, starchlike substances that are easy to digest, as well as a bitter substance (taraxacin) that improves digestion through the stimulation of stomach secretions. Because taraxacin does stimulate these secretions, however, dandelion is contraindicated if you have heartburn or other kinds of digestive pain.

☞ Directions: Eat young spring dandelion greens either raw, or lightly sauteed with olive oil, lemon, and garlic. To make a tea of the root, place 1 ounce of the dried chopped root in 1 pint of water and simmer for twenty minutes. Cool and strain. Drink the pint in 3 doses throughout the day. Do this periodically.

YELLOW DOCK: Yellow dock *(Rumex crispus)* has been used in European medicine since the time of the ancient Greeks as a bitter tonic, laxative, liver stimulant, and dressing for wounds. American Indians used North American species of yellow dock in similar ways. It is still used in folk medicine today by some residents in the Appalachian mountains and in the rural Midwest.

Yellow dock root stimulates intestinal secretions and promotes bile flow, which aids fat digestion and has a light laxative action. Long considered a blood purifier, yellow dock may also be effective in treating a number of conditions that stem from liver dysfunction. (Yellow dock has strong laxative properties, so it should be taken in low doses.) It is contraindicated in pregnancy because the constituents it contains that stimulate the bowels may also stimulate the smooth muscle of the uterus.

continued on page 88

Food for Thought

If a material is readily available, folk medicine usually finds a use for it. Thus, it is no surprise that foods of all sorts have always been a very important part of traditional folk remedies. In addition to their availability, foods have certain obvious effects on health and body functions. There are foods that are irritants (such as mustard, pepper, and hot peppers), foods that are stimulants or soporifics (which make you sleepy), foods that increase the flow of urine, and foods that act as laxatives. In short, there are many biological activities that can be observed in connection with foods.

All these reasons make a variety of foods natural candidates for the folk medicine chest—and many a "Doctor Mom" was—and still is—a walking encyclopedia of this information. For example, here's a set of remedies provided by one African-American woman from Maryland: Place the lining of a raw egg on a boil and smooth it around the edges. This will draw the boil to a head. Carry an Irish potato in your pocket to relieve hemorrhoids. Put a poultice of crushed onions on the chest to reduce fever, or, for a child with fever, place the onion poultice on the wrists. To help ease asthma, boil and steep dried field mullet leaves, add cream and sugar if you like, and drink. Or you can smoke field mullet and smell or inhale its vapors. In these examples, we find not only a variety of foods, but also a combination of natural and magical remedies. The egg lining, the mullet tea, and the mullet vapors seem to have a direct, physical connection to what is being treated. The Irish potato in the pocket has, at most, a distant and apparently magical connection to hemorrhoids. The onion poultice seems physical, but when placed on the wrists, it's a little less so. This is typical of folk medicine where modern distinctions between "natural" remedies and "magical" ones are not consistently made.

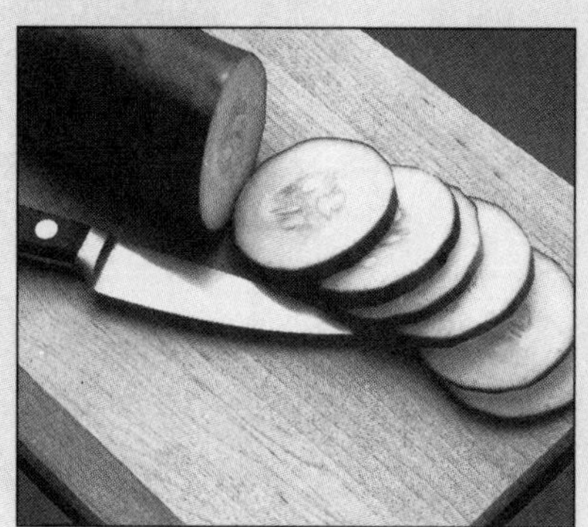

Cucumbers can cool a fever.

Some food remedies sound like pure commonsense, such as the Georgia folk cure for obesity that prescribes eating lean meat, rye bread, and leafy vegetables. Much of folk medicine is dietary, and, as medical researchers are coming to realize, many of our ills result from poor or unbalanced diets. But most traditional food remedies go far beyond anything found in contemporary medical advice. Many medicinal foods are intended as "tonics" to "build up" strength. For example, from Georgia comes a recipe for minced rabbit and celery that's supposed to increase vigor and improve digestion. And many people have heard of taking sulfur and molasses in the spring to "purify the blood." Foods are also recommended for strengthening the mind. Fish has a reputation for being "brain food," but the Pennsylvania German tradition recommends pig brains pickled in vinegar for the same purpose. It is also common in folk tradition to find that no part of an animal or plant that is remotely edible should be wasted!

In folk medicine, colds and respiratory infections are among the illnesses most frequently treated with food preparations. Most remedies involve smearing fat—such as goose grease, mutton tallow, or beef suet—on the patient. Sometimes these fats are mixed with irritants such as mustard. Similarly, salt pork (which is largely fat) was frequently recommended as a poultice and occasionally covered with pepper as an irritant. Salt pork was applied to sore throats—and recommended as a food for cold sufferers. From Georgia comes a remedy for croup in which hog lard mixed with sugar and turpentine is either applied as a poultice or swallowed! Onion syrup, which is made by roasting an onion, is a cough treatment still used in many American homes, often with honey added. Whooping cough is a very severe, sometimes fatal, childhood illness that is very difficult to treat. Because of this, remedies for the illness have often been exotic, such as drinking mare's milk or consuming toad soup (from Georgia).

Dressings

Foods and other ingredients have often been used as poultices or wound dressings in folk medicine. Some dressings from the Pennsylvania German tradition were made with onion, dog fat, skunk fat, unsalted butter, a squill (a bulbous plant with numerous medicinal uses) fried in fat, homemade soap soaked in vinegar, a cloth saturated with vinegar, and spiderwebs. A simpler dressing from the same tradition was to salt the wound (to disinfect) and then bind it with a slice of bacon to "draw out" any infection. As strange as this may sound, it is similar to a practice that has been shown to be medically effective. In hot, moist climates there are insects whose larva hatch in human skin, causing a painful swelling from which the insect eventually emerges. Bacon placed over these swellings has been shown to bring the larva to the surface promptly where they can be grasped with tweezers and removed, reducing the risk of infection!

A variety of vegetables were used to "draw out" fevers. For example, in Maryland it was said that a dressing of pulse (a medicinal plant) and beaten horseradish or cucumbers tied to the feet could relieve fevers. Other remedies are more medically sound. For instance, wrapping a feverish patient in wet collard leaves or peach tree leaves dipped in salty vinegar makes medical sense. Wet leaves would provide evaporative cooling that will temporarily reduce the fever.

Practically every food imaginable has been used medicinally, and nearly every ailment has one or more food remedies that can be employed, whether in the form of wound dressings or magic rituals. Many of these ideas were once ridiculed by official medicine. Today, many of these remedies have joined conventional medical wisdom. Other food remedies never will, but that will not prevent them from being used in folk tradition.

An Endangered Species

"Goldenseal is the king and queen of herbs that the Good Lord put in the ground," according to traditional Appalachian herbalist Tommie Bass in *Herbal Medicine Past and Present* (Volume II), by John K. Crellin and Jane Philpott. The Cherokee Indians mixed powdered goldenseal root with bear grease and slathered their bodies to protect themselves from mosquitoes and other insects. Pioneers adapted the herb and used it to treat wounds, rashes, mouth sores, morning sickness, liver and stomach complaints, internal hemorrhaging, depressed appetite, constipation, and urinary and uterine problems.

Goldenseal formerly abounded in the eastern forests of this country, but, due to overharvesting (it takes about five years for the root to get large enough to harvest) and loss of habitat, it was recently declared an endangered species. Goldenseal is contraindicated in acute colds and flu (it can make them worse) and is ineffective when used to mask the presence of drugs in urine specimens. Unfortunately, these are the two most common modern uses, and such misuse is probably contributing to the extinction of the plant.

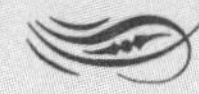

☞ Directions: Place 2 tablespoons of chopped dried yellow dock root in 1 pint of boiling water. Simmer for twenty minutes. Cool and strain. The dose is 3 tablespoons three times a day. Try the treatment for a week or two.

STINGING NETTLE: In Appalachian folk medicine, nettle *(Urtica dioica)* is a traditional spring tonic. It is taken as a tea or tincture after a long winter of sedentary habits and a lack of fresh fruits and vegetables, common in all agrarian communities in regions with cold winters. Preparations are used today in European medicine to treat arthritis and enlarged prostate. Modern research shows that nettle has an anti-inflammatory effect. The herb is also highly nutritious—an ounce of nettle contains more than the minimum daily requirement of calcium, two thirds of the requirement of magnesium, and more than one third of the requirement of potassium.

☞ Directions: Place 1 ounce of dried nettle in 1 quart of water and simmer until one third of the liquid is evaporated. Cool and strain. Drink the remaining liquid in 3 divided doses. Also, try this method, told to traditional Appalachian herbalist Tommie Bass by a local American Indian: Place 1 inch of dried nettle in the bottom of a 1-pint bottle and fill the bottle with whiskey. Let the bottle sit for a week, shaking it daily. Then take 1 tablespoon of the mixture three times a day. Take for two to three weeks.

RED CLOVER: Red clover tea *(Trifolium pratense)* is another traditional spring tonic among residents in the Appalachians. Some of red clover's constituents are thought to stimulate the immune system. Another one of its constituents, coumarin, has blood-thinning properties. Thus, red clover should not be used with pharmaceutical blood-thinning medications, including aspirin. Red clover also has a high mineral content: An ounce of the flowering tops contains half the minimum daily requirement of calcium, about a fourth of the requirement of magnesium, and a third of the requirement for potassium.

☞ Directions: Add 1 ounce of red clover tops to 1 quart of water. Simmer until one third of the water is gone. Cool and strain. Drink the liquid in 3 doses daily for two to three weeks.

BONESET: Boneset *(Eupatorium perfoliatum)* was without a doubt the most famous of the bitter tonics in the early American colonies. (A bitter tonic was a tonic used to stimulate digestion.) Medical botanists Walter and Memory Lewis, in their book *Medical Botany,* state that boneset "was always found in the well-regulated household."

Boneset earned its name because, as a hot tea, it reportedly cured "breakbone fever," an old term for influenza. It is usually taken as a cold tea in small doses. High doses can induce vomiting; it was used for this purpose by physicians of the 19th century.

☞ Directions: To use as a bitter tonic, place 1 tablespoon of dried boneset leaves in a cup and cover with boiling water. Let stand until the water is room temperature. Strain and drink in 3 divided doses during the day, away from meals.

ELDER: The berries and flowers of the black elder *(Sambucus nigra)* have been used as a blood purifier and flu remedy. In British folk herbalism it was taken in the form of elderberry wine. The berries of the North American variety of the plant, *Sambucus canadensis*, were used for the same purposes by the Houma Indians of Louisiana. European settlers brought elderberry plants with them to the American colonies.

Elder was an official medicine in the *United States Pharmacopoeia* from 1820 to 1905. It was recommended as an "alterative," an old medical term for blood purifier. The elderberry that bears blue fruit is perfectly safe to eat, although large quantities of the raw berries can cause some indigestion and act as a laxative. Cooking the berries before eating them cancels this action. The leaves, bark, and root, on the other hand, are slightly toxic and should not be ingested. Don't use the elder plant that bears red berries. This plant is of a different species.

☞ Directions: Fill half of a 1-quart pot with elderberries. Add water until the pot is nearly full and bring to a boil. Simmer on the lowest heat until one third of the water has evaporated. Strain and store in the refrigerator. Add 1 teaspoon to a cup of water and drink three times a day. Do this for two to three weeks.

SASSAFRAS: Sassafras *(Sassafras albidum)* was used as a spring tonic in the eastern parts of the United States, throughout New England, among the Pennsylvania Germans, and through Appalachia all the way to northern Georgia and Alabama. Colonists learned the use of sassafras from the Indians. Spanish colonists used it as a universal remedy and shipped samples back to Spain. The plant was considered such an important medicine by colonists in Virginia and Massachusetts that boatloads of it were shipped back to England after the year 1602.

Epazote

One of the most frequently used folk medicines in the American Southwest is epazote, (*Chenopodium ambrosiodes anthelminticum*). Like most traditional blood purifiers, it is used for a variety of conditions, including stomachache, cough, toothache, and worms. Colonists learned about the plant from American Indians in the region, who used epazote as a spring tonic. The oil of the plant was an official medicine for worms in the *United States Pharmacopoeia* from 1820 to 1947. Use for longer than a week as a blood purifier is not recommended.

☞ Directions: Place 1 ounce of epazote leaves in a 1-quart jar and fill with boiling water. Cover the jar and let the water cool to room temperature. Take 2 or 3 cups a day for up to seven days.

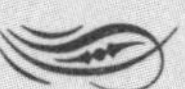

Sassafras has a wide variety of active constituents, several of them with cancer-preventing properties. It also contains the constituent saffrole, which has been found to cause cancer in mice when given in large doses. Saffrole is not soluble in water and is not present in significant quantities in traditional teas. However, the U.S. Food and Drug Administration banned the interstate marketing of sassafras for sassafras tea in 1976 because of its saffrole content.

☞ Directions: Place 1 ounce of sassafras root bark in 1 quart of water. Cover, bring to a boil, and simmer on the lowest heat for fifteen minutes. Let the water cool to room temperature. Strain and drink 1 cup a day for seven to fourteen days.

SARSAPARILLA: Sarsaparilla *(Smilax officinalis)*, which grows mainly in the semi-tropical areas of North America, was one of the most important "new" plants discovered in the colonies by the Europeans, and it was shipped in large amounts back to Europe as a blood purifier and treatment for syphilis. It is still used today as a blood purifier in the folk medicine of Pennsylvania Germans and throughout Appalachia. In some parts of the mountains, it is considered a second-best substitute for the more potent sassafras. The German government has judged that no scientific evidence exists to support the use of sarsaparilla for any medical condition. Use for longer than seven to fourteen days is not recommended.

☞ Directions: Simmer 1 ounce of dried and chopped sarsaparilla root in 1 quart of water for twenty to thirty minutes. Strain and drink 1 or 2 cups a day for up to seven days.

YERBA MANSA: In Beatrice Roeder's *Chicano Folk Medicine from Los Angeles,* folk scholar Laura Curtin, as expert on Southwestern traditional medicine, states: "No other plant enjoys so wide a medicinal fame or has a higher repute," than yerba mansa *(Anemopsis californica)*. Spanish settlers learned the plant's uses from the Maricopa, Pima, and Tewa Indian groups. "Yerba

Good for Molasses

New Englanders, Indiana farmers, and the people of Appalachia have long used molasses as a "blood builder," either alone or added to blood-purifying teas and foods. Why? Molasses is one of the most mineral-dense foods available to us. Two tablespoons of blackstrap molasses, the most concentrated form, contain 340 milligrams of calcium, 6.5 milligrams of iron, 85 milligrams of magnesium, 1000 milligrams of potassium, .75 milligram of copper, and 1 milligram of manganese, all significant portions of the recommended dietary allowance.

mansa" is short for "yerba del indio manso," or "herb of the tamed Indians." American physicians of the Eclectic school began using it in 1877, and continued to do so until the 1940s. These physicians recommended the plant as a remedy for treating conditions of the mucous membranes—conditions that involved a stuffy sensation in the head and throat, a cough with expectoration, or mucous discharges from the bowels or urinary tract.

☞ Directions: Place 1 ounce of yerba mansa in 1 quart of water, bring to a boil, and simmer for twenty to thirty minutes. Let stand until cool. Drink 1 to 3 cups each day for a week or two.

EAT GREENS: Pennsylvania Germans make a ritual of "thinning the blood" in the spring by eating "blutreinigungsmittel," which include such greens as dandelion *(Taraxacum officinale)* and plantain *(Plantago major)*. Farmers in Indiana purify the blood by consuming the greens of the two plants lamb's quarters *(Chenopodium album)* and wild mustard *(Brassica kaber)*.

☞ Directions: Be sure to collect the greens in areas that have not been sprayed with pesticides! Eat them raw in salads or stir fry them with a little olive oil, garlic, and lemon. Eat as often as desired.

BEETS: American folk remedies list several sources that mention beet juice as a blood purifier. One source states that only raw beets should be used because cooking them destroys whatever blood cleansing properties are present. The contemporary Amish use beet juice as a "blood builder," sometimes mixed with red grape juice. Beets contain betaine, which has beneficial effects on the liver, and several other constituents with anti-inflammatory and immunostimulant properties. Beets are eaten instead of juiced in Appalachia, however.

☞ Directions: Purchase beets (home grown or organically grown, if possible) and juice them in a juicer. Drink an 8-ounce glass each day for a few weeks. You can eat beets whole, too.

HONEY AND CIDER VINEGAR: Honey and cider vinegar is a traditional New England blood strengthening remedy. The remedy was popularized by Dr. D.C. Jarvis in his book, *Folk Remedies: A Vermont Doctor's Guide to Good Health.* Jarvis theorized that the remedy works by neutralizing destructive acids in the blood, helping to prevent a wide variety of diseases. And although this has never been proven to be true, honey-cider vinegar is still used as a sort of cure-all.

☞ Directions: Put 2 teaspoons of honey and 2 teaspoons of apple cider vinegar in a glass of water. Mix. Drink 1 or 2 glasses a day. Jarvis recommends doing this on an ongoing basis.

Blood-Purifying Formulas

Several blood purifying herbs are often combined in the folk medicine of the eastern United Sates. Simple combinations of two or three of the single herbs listed in this section, such as burdock with sassafras, sassafras and sarsaparilla, and dandelion and sarsaparilla, appear in old folk remedy books as well as contemporary folk medicine. Two traditional formulas are shown below (see "Formula #1" and "Formula #2").

FORMULA #1: The following blood purifying tonic formula comes from a collection of American folk remedies, called *American Folk Medicine,* by folklorist Clarence Meyer.

☞ Directions: Combine 1 ounce of sarsaparilla root *(Smilax spp.),* 1 ounce of yellow dock root *(Rumex crispus),* ½ ounce of celandine herb *(Chelidonium majus),* 1 ounce of red clover flowers *(Trifolium pratense),* ½ ounce of dandelion root *(Taraxacum officinale),* ½ ounce of queen of the meadow tops *(Eupatorium purpureum),* ½ ounce elder flowers *(Sambucus canadensis, S. nigra),* and ½ ounce of prickly ash bark *(Zanthoxylum americonum).* Boil the mixture in 4 quarts of water until the water is reduced to 3 quarts. Strain when cool; add a cup of molasses. Store in the refrigerator. The dose is one fourth of a cup three times a day. If some of the herbs are unavailable at the health food store or herb shop, it is alright to omit a few from the recipe.

FORMULA #2: Another good blood-purifying recipe from old New England is as follows:

☞ Directions: Take 1 ounce of chopped burdock root, 1 ounce of yellow dock root, 1 ounce of sarsaparilla root, ½ ounce of red clover blossoms, 2 ounces of licorice root, and ½ ounce of coriander seeds. Mix them well. Add 2 tablespoons of the mixture to 1 pint of water and boil for five minutes. Let stand until cool. Strain and drink half a cup two to three times a day, away from meals. Take for two to three weeks.

Boils and Carbuncles

Boils can occur on any part of the body that has hair follicles. Thus, only the lips, palms, and soles of the feet can be spared

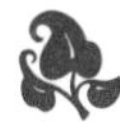

Boils—furuncles is the medical term—are tender, inflamed swellings centered around hair follicles in the scalp or skin. They result from infection by various strains of *Staphylococcus* bacteria. Carbuncles are clusters of boils, often appearing on the nape of the neck. Boils and carbuncles may appear on otherwise healthy individuals, although diabetes mellitus, debilitating diseases, and old age may predispose a person to the condition. Boils do not normally present a health hazard, but carbuncles may be accompanied by fever and exhaustion. Boils on the nose or in the central area of the face require prompt medical attention and treatment with antibiotics, however, because the bacterial infection can spread easily from that area to the brain.

Conventional and traditional treatment for simple boils is identical: Applications of moist heat until the boil comes to a head and drains spontaneously. Surgical incision or squeezing can spread the infection internally and should be avoided. For more serious or recurrent infections, the conventional treatment is antibiotic therapy. Besides the use of poultices and disinfectant washes, traditional medicine and folk remedies also center on purifying the blood through building up the strength of the immune system to resist bacterial infection.

Remedies

CHAMOMILE POULTICE: The folk medicine of the American Southwest recommends a poultice of hot chamomile tea *(Matricaria recutita)* for treating boils. Chamomile contains essential oils that have antiseptic, antibacterial, and anti-inflammatory properties.

☞ Directions: Place ½ ounce of chamomile flowers in a 1-pint canning jar and cover with boiling water. Cover the jar tightly and let stand for fifteen minutes. Strain the liquid and apply the hot mash directly to the boil. Cover with a cloth, and keep the cloth moist with the strained liquid. Do this remedy every two to three hours for twenty minutes at a time, until the boil comes to a head and drains.

SLIPPERY ELM POULTICE: An Appalachian remedy for boils combines hot water with slippery elm to make a paste. When mixed with water, shredded or powdered slippery elm bark *(Ulmus fulva)* makes a thick, sticky mass that can easily be applied to the skin. The mucilage in the bark soothes the tissues and the heat from the hot water draws blood to the area.

☞ Directions: In a pot, bring ½ cup of water to a boil. Turn off the heat and, stirring, add enough slippery elm bark powder to make a thick paste. Apply the paste directly to the boil, and cover with a cloth. Repeat every one to two hours until the boil comes to a head and drains.

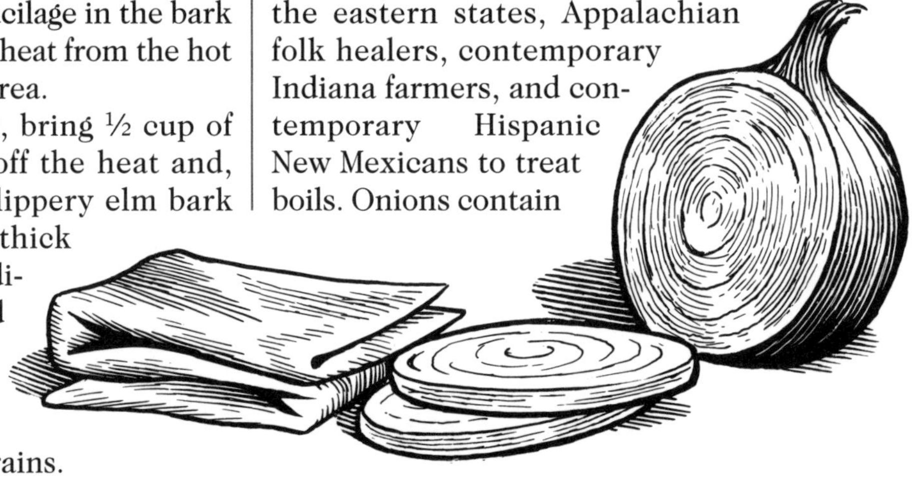

CORNMEAL POULTICE: A folk remedy of the Aztecs—which survives today in the folk medicine of the American Southwest—was to apply a poultice of cornmeal and hot water to the boil. The same method was used by the Cherokee Indians, who passed the remedy along to the Appalachians. The remedy is still used today in rural Indiana. It is the texture of the corn and its ability to hold the heat of water—not the medicinal properties of the corn—that are responsible for the value of this treatment.

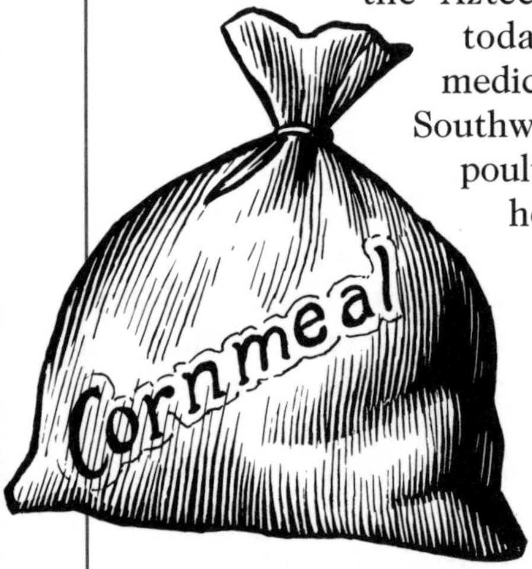

☞ Directions: In a pot, bring ½ cup of water to a boil. Turn off the heat and add cornmeal to make a thick paste. Apply the mixture to the boil, and cover with a cloth. Repeat every one to two hours until the boil comes to a head and drains.

ONION POULTICE: Onion *(Allium cepa)* poultices were used among eastern American Indian tribes, European colonists of the eastern states, Appalachian folk healers, contemporary Indiana farmers, and contemporary Hispanic New Mexicans to treat boils. Onions contain antiseptic chemicals and irritating constituents that draw blood and heat to the affected area.

☞ Directions: Place a thick slice of onion over the boil and keep in place by wrapping with a cloth. Change every three to four hours until the boil comes to a head and drains.

FLAX SEEDS AND OIL: Poultices made of flax seeds or flax oil are recommended in the folk literature of New England, Appalachia, and Indiana. If flaxseed (linseed) oil is used instead of the seeds, it must be mixed with flour or cornmeal. Although flax seeds and flax oil are sometimes used medicinally for their essential fatty acid content to prevent inflammatory diseases, this probably has no local effect when applied topically. Any effect probably comes from the texture of the poultices rather than their constituents.

☞ Directions: Grind 1 tablespoon of flax seeds. Add the seeds to ¼ cup of boiling water. Let the mixture become gelatinous. Cover the boil with a cloth, and then spread the flaxseed mush over it, as hot as can be tolerated. Cover the mush with another cloth. Leave the poultice on for one to two hours, until the mush completely dries. Repeat four times a day until the boil comes to a head and drains.

EGG SKIN POULTICE: A 19th century remedy for treating boils in the eastern United States was to apply the soft outer skin of a hard-boiled egg directly to the boil. It is now a commonly used remedy in contemporary New England, Appalachia, and southwestern Colorado.

☞ Directions: Hard boil an egg. Crack off the shell and carefully peel the outer skin off the egg. Wet it and apply the egg skin directly to the boil and cover with a clean cloth.

PORK POULTICE: Salt pork or bacon poultices are commonly used to treat various skin afflictions throughout New England and Appalachia. To treat a boil, you can try using a pork poultice. The poultice does not need to be hot, but the meat used should be fat meat. It is probably the constituents in the fat and the salt used to preserve the meat that bring the boil to a head.

☞ Directions: Roll some fatty pork or bacon in salt and place the meat between two pieces of cloth. Apply the poultice to the boil. Repeat throughout the day until the boil comes to a head and drains.

BREAD AND MILK POULTICE: Poultices made of bread and milk have been used to treat boils in New England, Appalachia, Indiana, and among Hispanics in southwestern Colorado. It is the drawing nature of the mixture and the heat of the poultice that make this remedy work.

☞ Directions: Heat 1 cup of milk and add 3 teaspoons of salt. (Add the salt slowly so it will not curdle the milk.) Simmer the mixture for ten minutes. Thicken the mixture by adding flour or crumbled bread pieces. Divide the mixture into four poultices and apply one poultice to the boil every half hour. The poultice may also be applied before bedtime, held in place with a cloth, and kept on overnight.

continued on page 98

A Gypsy Formula

A gypsy formula from Spain for treating boils combines several of the remedies already described above: Make a tea of burdock and stinging nettle leaves and add 2 crushed garlic cloves. Drink a cup three times a day on an empty stomach, before meals. This tea from across the Atlantic is remarkably similar to one used in the contemporary herbalism of the Pacific Northwest that uses burdock and nettle without the garlic.

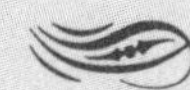

The Dead Lend a Hand

Although this may seem contradictory, folk medicine everywhere attributes special curative powers to corpses. Several reasons have been offered for this odd notion. In folk medicine, many remedies are opposites of their symptoms—such as when fullness is treated with bleeding or when irritating mustard plasters are applied to sore muscles. In the case of the corpse, it is believed that death may bring about health. It is also believed that the dead form a connection to the spiritual domain, and spirits are thought to be endowed with supernatural power.

The corpses that historically have received the most attention in folk medicine are those of executed criminals or suicides. This has led many scholars to suggest that, in folk medicine, untimely death is the major source of power. Many people believe humans have a preordained life span. When death occurs prematurely, they imagine the vital, spiritual energy remains potent, at least until the time a person would have died naturally.

As is common throughout folk belief, powers that are effective in healing also have other uses—sometimes rather strange ones. The hand is the most common body part of the corpse used in healing. This use of the hand comes from a grisly and ancient idea called "the hand of glory." The hand of glory was a charm used by burglars, who believed it would make them invisible and prevent the occupants of a house from hearing any sounds they made. (In some versions, it was said that the charm would actually paralyze its victims.)

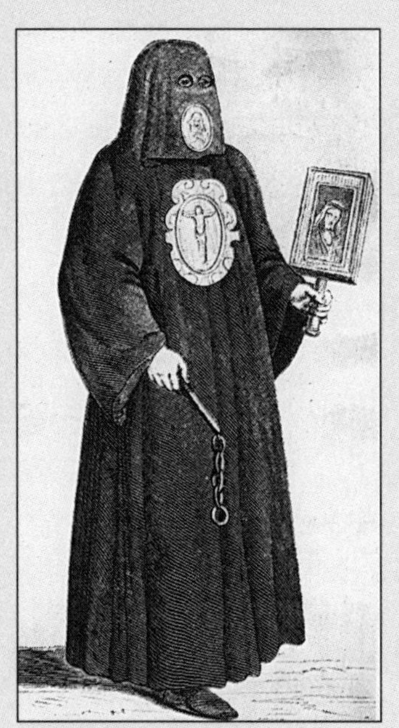

Hangmen were considered to be important healers.

The hand of glory was made by preserving the hand of a hanged criminal. Then a candle made from a corpse's fat would be placed in the hand and lit, or the fingers of the hand itself, soaked in fat, would be burned as candles! Most uses of the executed corpse were intended to heal rather than steal, however.

In Europe, the hangman was widely considered to have supernatural powers. This may have been because executions are a kind of sacrifice and, in a sense, the hangman represents God's authority in ending a life. Many hangmen advertised themselves as healers, and it was common for them to sell bits of clothing that belonged to the hanged criminal for magical and medical purposes. (Hangmen inherited the deceased's clothing as part of the payment for their grisly task.) Splinters from the gallows and the hangman's rope were also sold for healing purposes. Some hangmen would even permit parts of the hanged corpse to be taken.

In Pennsylvania and Ohio, the medicinal use of the hangman's rope was reported in both German and English tradition as a remedy for "fits" (seizures) and headache. The headache cure required that the noose be put around the patient's head! The use of gallow wood as a treatment for fever was recorded in *Natural History,* which was written in the first century A.D. by the Roman scholar and scientist Pliny the Elder. The use of gallow wood to treat fever continued in folk medicine. For example, in 1883, the remedy was published in the Philadelphia, Pennsylvania, magazine *The Casket.*

In addition to the executions, suicides also have an important place in the folklore of premature death. In both Pennsylvania and Ohio the hanging rope of a suicide was believed to cure epilepsy.

Use of the dead in American folk medicine has its roots in European tradition. In this country, however, there were actually very few healing beliefs that involved a hanged corpse. This is probably because public hangings were practiced for a relatively brief time in America, and today only Delaware, Montana, New Hampshire, and Washington retain hanging as an official method of execution. Still, folklorists have found among Pennsylvania Germans the belief that a wen (a large sebaceous cyst) will go away if it is passed across the head of a recently hanged man.

In America, however, the most common "corpse medicine" involves ordinary dead bodies. Treatments often take place at wakes or viewings rather than executions. Remedies are usually for warts, goiters, wens, or tumors—things that need to be "taken away." Since the dead are "going away," these cures involve a sort of magical transference. According to folklorist Vance Randolph, the people of the Ozark region often would attend viewings to treat goiters.

From the Midwest come two similar stories of such treatments. One account includes instructions for a cure: A fourteen-year-old girl went to where a corpse was laid out and rubbed her goiter three times with the corpse's hand, then returned the hand to its exact original position. Her goiter was said to be gone in a year. Another account explains that to rid yourself of a goiter you must use the hand from the same side of the corpse's body that your goiter is on. The remedy goes on to describe a person who used the left hand of a corpse to treat two goiters, one on each side. Only the goiter on the left side went away, confirming the tradition. This use of the dead hand for goiter seems very widespread and fairly current. Folk medicine scholar Wayland Hand tells of a woman with a noticeable goiter who, while waiting for a traffic light to change, was approached by a stranger who recommended that she treat the goiter by touching it with the hand of a corpse. This happened in California in the 1960s, and similar treatments have also been recorded in New York, Pennsylvania, Indiana, and Illinois.

Related beliefs for treating external tumors are widespread. However, sometimes the cure is a bit more complicated, as in this Pennsylvania German version: A string is tied around a dead man's finger. Then, the sting is removed and tied around the tumor. As the string rots the tumor will disappear.

Other medicinal uses of the dead include placing a corpse's finger in the mouth for toothache (Alabama) and the general use of the dead man's hand to improve the complexion—by running the hand over moles, blackheads, and birthmarks.

Blood Purifiers

A common approach in folk medicine to treat or prevent boils is to "purify the blood." The idea behind this remedy is to build the body's resistance to the boil from the inside out. (See the introduction on blood purifiers, page 82.) Some traditional blood-purifying herbs specifically used to treat boils are burdock and garlic. Appalachians recommend sassafras. Yerba mansa is the herb of choice in the folk medicine of southwestern American Indian tribes; it is also recommended by Hispanics residing in that area. Eclectic physicians of the last century prescribed ingesting echinacea to treat boils.

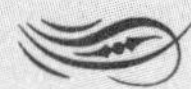

BURDOCK: Burdock *(Arctium lappa, A. minus)* is considered a universal remedy for treating boils in contemporary European and North American herbalism. Drinking burdock tea to treat boils is a remedy still practiced today in Appalachia and in parts of rural Indiana. The constituents in burdock bring circulation to the surface of the skin and induce a light sweat. This increased circulation and corresponding movement of fluid and lymph at the surface of the skin may be responsible for the treatment's healing effect.

☞ Directions: Place 1 ounce of dried and ground burdock root in 1 quart of water. Bring the water to a boil and simmer on low heat for thirty minutes. Drink 4 cups of the hot tea each day until the boil comes to a head and drains. Along with this remedy, you can apply a poultice of fresh boiled burdock leaves directly to the boil.

NUTMEG: A popular remedy for treating boils in New England, Appalachia, and parts of the American Southwest is eating nutmeg *(Myristica fragrans).* Nutmeg is also sometimes applied directly to the boil as a poultice. Nutmeg stimulates the body's circulation, which conceivably could assist the body in fighting the infection of the boil.

☞ Directions: Grind nutmeg. Stir ½ teaspoon into a cup of hot water and drink. Do this three to four times a day for up to three days.

CHRYSANTHEMUM FLOWERS: Drinking chrysanthemum flower tea is a Chinese folk remedy for treating boils that is still used in contemporary Chinese medicine today. The tea may also be applied as a compress. Chrysanthemum *(Chrysanthemum indicum flos)* flower tea is a common beverage among Asians in the United States and can usually be purchased in any Chinese or Korean food or herb shop. The Chinese name for the tea (and the herb) is yeh-chu-hua. Chinese and Japanese researchers have found constituents in chrysanthemum tea that inhibit *Staphylococcus* bacteria, the strain of bacteria that causes boils.

☞ Directions: Brew chrysanthemum flower tea according to the directions on the package. Dip a cloth in the hot tea and apply it to the boil every one to two hours. You can also drink 3 to 4 cups of the tea each day.

FIG POULTICE: Last century, fig poultices were used to treat boils in the folk medicine of the eastern United States. As of the 1980s, it remains a practice among residents of rural Indiana.

☞ Directions: To make a poultice, wash and peel ripe figs. Split one open and apply it directly to the boil and cover the area with a clean cloth or gauze. Leave it on as long as you like.

CUPPING: Applying suction to a boil with a cup or a jar has been a universal remedy for treating boils in traditional medicine from China, throughout Central Asia and the Middle East, in Medieval Europe, and among elders today in New England and Indiana. Cupping is the application of suction over specific area in the body. Practitioners warm air in a glass jar, then overturn it onto the body area to be treated. As the air cools, it contracts, causing the suction. The benefits of cupping come both from the moist heat and the suction.

☞ Directions: Boil a cup in a pot of water for a few minutes. Dump the water, and, let the cup cool a bit before applying it to the patient's skin. Using tongs, press the hot cup over the boil. The cup should cover the boil completely.

As the cup cools, a suction will form. (The suction probably brings blood and circulation to the area, which helps to hasten healing.) Alternately, you can try heating the air inside the cup with a candle. Apply as directed above.

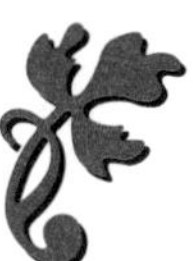

Breast Conditions

The most common folk remedies for the breast are herbs and foods to help increase milk production for nursing, to decrease milk after weaning, or to ease nipple discomfort

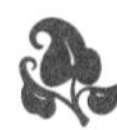

Today breast cancer is a major concern. It is the most common form of cancer in women, with 140,000 new cases diagnosed each year. Breast cancer was relatively rare until the last hundred years; thus, it was not a major concern to our ancestors of the last century. Scientists theorized that breast cancer could be directly related to our 20th century Western diet. After all, breast cancer is not common among those societies eating more traditional diets. Breast cancer was classified as a "Western disease" by medical researchers in the late 1970s.

Beware of Goat's Rue

Goat's rue (*Galega officinalis*) is a traditional remedy for increasing lactation, brought to North America by European colonists. (Extracts of goat's rue are still sold today in Europe for this purpose.) The plant's ability to increase milk is questionable, however. American physicians of the last century—even those who recommended herbal medicines—questioned its value and dropped mention of it from their medical texts by the 1920s. Veterinary studies in the 1940s showed that it did not increase milk production in goats; in fact it caused a type of poisoning in sheep. After a German government regulatory committee reviewed herbal medicines, it declined to approve goat's rue as a medicine for any purpose. The benefits of trying goat's rue, if any, appear not worth the risks of toxicity or illness.

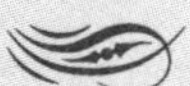

Though there are no folk remedies capable of curing breast cancer, there are remedies for treating other maladies of the breast. The most common folk remedies for the breast are herbs and foods to help increase milk production for nursing, to dry up the milk after weaning, or to ease the discomfort of cracked or caked nipples.

Because getting adequate nutrition to provide breast milk is a challenge for new mothers, many traditional folk remedies emphasize improving the mother's nourishment. After all, the mother may have to produce as much as a quart and a half of milk a day—milk that includes 20 grams of protein, 50 grams of fat, and 2 to 3 grams of calcium. Increasing liquid intake, either by drinking more water or by taking in more gruels and teas, is a common folk treatment.

Cracking and caking of breasts can also be a problem among nursing mothers. Care must be made to distinguish between normal cracking and infection (mastitis), however. An unattended breast infection can progress to an abscess and more serious infection. Mastitis that appears in the first months after a hospital birth should receive prompt medical attention because of the danger of antibiotic-resistant staphylococcal infection. Folk treatments for cracked and caked nipples include heat applications, soothing ointments and other substances, and bitter herbs applied directly to the nipples.

Remedies

HERBS TO INCREASE MILK

FENNEL SEEDS AND BARLEY WATER: In *American Folk Medicine,* a collection of folk remedies by Clarence Meyer, the combining of fennel with the water from cooked barley is recommended. The barley water probably contains some of the mineral nutrition of the grains. Good nutrition may help increase a mother's milk production.

☞ Directions: Prepare the barley water first by simmering a cup of barley in 1½ quarts of water for forty minutes on very low heat in a covered pot. Strain out the barley and save the water. To prepare the tea, place 1 teaspoon of fennel seeds in a cup. Bring 1 cup of barley water to a boil, and pour over fennel seeds. Let the water stand until it reaches room temperature. Strain. Drink only a few cups a day.

ANISE: A tea of anise seeds *(Pimpinella anisum)* was used in the eastern states in the 1800s as a method to increase milk production in nursing mothers. The practice survives today in the folk medicine of the Appalachians. Modern science has not proven that anise increases milk flow, but it was recommended by the Eclectic physicians of the last century for this purpose (see "Eclectic Medicine," page 29). Anise contains the essential oil anethole, which has shown to increase milk production in animal studies.

☞ Directions: Grind up 1 to 2 teaspoonfuls of anise seed in a coffee grinder, and place the powder in a cup. Fill the cup with boiling water, cover, and let stand for ten minutes. Drink 2 to 3 cups a day while nursing.

DILL SEED: Dill seed *(Anethum graveolens)* is used today in the folk medicine of the Appalachians to increase milk production in nursing mothers. Like anise, it contains the essential oil anethole, which has been shown to increase milk production in animal studies.

☞ Directions: Place 1 tablespoon of dill weed or 1 teaspoon of the ground (or crushed) seeds in a cup. Fill the cup with boiling water and cover. Let stand for twenty minutes. Strain. Drink 2 or 3 cups a day while nursing.

HOP TEA: A folk remedy from upstate New York is hop *(Humulus lupulus)* tea. Hop tea is reportedly used to increase milk production in the nursing mothers of twins, who have to produce more milk. If you have drunk beer, you will be familiar with hop's bitter taste. This bitterness makes hop an excellent digestive aid. Hop also contains chemicals that depress the central nervous system, making it a useful sedative. Its sedative properties may help nursing mothers relax.

Besides hop tea, folk practitioners have recommended hop to nursing mothers in the form of beer. But be-

continued on page 105

Helpful Herbs

Aromatic herbs such as fennel (*Foeniculum vulgare*), anise (*Pimpinella anisum*), and dill (*Anethum graveolens*) have been used in European folk medicine since antiquity to increase breast milk production. The use of these herbs came to North America with the colonists and persists today in the folk medicine of the Appalachians. Although modern science has not studied the plants' ability to increase breast milk production in humans, all three of these spices contain the essential oil anethole, which has been shown to increase milk production in animal studies. These common cooking spices may also improve a nursing mother's digestion.

Powwow and the Pennsylvania Dutch

In the rolling hills of eastern Pennsylvania lives a group of people often referred to as the "Pennsylvania Dutch." They are descendants of German, Swiss, and Alsatian immigrants who settled in the area in the eighteen and nineteen hundreds. The term "Pennsylvania Dutch" comes from the English colonists' mispronunciation of the German dialect words for German—"deutsch" or "deitsh."

The best known Pennsylvania Dutch people today are the Amish, although they only represent about 10 percent of the group. The Amish are among the "plain Dutch," members of the very conservative, very spiritually oriented religious groups that also include the Mennonites, the Brethren, and the Dunkers. They wear plain, old-fashioned clothing and mostly avoid using electricity, automobiles, and telephones. The other 90 percent of Pennsylvania Dutch have blended into the American mainstream. Yet the geographic concentration of the "plain Dutch" groups, plus their influence, has allowed a very distinct Pennsylvania Dutch folk culture to persist.

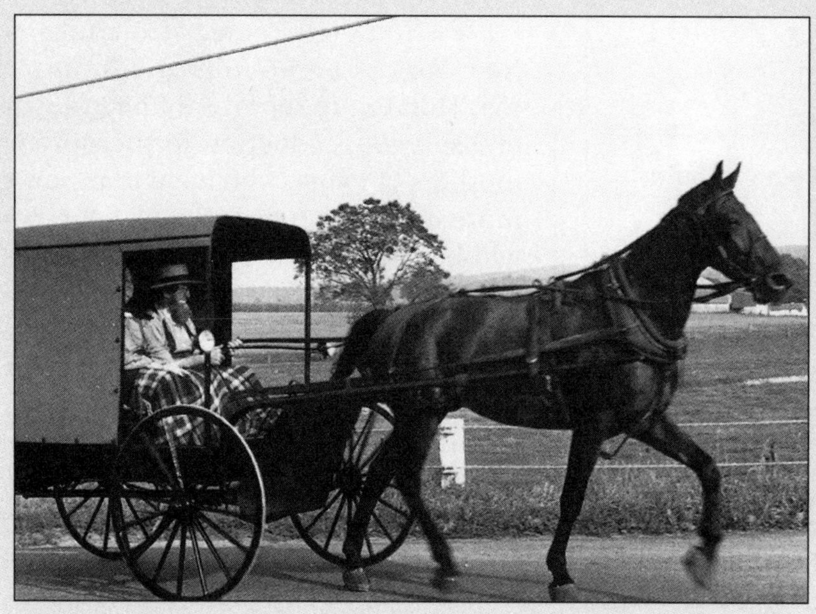

Powwow tradition is found throughout the Pennsylvania region.

This culture includes a German dialect that is spoken by about 175,000 people (and understood by twice that many) and a primarily religious folk healing tradition commonly called "powwow" (also known as "brauche" or "braucherei" in dialect). Although powwow is an Algonquin Indian word, the healing tradition is not connected with the American Indians. (English colonists probably applied the word to the tradition in insult.) Today the powwow tradition is found throughout the region, among people of all sorts of religious backgrounds—including those with no Pennsylvania German ancestry.

Powwow uses whispered prayers and Bible verses accompanied by "laying on of hands"; it has connections with "natural healing" and the use of herbs as well. Many individuals who practice powwow know one or a few of the traditional "charms." A charm is used for a specific purpose, such as removing a wart or stopping blood. Most charms end with "the Three Highest Names," because, to the believer, they are prayers. For example, a charm to stop bleeding is:

Jesu Christ, dearest blood!
That stoppeth the pain and stoppeth the blood.
In this help you [patient's first name],
God the Father, God the Son, God the Holy Ghost.
Amen

Other verbal charms are not so much thought of as prayers. For example, the following treatment for a wen (an old term for a cyst) is directly connected to the astrological idea that things you want to decrease and disappear can be magically connected to the waning moon. Thus, to rid yourself of a wen, you must look over the wen, directly towards the moon, and say: "Whatever grows, does grow; and whatever diminishes, does diminish." This must be said three times in the same breath. Although this remedy is not said as a prayer, the use of three as a magic number in European-American culture is directly related to the Christian Trinity.

Some powwow healers (called "powwows") know a vast variety of these charms and are often sought out for healing; others know few remedies and are only consulted occasionally. Some powwows work full time, while others keep some other occupation. Although most powwow healers do not charge, many accept "free will offerings" in whatever amount the patient wishes to contribute. (There is a widely held belief that charging would be wrong because the gift of healing is God-given. Charging might also give rise to accusations of practicing medicine without a license.)

Powwow Witchcraft

The idea that some sickness is supernaturally caused by witchcraft or sorcery has been believed all over the world. Most people know about the witchcraft trials in Europe and the colonies—especially in Salem, Massachusetts—in the 17th and 18th centuries. Similar violence has continued, occasionally right up to the present.

In the 1920s, a powwow practitioner named John Blymire fell ill. Another powwow, who was reputed to be a "witch doctor," diagnosed Blymire's illness as being magically induced by a third powwow. The traditional remedy was to steal the accused sorcerer's copy of Hohman's *The Long Lost Friend*. During the attempted theft of the book, the accused man was killed. The ensuing murder trial, in York, Pennsylvania, was called a "witchcraft trial" in newspapers of the time, although the judge refused to allow the subject of witchcraft to be mentioned—insisting that such beliefs were impossible in the 20th century. John Blymire was found guilty of first-degree murder and sentenced to life in prison. But, thanks to good behavior in prison, he was paroled in 1953 and lived out the remainder of his life in peace.

Powwow and the Pennsylvania Dutch

Although powwow is mainly an oral tradition, it is also recited from "charm books." These small booklets of prayers and rituals for healing are often accompanied by handy recipes and instructions for household and farm activities. The most popular of these books is *Der Lang verborgene Freund*, published in 1820 in Reading, Pennsylvania, by a German immigrant named John George Hohman. The remedies in this collection range from cures for fevers or epilepsy to ways to make chickens lay more eggs to "relieving persons or animals bewitched." In addition, Hohman's book includes recipes for liniments and the medicinal uses of such common household materials as milk, bread, cloves, wine, and ashes.

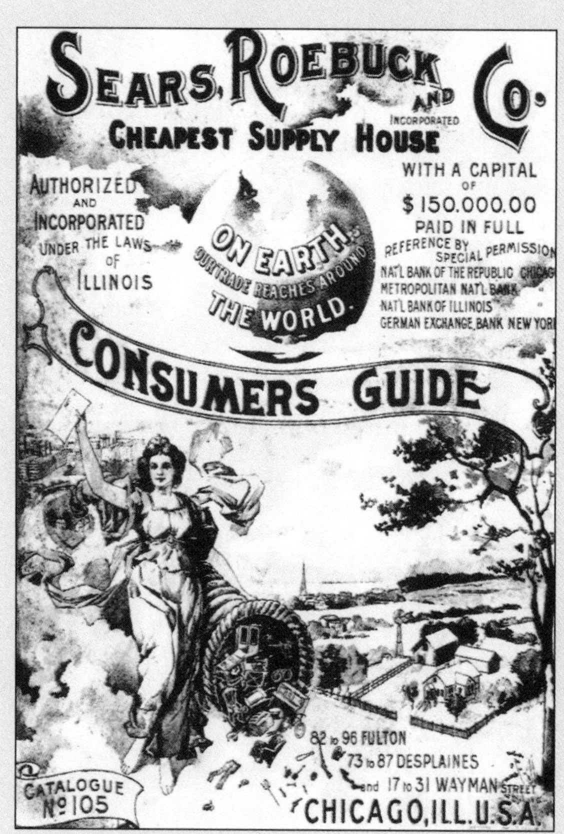

Powwow "charm books" were once sold through the Sears Roebuck catalogue.

The book was translated into two English versions in the mid-19 century, *The Long Lost Friend* (1856) and *The Long Forgotten Friend* (1863). All three versions of the book remain in print today and are accompanied by editions of several older European charm books and handwritten books compiled by individual powwow healers. Not only have these books supported continuity in the powwow tradition, they have also helped powwow to spread its influence to other parts of the country—especially since the books were sold through the Sears Roebuck catalogue around the end of the 19th century!

Powwow has generally been frowned upon by Pennsylvania Dutch ministers and has therefore been long separated from church influence. As in many other folk healing traditions, this separation allowed powwow to hang onto ideas rejected by the churches around it. For example, the idea that disease can be caused by witchcraft remains common in powwow, and many powwow remedies appear magical. Because of this, the powwow healer is often somewhat feared as well as respected. However, because powwow healers usually consider their healing a religious vocation, the remedies often parallel more mainstream forms of contemporary religious healing. There are today, in fact, many in Pennsylvania who use the terms "powwow" and "faith healing" interchangeably.

cause beer contains only small amounts of hop, it is possible that any of the beer's benefits to nursing are entirely due to the increased liquid ingested. Besides, beer drinking is not recommended to nursing mothers.

☞ Directions: Place 1 teaspoon of the herb in a cup and fill with boiling water. Cover the cup and let stand for ten minutes. Strain. Drink 2 or 3 cups a day as long as you continue nursing.

ALFALFA: Eclectic physicians in the first decades of this century performed experiments with alfalfa *(Medicago sativa)* that verified its ability to increase milk flow in humans. Today, alfalfa is recommended by the Amish to increase breast milk production in nursing mothers.

Alfalfa is unusually rich in mineral nutrition. An ounce of the herb contains 300 milligrams of calcium, 76 milligrams of magnesium, and 400 milligrams of potassium. But an amino acid in alfalfa called canavanine may cause or exacerbate autoimmune diseases, especially systemic lupus erythematosus. All recorded cases of these conditions in animals or humans were the result of eating alfalfa leaves or alfalfa sprouts, however. Though the amount of the amino acid in a tea made of alfalfa is negligible, as a precaution, those with pre-existing autoimmune diseases should avoid consuming any form of alfalfa.

☞ Directions: Place 1 ounce of dried alfalfa leaves in a pot and cover with 1 quart of water. Bring to a boil, and then simmer on low heat for forty to sixty minutes. Strain. Drink 3 or 4 cups of the tea during the day as long as you continue nursing.

Salves for Sore Breasts

Salves for sore breasts commonly appear in the folk collections of the eastern states. The salves are commonly made of a mixture of bitter herbs and various kinds of oil. The herbs recommended for this type of use include chamomile (*Matricaria recutita, Anthemis nobilis*), hop (*Humulus lupulus*), and elder flowers (*Sambucus spp.*).

Salves are made by heating an herb with fat until the fat absorbs the plant's healing properties. A thickening agent, such as beeswax, is then added to the strained mixture to give it a thicker consistency. The salve is allowed to cool to room temperature (or refrigerated) and then applied to cracked nipples.

CHICKWEED: An Amish herbal treatment to increase breast milk production is drinking chickweed *(Stellaria media)* tea. An ounce of the dried herb contains 400 milligrams of calcium, 8.4 milligrams of iron, 176 milligrams of magnesium, and 280 milligrams of potassium. Thus, chickweed is very nutritious, a factor that is likely to contribute to increasing milk flow.

☞ Directions: Place 1 ounce of chickweed in 1 quart of water. Bring the water to a boil, and then simmer on the lowest heat for one hour. Strain and drink the liquid throughout the day. Continue doing so for two to three weeks.

OATMEAL GRUEL: The Amish also recommend an oatmeal gruel to help increase milk flow. Oatmeal is a nourishing cereal that contains starches, proteins, vitamins, minerals, and dietary fiber. In fact, two cups of oats contain 52 grams of protein, 8 grams of essential fatty acids, 14.8 milligrams of iron, 552 milligrams of magnesium, 1 milligram of copper, 12 milligrams of zinc, 15.2 milligrams of manganese, and 194 milligrams of folic acid—values that are either over or near the recommended dietary allowance for each of these nutrients.

☞ Directions: To make an oatmeal gruel, place 1 cup of oats in 3 cups of water and simmer for forty minutes in a covered pot. Add molasses or honey to taste. (Also, you can pour off the liquid and put it aside to drink during the day.) The Amish recipe recommends eating the gruel two to three times a day as long as you continue nursing.

DECREASING MILK

GARDEN SAGE: Since antiquity, European folk medicine has recommended using garden sage *(Salvia officinalis)* to decrease milk flow. It was introduced to North America with the colonists, who brought their garden plants with them. A hardy plant, garden sage has become naturalized here and is cultivated as far north as Canada.

Garden sage decreases a mother's milk flow, so it's a useful herb to take while weaning infants. Physicians of the last century adopted garden sage for this purpose. Though it is not commonly practiced in contemporary North American medicine, midwives in upstate New York still recommend sage to help slow milk production. (Note that this is garden sage and not one of the many desert sage species.)

☞ Directions: Place ½ ounce of sage leaf in a 1-quart jar and fill with boiling water. Cover the jar tightly and let stand until the water cools to room temperature. Use the tea to bathe the breasts and nipples during weaning. Also, drink 3 cups of the cool tea a day for a week or two.

NIPPLE DISCOMFORT

CHAMOMILE FOMENTATION: Chamomile's *(Matricaria recutita, Anthemis nobilis)* medicinal properties are derived from its essential oils. Chamomile can be used as an anti-inflammatory to reduce swelling and infection. A traditional treatment for cracked nipples from New England residents is a hot application of chamomile tea.

☞ Directions: Boil a few handfuls of chamomile flowers in a half-and-half mixture of milk and water. Let the mixture cool a bit, then soak a piece of flannel in it. Use the cloth to apply the mixture to the breasts. Do this every twelve hours, as long as needed. The heat increases circulation to the area (which helps to reduce swelling and inflammation), and the tea-milk mixture is soothing to cracked skin.

BAYBERRY TEA WASH: Massachusetts folk herbalist Samuel Thomson introduced bayberry *(Myrica cerifera)* into medical practice in the early 1800s. His theories on herbalism spread among farmers from New England to the Midwest and eventually as far west as Utah. Bayberry was used throughout these regions as a wash for sores and external ulcers that would not heal. And, sometimes, it was used as a wash for sore and cracked nipples. Bayberry has never been approved as an official medicine to treat this condition in the United States or Germany, however.

☞ Directions: Place ½ ounce of bayberry in 1 pint of water. Bring the water to a boil and simmer, covered, for twenty minutes. Strain and soak a cloth in the tea. Use the damp cloth to wash the nipples each day as needed.

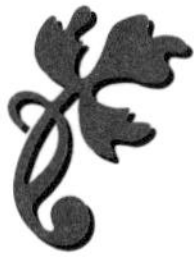

Burns and Sunburns

Although they can be quite painful, many burns are minor and can be easily treated with simple remedies at home

Burns are medically classified in two ways: by the depth of the burn and by the amount of body area the burn covers. Deep burns and burns covering large surface areas require medical examination. The most superficial burn is the first-degree burn, which is typical of a simple sunburn. A second-degree burn penetrates deeper into the skin and is usually accompanied by blisters. Third-degree burns involve deep tissue destruction. Third-degree burns may not blister, so they at first may appear to be less serious than they are. Often the skin looks whitish or charred. The chief risk of second- and third-degree burns is infection, and the more surface area that is affected, the more serious the risk. Infection may enter through ruptured blisters or through seemingly intact skin that has been burned. Folk remedies are inappropriate for these burns, and some could actually promote infection. Conventional treatment for simple superficial burns includes cooling the tissues as soon as possible to reduce inflammation and blistering, and applying soothing ointments. This is the same strategy used by folk healers throughout the world. Some of the folk remedies below, such as aloe vera and plantain leaf, are disinfectants and probably helped to save lives endangered by infected burns in the past.

Remedies

BUTTER AND CREAM: A kitchen burn remedy that comes in handy in most houses is butter, which is mentioned in the folk literature of New England, North Carolina, Northern Georgia, Indiana, and the San Luis Valley of Colorado. Butterfat contains fats that have antimicrobial properties. Thus, butter may help disinfect as well as soothe a burn. An alternative to butter, in the folklore of the Amish dairy farmers, is to dip the burned area in cream.

☞ Directions: After dipping a minor burn in cold water and drying it, apply butter or cream.

BAKING SODA POULTICE: Baking soda, sometimes used in combination with other substances, is mentioned as a burn remedy in folk remedy sources from New England and Indiana and among the Seventh Day Adventists.

☞ Directions: To treat a minor burn, mix baking soda and enough raw egg whites to form a paste. Place the mash directly on the burn and cover with gauze.

BAKING SODA BATH: The Seventh Day Adventists recommend a baking soda bath for treating sunburn.

☞ Directions: Fill a tub with 94–98°F water. Add a cup of commercial baking soda. Soak in the tub for thirty to sixty minutes. Let the skin dry naturally, without using a towel.

VINEGAR: Vinegar washes are recommended in folk remedies from New England and New Mexico. Vinegar is both astringent and antiseptic, and, like cool water, it helps to prevent blisters.

☞ Directions: Apply vinegar to the burn every few minutes. Dilute the vinegar if the skin is very sensitive.

ALOE VERA: The juice of the aloe vera plant has been used as a burn remedy by practically every culture. Aloe vera is recommended as

Everything Oily

Conventional treatment for a minor burn is to first dip the burned area in cold water, dry it, and then cover the area with an oily salve or ointment. Oily substances used in the folk medicines of various cultures have included, besides butter: egg yolks, lard, olive oil, bear fat, chicken fat, goose "grease," skunk oil, mutton tallow, deer tallow, cocoa butter, petroleum jelly, fish oil, axle grease, and, believe it or not, kerosene.

a remedy for burns—from sunburn to serious third-degree burns—in the folk literature of American Indians, New Englanders, the Amish, Indiana residents, Gypsies, residents of northern Georgia, and Chinese immigrants. Aloe vera gel also acts as a disinfectant and reduces bacteria in burns.

☞ Directions: For a small burn, break off a leaf, slice it down the middle, and rub the gel on the skin. To make a poultice of aloe, place the cut leaf on the burned area, and wrap the area with gauze. You can also apply store-bought aloe gel or juice. An alternate formula is to extend the aloe vera sap with olive oil. Here's how: Add 8 ounces of extra virgin olive oil to 2 ounces of fresh squeezed aloe vera sap. (Place the sap in a large bowl and add the oil a few drops at a time while stirring.) Apply directly to the burn area.

PLANTAIN: Plantain *(Plantago major)*, a popular remedy for wounds, bites, and stings, is also recommended for treating burns in the folk literature of the Seneca Indians. Contemporary New Englanders and Hispanics of the American Southwest also encourage its use. The plantain leaf contains at least 15 constituents with identified anti-

Physiomedicalist Medicine

The most influential folk herbalist in United States history is Samuel Thomson (1769-1843), a self-educated "doctor" from New Hampshire. Thomson advocated the use of simple herbal remedies and severely criticized the methods of the medical doctors of the day. By the 1840s, his "Thomsonian" movement had claimed as many as a million adherents—about 20 percent of the American population at the time—who purchased his books of home remedies or ordered his herbal remedies through the mail. Emerging from this folk movement around 1840 came the Physiomedicalist school of medicine, which included doctors who used Thomson's philosophy and methods. Physiomedicalist medicine in the United States passed away with the death of its most prominent adherent, William Cook, M.D., in 1899. However, an English doctor named A.I. Coffin, who had studied with Thomson in the 1820s, and also with American Indian doctors, had spread the movement to England. He lectured in small towns across that country, and the resulting folk movement that sprang up there was similar to the Thomsonian herbalism of the United States. Physiomedicalism profoundly influenced British herbalism from that time on. Today, herbalists are licensed in England, and their training and approach remains strongly influenced by Physiomedicalism.

inflammatory properties, 17 constituents with bactericidal properties, 6 analgesics, and 5 antiseptics. It also contains the constituent allantoin, which promotes cell proliferation and tissue healing.

☞ Directions: Crush some fresh plantain leaves and rub the juice directly onto the burn area.

TOBACCO: An American Indian treatment for burns is to wash the area in tobacco tea. Indiana medical folklore suggests applying a wad of chewing tobacco to the burned area.

☞ Directions: Remove the tobacco from a package of cigarettes and add it to 1 quart of water. Boil the water until the volume is reduced to 1 pint. Strain and let cool to room temperature. Wash the burn area with the tea as often as you'd like.

POTATO POULTICE: Some residents of New England, Indiana, and North Carolina have reported using potato poultices in treating burns. The same use is widespread in the folk medicine of India and has even attracted the attention of researchers there. Potato poultices were tested on severe burns in a 1990 clinical trial at a children's hospital in Bombay, India. A control group received a conventional treatment with an ointment of silver sulfadiazine. The test group also received the sulfadiazine, in addition to a dressing of potato peels. The patients in the latter group showed faster healing than the control patients. Potato treatments without the conventional antibiotic ointment may promote infection on the open wounds of severe burns, however. (A 1996 trial at a burn unit in Maharashtra, India, compared the efficacy of potato treatments to honey-impregnated gauze. The honey treatments were much more effective and prevented infection, whereas the patients receiving potato poultices showed persistent infections in their burns within the first week of the trial.)

Fire Doctors and Special Prayers

In Appalachian and southern culture, it is believed by some that certain individuals—called "fire doctors"—have the ability to "talk" fire out of a burn. The belief is so strong that some individuals with serious burns will refuse any other medical treatment. In Louisiana folk medicine, the "fire passages" of the Bible are recited by the fire doctor. The identity of the passages is closely guarded and passed on from one healer to another only at the time of a fire doctor's death. In *The Frank C. Brown Collection of North Carolina Folklore*, one prayer recited by a northern Georgia fire doctor is: "The mother of God went over the fiery fields. She had in her hand a fiery brand. The fire did not go out; it did not go in. In the name of the Father, the Son, and the Holy Ghost. Amen." The prayer is repeated three times; the fire doctor blows on the burn and wets the area each time.

Manure Rx

One remedy, though perhaps unappealing and unsanitary, is to apply manure or excrement to a burn. Although the texture of manure may be soothing to the burn, if there is any break in the skin, the risk of infection is very high. In *Country Folk Remedies: Tales of Skunk Oil, Sassafras Tea and Other Old-Time Remedies Gathered by Elisabeth Janos*, New England folklorist Elizabeth Janos relates one folk narrative: "I took about two cups of chicken manure and the same amount of pure lard. I boiled them together for about fifteen minutes, then let it cool. It makes a somewhat smelly yellow salve. I used it on him three to four times a day. In about two weeks he was healed, and no scar was left." Cow manure is used by other New Englanders, and dog excrement is used by Mexican Indians.

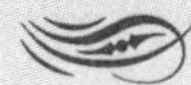

☞ Directions: Apply a poultice of grated raw potato directly to the burn and hold it in place with a cloth. Change the poultice every one to two hours until the burn heals. This treatment is not appropriate for burns with broken skin or ruptured blisters.

HONEY: Honey is a universal folk remedy to disinfect wounds and burns throughout the world. It is highly regarded in the folk literature of the Amish, Chinese immigrants, Indiana residents, and residents of the American Southwest. Honey naturally attracts water, and, when applied to a burn or wound, draws fluids out of the tissues, effectively cleaning the wound. Furthermore, most bacteria cannot live in the presence of honey. Honey is sometimes applied to gauze and used to dress severe burns in conventional medicine. In the early 1990s, physicians at a hospital in Maharashtra, India, performed clinical trials comparing honey-impregnated gauze with three different conventional burn treatments, and the honey treatment was superior in each case.

In a 1991 study, the doctors compared the honey-gauze to gauze treated with silver sulfadiazine. In 52 patients treated with honey, 91 percent of wounds were sterile within seven days. In the 52 patients treated with silver sulfadiazine, 93 percent of wounds still showed signs of infection after seven days. The burns of the honey-treated patients began to heal in seven days, while, for the other group, healing began on average in 13 days. Of the wounds treated with honey, 87 percent healed within 15 days; only 10 percent of the wounds healed in the control group during that time. Important: The honey also provided greater pain relief and resulted in less scarring.

☞ Directions: Apply honey to a piece of sterile gauze, and place directly on the burn, honey side to the skin. Change the dressing three to four times a day. Be sure to seek medical attention for serious burns.

PINE BARK AND PINE PITCH: A remedy among American Indians of the eastern forests is pine bark *(Pinus spp.)*. Pine pitch, which is the congealed sap, has both anti-inflammatory and bactericidal properties.

☞ Directions: First place an oil, such as olive oil, on the burn. Spread pine pitch on a cloth and cover the burn with the cloth. Also, you can boil pine bark until it becomes soft. Then place the bark on the burn and cover with a clean piece of cloth or gauze. You can do this off and on until the burn heals.

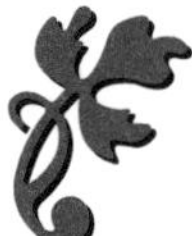

Catarrh

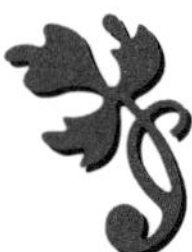

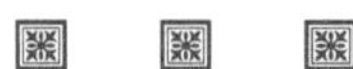

In folk medicine, as you shall see, the best treatment for catarrh is to encourage the flow of fresh mucus

As an organ of breathing, the nose moisturizes incoming air and filters out any foreign materials. Small glands within the lining of the nose secrete mucus, a sticky substance that lubricates the walls of the nose and throat. Mucus humidifies the incoming air and traps bacteria, dust, and other particles entering the nose. Many disease-causing bacteria are either dissolved by chemical elements in the mucus or transported to the entrance of the throat by tiny hairs called *cilia.* In the throat, any remaining bacteria are swallowed and killed by acids and other chemicals produced in the stomach. This efficient line of defense protects the body against the billions of bacteria continually entering the nose.

Although it may be a source of discomfort during a cold, cough, or bout of bronchitis, mucus is an essential part of the body's defense system. Because it contains antibodies to each organism that has ever attacked an individual's body, mucus is a personally tailored, genetically engineered antibiotic paste that washes away or kills infectious organisms. Thin, liquid mucus that flows freely is a sign of good health, healing, and the defeat of invading organisms or other irritants to the mucous membranes. Thus, it is rarely wise to use decongestants during the acute stages of a cold. A better strategy is to drink plenty of liquids to help thin the mucus even more, therefore increasing the efficiency of its flow and reducing cold discomfort.

Mucus usually flows properly during the early stages of a cold or infection. If the body's initial response to the organisms does not succeed in eliminating them, however, the invaders can take up long-term residence in the mucous membranes, causing chronic inflammation, ulceration, and scarring of the membranes. The result may be catarrh—chronic, thick mucous secretions that do not flow freely or efficiently and are coughed up or otherwise eliminated only with difficulty. The best treatment for this condition is not to suppress the mucus but to encourage the flow of fresh mucus to the infected membranes. Thus, in traditional systems of medicine, such as in the Chinese, Ayurvedic, Arabic, and naturopathic systems, and also in folk medicine, the most common treatment for chronic mucus conditions is to give expectorant, mucus-producing herbs. Most of these herbs also contain antimicrobial substances that may kill the invading organisms causing the infection.

Some traditional remedies, such as goldenseal, are drying and astringent to the mucous membranes and reduce mucous flow rather than increase it. Remedies like these should never be used in the acute first stages of a nasal or bronchial infection.

Any fever that arises while you have a chronic mucous condition warrants medical attention.

Remedies

FENUGREEK: Fenugreek seeds *(Trigonella foenum-graecum)* have been used medicinally throughout the Mediterranean region since the time of the ancient Egyptians. The ancient Egyptians used fenugreek to stimulate uterine contractions and promote childbirth, an effect that has been verified in modern animal trials. (Thus, it is not appropriate for use in medicinal amounts during pregnancy.) The seeds remain an important medicine in both Ayurveda (the traditional medicine of India) and Arabic medicine. The Prophet Muhammad said of the seeds: "If you knew the value of fenugreek, you would pay its weight in gold." The common name comes from the Latin "foenum Gracium" or "Greek hay."

The main use of fenugreek seeds in traditional medicine is as an expectorant, antiseptic, and digestive stimulant. The Amish recommend fenugreek seed tea to treat chronic mucus. The seeds contain a variety of antiseptic and anti-inflammatory constituents. Modern research shows that the seeds also have properties that can lower blood sugar, however, so if you are diabetic and taking medications, don't take a medicinal amount of fenugreek without consulting your physician.

☞ Directions: Crush 1 ounce of fenugreek seeds in a coffee grinder or with a mortar and pestle and place in a 1-pint jar. Fill with boiling water. Cover and let stand until the tea reaches room temperature. Drink the pint in 4 doses during the day. Drink on an empty stomach.

SALT WATER: Another recommendation from the Amish for clearing chronic nasal mucus is to sniff salt water up the nose. Salt is a powerful antimicrobial agent. Its medicinal use as a wash for wounds or infections goes back to prehistory. It was probably first used when primitive peoples living by the sea observed the mild disinfectant properties of sea water.

☞ Directions: Place 1 tablespoon of salt in a pint of warm water and stir. Take some into the hand and sniff it up the nose.

SPEARMINT AND PEPPERMINT: A mucus remedy shared by both the Amish

continued on page 117

Wild Animal Magic

While folk medicine uses domestic animals for both natural and magical purposes, wild animals are almost always used for magical reasons. This may be because many wild animals are more difficult to obtain. This seems especially likely because those wild animals that *are* easily accessible, especially insects and spiders, have more often been put to natural uses.

BIRDS: Birds' nests, which are relatively easy to find, have been linked magically with headache. Folklorists in several different parts of the United States have discovered the belief that if discarded human hair is used by birds to build a nest, its former owner will get a headache. The reverse effect—and opposite logic—is also found. It is believed by some that headaches can be prevented by placing your first pulled tooth in a bird's nest.

MUSKRATS: Another readily accessible wild animal is the muskrat, widely trapped for its fur. In Maryland, a fresh muskrat skin was used to prevent colds by sewing the bloody side of the skin to red flannel. The flannel side was then worn next to the skin until it fell off of its own accord. The effect was said to be enhanced by first rubbing the patient with goose grease.

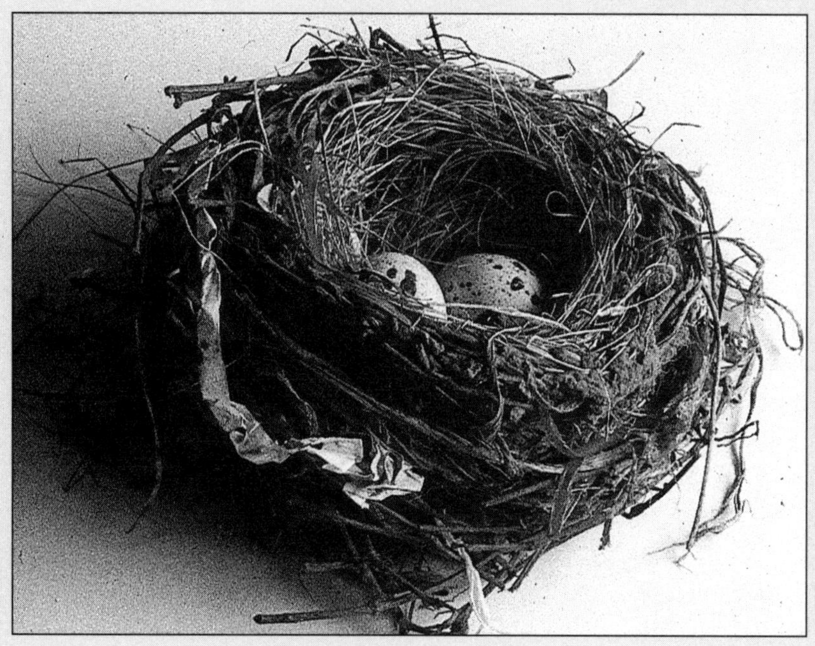

If it ends up in a nest, it could come back to hurt—or help—you.

MOLES: Of all the wild mammals used in folk medicine, the lowly mole has perhaps the longest and most peculiar history. Moles are small rodents that live underground and eat insects. In ancient times the mole was venerated from India to Europe as spiritually powerful. In Greece, the name of the god of healing, Asclepias, is derived from the ancient Greek word for mole. This veneration is in part due to the mole's ability to live so completely underground—which is unique among mammals—and the fact that the powers of fertility and mystery have been attributed to the underground world. For these reasons, the mole occupies a special place in occult folk medicine. One means of acquiring the power to heal is to hold a mole tightly in your hand and suffocate it. Some people

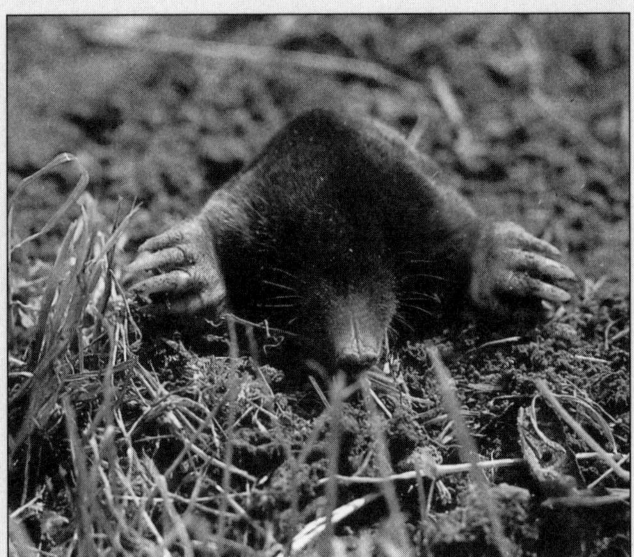

In folk medicine, the mole is used to cure.

Mysterious Little Creatures

Although we may not think of them in this way, earthworms are a kind of wild animal. And they are readily available—as anyone who has ever collected fishing bait or dug up a garden plot knows. Earthworms are mysterious little creatures, which is a plus in folk medicine. Although most people today may find the idea disgusting, a common topical remedy was once made by cooking earthworms in a skillet and saving the oil.

No more appetizing is this remedy for quinsy (severe tonsillitis), which was reported in the 1930s in Pennsylvania: Fill a flannel cloth with live earthworms and pin it around the patient's neck. The worms will draw out the soreness and die. Earthworms are also said to die when they come in contact with the left side of a seventh son of a seventh son, an indication of the great power bestowed by this birth order.

believe that, as the mole dies, its power is transferred to the one who holds it. This belief can still be encountered in many rural parts of the United States. Most remedies that use moles involve injury or death to the animal. A tooth extracted from a live mole and worn around the neck is said to prevent toothache (a belief also common in ancient Greece and Rome). A mole's foot worn around the neck as an amulet is supposed to prevent the pain of teething. In North Carolina, the string holding the mole paw must be black, and, in some cases, the paw is supposed to be bitten off a live mole. The use of "moleskin" to protect sore and blistered skin is the one connection that exists between moles and contemporary medicine. Fortunately the moleskin purchased in pharmacies today is a kind of cotton twill, not the result of animal sacrifice!

SNAKES: Snakes, and the oil rendered from them, have long been prominent in American folk medicine. So much so that the term "snake oil" is synonymous with fraudulent and useless remedies. This is due to the practices of quacks and medicine peddlers in the late 19th century (see "Patent Medicines," page 80). Snakes and snake oil, however, have also been important in authentic folk traditions. According to some African-American traditions, snake bones can be used as an amulet to cure toothache. In Colorado, it is said that

Wild Animal Magic

if a person with a goiter wears a snake around his neck, the snake will take the goiter when it crawls away. (The exact type of snake was not specified but, presumably, it would have to be of the non-poisonous variety.)

After snake oil, snakeskin is the most widely used part of the snake in folk remedies. In Maryland, it is said that snake-skin worn around the foot will ease cramps. Snake-skin has been worn in many parts of the country to alleviate rheumatism. And one odd medicinal function for snakes reported from southern Illinois says that rheumatism can be frightened out of a patient either by a tornado or by a water moccasin snake!

TOADS: Toads, widely and mistakenly believed to cause warts, figure very prominently in traditional remedies. Many of these treatments seem to involve magical transfer of an illness to a toad or to a toad's body part. The following remedy for a foot wound that won't heal comes from Pennsylvania: Tie a linen thread around the foot of a toad, cut off the foot, and tie it to your sore leg. Leave the thread in place until it falls off, and the wound will be healed. In Georgia, local legend has it that whooping cough can be cured by tying a toad to the patient's bedpost. And in the folk medicine of California, asthma is thought to be cured by having the patient spit into a toad's mouth. In North Carolina, some think malaria can be relieved by blowing into a toad's mouth. Finally, in Utah, it is said that toads can suck cancer right out of the body.

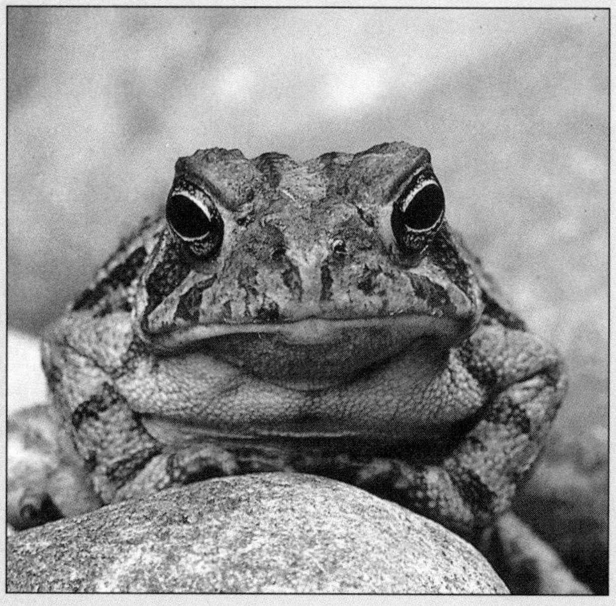

Toads are used to remedy various illnesses.

EELS: Even though fishing has been popular for food and sport through the centuries, fish remedies are relatively scarce in folk medicine. Those folk remedies that do involve fish often focus on eels. The Pennsylvania Germans say alcoholism can be cured by drinking whisky through which a live eel has passed. The Pennsylvania Germans also tie an eel skin around the arm to remedy a nosebleed. The most common use of eel skin is for treating joint pain, however. In Pennsylvania, it is believed that the skin of an eel, especially one caught in March, will provide relief when applied to a sprain. In Georgia, eel skin is combined with the widely used copper bracelet to cure arthritis.

and residents of the southern Appalachians is to inhale the vapors of peppermint *(Mentha piperita)* or spearmint *(Mentha spicata)*. The oils of these plants have antiseptic and anti-inflammatory properties, but much of the relief the mints have to offer may come from their menthol content. Menthol acts as a decongestant. Peppermint contains more menthol than spearmint and might be the better remedy here.

☞ Directions: Place ½ ounce of dried mint leaves in a bowl. Pour in enough boiling water to cover the leaves. Inhale the steam. Be careful not to burn your nose.

WILD BERGAMOT AND THYME: American Indians inhaled the steam of the upper parts of the wild bergamot plant *(Monarda fistulosa)* as a mucus remedy. Other *Monarda* species, including horsemint *(Monarda punctata)* and beebalm *(Monarda menthaefolium)* have been used as cough medicines and antiseptics. All three plants contain large amounts of the constituent thymol, which has anti-inflammatory, antiseptic, and expectorant properties. Thymol is present in large amounts in the kitchen spice thyme *(Thymus vulgaris)*, which has been used in the same way in traditional European folk medicine.

☞ Directions: Place ½ ounce of dried *Monarda* or thyme leaves in a bowl. Pour in enough boiling water to cover, and inhale the steam. Be careful not to burn your nose.

PLEURISY ROOT: A treatment for mucus conditions that appears in folklorist Clarence Meyer's *American Folk Medicine* is a tea of pleurisy root *(Asclepias tuberosa)*. The plant, a relative of milkweed, is native to North America and was used by members of the Cherokee, Delaware, Mohegan, Omaha, and Ponca Indian tribes as an expectorant. The colonists learned its use from the Indians. It was eventually adopted by all the North American schools of medicine, and it was listed in the *United States Pharmacopoeia* from 1820 until 1900. Pleurisy root can cause nausea or vomiting in larger doses, so use it only in the amounts described below. Don't use pleurisy root at all if you are pregnant.

☞ Directions: Place 1 ounce of pleurisy root and ¼ ounce of dried ginger in a 1-pint jar. Fill with boiling water. Cover and let steep for twenty minutes. Strain and sweeten if desired. Take 1 tablespoon doses three to four times a day for up to a week.

ROSEMARY: A folk remedy of Mexico and the Hispanic Southwest for treating a runny nose is rosemary *(Rosmarinus officinalis)*. Rosemary contains at least ten different expectorant constituents. Its constituent rosmarinic acid, which is also found in peppermint, spearmint, thyme, and some *Monarda* species, has powerful antiseptic and anti-inflammatory properties.

☞ Directions: Crush ½ ounce of rosemary leaves and place them in a 1-pint jar. Fill with boiling water, cover, and let stand for twenty to thirty minutes. Drink the pint in 4 doses during the day. Drink on an empty stomach.

GOLDENSEAL: Probably the most famous remedy for treating a runny nose in the history of United States folk medicine is goldenseal *(Hydrastis canadensis)*. Colonists learned its use from the American Indians. It was a household medicine in the colonies before independence and was entered into standard medical practice by the early 19th century. Physicians of the Eclectic, Physiomedicalist, and homeopathic schools of medicine of the 19th century considered it to be a "mucous membrane tonic" and prescribed goldenseal for chronic (but not acute) mucous membrane discharges. (They avoided prescribing it for the acute phase of mucous membrane infection because strong astringent constituents in goldenseal can suppress the healthy mucous discharge.)

Professional medical herbalists in North America use the plant for the same purpose today. Goldenseal is one of the top ten herbs purchased in health food stores. To the public, it has a reputation as an antibiotic, because of its constituent berberine. Thus, the public buys goldenseal because they think it will work like an antibiotic: It will be absorbed into the bloodstream and reach the site of the infection. And although berberine is a broad-spectrum antimicrobial agent, it is very poorly absorbed in the gut and offers no protection against infection. It only works if it comes in direct contact with the mucous membranes. Thus, goldenseal was applied topically, as snuff or as tea, directly to mucous membranes in North American folk traditions and 19th century medicine.

☞ Directions: Place 1 teaspoon of goldenseal powder in a 1-pint jar and fill with boiling water. Cover and let cool to room temperature, shaking the bottle from time to time to mix its contents. To treat nasal mucus, sniff a handful of the tea up the nose. Also, swish 1 ounce of tea around the mouth, gargle, and swallow.

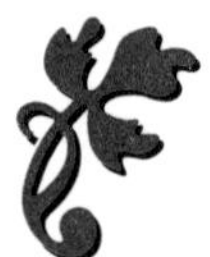

Cold and Flu

The common cold is aptly named. It is so common, in fact, that all human beings from every region of the globe experience it at one time or another during their lives

A simple common cold is a collection of familiar symptoms signaling an infection of the upper respiratory tract, which includes the nose, throat, and sinuses. At least five major categories of viruses cause colds. One of these groups, and perhaps the most common, the rhinoviruses, includes a minimum of 100 different viruses. The viruses that cause a cold reproduce in the mucous membranes. The viruses do not penetrate deeper into the body—into the gastrointestinal tract, for example—because they cannot survive at the higher body temperatures there.

Although we often say "colds and flu" in the same breath, influenza is a very different disease from the common cold. The influenza virus takes up residence mainly in the throat and bronchial tract. If you have the flu, you usually have a fever, and a fever is not usually present in a cold. The fever usually passes within three days, but the fatigue, muscle aches, and cough that result from the flu can linger for weeks. Influenza will not seriously injure a normally healthy person, but those with preexisting lung conditions, the elderly, and others with weakened resistance are especially prone to the flu's deadly effects.

Flu is known as the "Last of the Great Plagues" because it kills so many people worldwide each year, including about 20,000 Americans. And when highly virulent flu strains periodically erupt, the death toll can rise even higher. For example, a flu epidemic just after World War I killed more than 30 million people worldwide.

The conventional treatment for flu in those at high risk for fatal complications is immunization in late fall with a flu vaccine. Immunization is also recommended for those who care for such high-risk patients. The antiviral drug ribavarin can be taken as well; it may be effective in preventing severe pneumonia caused by the influenza virus.

Some patients request antibiotics from their doctors to treat a cold or flu episode, and unfortunately, many doctors comply. Antibiotic drugs are good only for bacterial infections and are ineffective against colds and flu. In fact, taking them inappropriately may promote the development of drug-resistant bacterial strains and may render the antibiotics ineffective later on when the patient really needs them. The drug resistant strains can also be passed on to others.

Sniffing Tea

Folk traditions frequently advise a cold or flu victim to sip hot fragrant teas. Most of the herbs in this section contain aromatic oils that have antibacterial, antiviral, antifungal, and anti-inflammatory actions. The oils escape with the steam of hot tea. (The steam also releases the oils' fragrance.) The steam delivers the oil's constituents directly to the surface of the mucous membranes, where they attack the invading organism causing the cold. Elder, ginger, yarrow, mint, thyme, horsemint, beebalm, lemon balm, catnip, garlic, onions, and mustard are all herbs that contain such aromatic oils.

Aspirin and other pain-killing drugs are also inappropriate treatments for cold and flu. Even though they may provide some temporary relief, they may suppress the immune system and can actually prolong the infection. And giving aspirin to children for colds and flu is a no-no. In rare cases, it can lead to the development of Reye syndrome, a serious and often fatal neurological disorder.

Remedies

ECHINACEA: Echinacea *(Echinacea angustifolia, Echinacea purpurea)* is, without a doubt, the most commonly used folk rem-

continued on page 121

Birth Order and Healing Powers

In the modern world, special abilities are attributed to those who have received specialized training. Physicians, with their many years of schooling, are a good example of these experts. Although healing has always involved learning, it has not always been a matter of mastering facts and technique. Folk healers, for example, differ from medical doctors in that they believe they have been led to their work by a Divine call. For that reason, the power given to folk healers has often been considered by the community as far more important than what they have actually studied or done.

For many healers, their calling is indicated by their circumstances of birth. Probably the best known birth indication of healing power is being the "seventh son of a seventh son." Women are healers in folk tradition, too, and seventh daughters are seen as having power also. Among Gypsies, seventh daughters are said to be especially talented fortune-tellers. Abilities often ascribed to seventh children include stopping blood flow, curing whooping cough, and curing thrush, which is a yeast infection of the mouth that was sometimes quite serious in infants before modern treatment was readily available.

For many healers, their calling is indicated by their circumstances of birth.

These were common medical emergencies, and respect for the healing abilities of seventh children was great. The powers of these children were not limited to healing, however, even though seventh sons were often nicknamed "Doc." Their talents could also be related to music. An example is Doc Watson, a gifted folk guitarist and singer, now quite famous, named for his birth order. In French tradition, a seventh child is said to have "the gift of the lily," which includes a kind of clairvoyance or second sight.

Being born after the death of one's father—sometimes called a "posthumous child"—was another circumstance of birth said to give healing power. In Illinois, folk tradition attributes the same healing powers to both posthumous children and those children who have never seen their father for other reasons. In Georgia, a belief has been recorded that connects the posthumous child with the power of seven, stating that "sore mouth among children," possibly a reference to thrush, can be cured by seven sips of water from the shoe of one who was born after her or his father died.

The most dramatic birth circumstance to convey healing power is being born with a "caul," or "veil." A caul is a portion of the amnion, the membrane that covers the fetus in the womb. Since ancient times, among both Romans and Jews, a baby born with this membrane adhering to its head has been believed to have special powers. It was also believed that the caul itself had supernatural powers and protected whoever owned it from demons. This belief made the caul a valuable commodity—one that was bought and sold up through the 19th century.

edy for treating colds and flu in the United States today. In fact, echinacea is the best selling medicinal herb in the country.

Echinacea was used as a remedy by the American Indians of the Great Plains states. The tribes residing in those areas used the herb for all manner of infectious diseases. Eclectic physicians, a now-defunct North American school of doctors who used herbs as medicines, adopted the use of echinacea in the mid-1880s. By 1920, it was the remedy they prescribed the most. The use of echinacea spread to Germany in the 1930s, where it remains an approved medicine today—used to treat colds, flu, and other conditions related to underlying deficiencies of the immune system.

Echinacea is also famous in the contemporary medical herbalism of Britain, Australia, and North America for its ability to "abort" a cold or flu. German clinical trials show that echinacea, taken preventively during cold and flu season, can reduce the frequency and severity of a viral infection. In fact, if echinacea is taken at the first onset of symptoms, the cold may never develop at all. Once a cold has set in, however, the other remedies in the section may be more beneficial.

☞ Directions: Purchase a tincture of echinacea at a health food store, herb shop, or drugstore. At the first sign of a cold or flu, take 1 teaspoon of the tincture every hour for three hours. If the infection persists, take 1 dropperful of the tincture every three hours.

Sweating It Out

Sweating is essential to cooling the body during a fever. Many traditional folk remedies use herbs for this purpose. These diaphoretic herbs have constituents that, when eaten, increase the blood circulation to the skin, which causes perspiration and ultimately lowers the fever.

It is essential to drink plenty of fluids when taking these herbs, however, or dehydration may result. Elder, ginger, yarrow, mint, boneset, pennyroyal, thyme, horsemint, beebalm, lemon balm, catnip, and garlic are all diaphoretic herbs. They're most effective when taken as hot teas. After drinking the tea, go to bed, wrap up in warm blankets, and sweat it out. Continue to drink plenty of fluids.

ELDER FLOWERS: Elderberry comprises about 13 species of deciduous shrubs native to North America and Europe. European settlers brought elderberry plants with them to the American colonies. The Paiute and Shoshone Indians in the Rocky Mountain region used the leaves and flowers of a North American species of elderberry to treat colds, flu, and fevers.

A tea made of elderberry flowers is approved by the German government as a medicine for colds, especially if a cough is present. The flower tea is also used to treat colds and flu in the folk medicine of contemporary Indiana. The Michigan Amish use the tea as well.

Recent research in Israel and Panama has shown that elderberry juice stimulates the immune system and also directly inhibits the influenza virus. Constituents in the plant's flowers and berries seem to have immunosuppressant properties that help inactivate the influenza virus, halting its spread. Elderberry has been shown to be effective against eight different strains of the flu virus. Drinking too much elderberry tea, more than indicated in the directions below, however, can leave you feeling nauseous. And, because of a documented diuretic effect, prolonged use may result in hypokalemia, or potassium loss. Avoid the use of elder during pregnancy and lactation.

☞ Directions: Place ½ ounce of elderberry flowers in a 1-quart canning jar and fill with boiling water. Cover and let steep for twenty minutes. Strain and pour a cup of the tea. Sweeten with honey. Take 1 cup once every four hours when you have a cold or flu. Wrap yourself up in warm blankets after drinking the tea to help induce sweating.

Starve a Cold?

"Starve a fever, feed a cold" is an aphorism of folk wisdom—one that you should try not to get confused. If you feed a fever or starve a cold, you may be making your fever worse and actually prolonging it.

During a fever, the body's metabolism goes into overdrive to produce white blood cells and antibodies to fight the infection. If you fast, your body doesn't have to produce digestive enzymes, freeing up the system to make more immune system components.

For a usually healthy person, fasting for 24 hours increases the activity of white blood cells by about 20 percent. So, at the first sign of fever, fast on liquids, carefully avoiding sugary juices, until your temperature returns to normal. And don't worry about starving—the body holds plenty of nutrients in reserve.

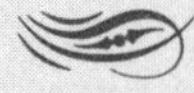

BONESET: The herb boneset *(Eupatorium perfoliatum)* got its name during an influenza epidemic in Pennsylvania in the 1700s. The flu was called "breakbone fever"; the word *breakbone* referred to the muscle aches and pains that accompanied the virus. Taking the herb, however, proved to "set the bones" and relieve the aches. The colonists learned the use of the plant from the Cherokee and Iroquois Indians and other eastern American Indian tribes.

The use of boneset for treating colds and flu spread to Europe. Today, some German medical schools continue to study its use. Boneset is frequently prescribed in Germany for treating acute viral infections, for which antibiotic drugs are not effective. The herb also continues to be used today in the folk medicine of Indiana and southern Illinois.

Constituents have been identified in boneset that are both immune-stimulating and anti-inflammatory. Do not overdo it with boneset, however, because it can induce vomiting if taken in large quantities. It was actually used for that purpose in the

18th and 19th centuries. Boneset is also know to have constituents that are allergenic. Boneset should be avoided during pregnancy and lactation.

☞ Directions: Place 1 teaspoon of dried boneset leaves in a cup and fill with boiling water. Let steep for fifteen minutes. Strain and drink the tea while it's warm. Go to bed immediately, wrapping yourself in blankets. Don't drink more than 1 cup every four hours and no more than 3 cups a day. Stop taking boneset if you begin to feel nauseous.

Hot Water Treatments

Treatments for colds and flu often emphasize using hot water for hot steam baths, gargles, and nasal irrigations. These remedies are mentioned in the folk literature of 19th century German immigrants as well as present-day Seventh Day Adventists. Such water methods have a sound basis in microbiology: The viruses that infect the mucous membranes cannot survive even at normal body temperatures. Thus, by washing the membranes with water even hotter than the body's core temperature, or flooding the membranes with steam, infecting viruses are killed.

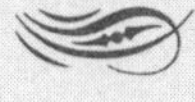

YARROW: The ancient Greeks used yarrow *(Achillea millefolium)* as a remedy for colds, flu, and fever. At least 18 American Indian tribes from all corners of North America used yarrow for the same purpose. The early colonists throughout North America used yarrow as a household medicine for a wide variety of ailments, usually conditions that were infectious or inflammatory in nature. The use of yarrow tea for colds and flu survives today in the folk medicine of North Carolina, Indiana, and upstate New York. Yarrow has documented anti-inflammatory, antispasmodic, diuretic, mild sedative, and moderate antibacterial activities.

☞ Directions: Place 1 ounce of dried or fresh yarrow in a 1-quart canning jar. Fill the jar with boiling water and cover tightly. Let steep for twenty minutes. Strain and pour a cup and sweeten with honey. Take 2 or 3 cups a day, bundling up in blankets and resting in bed after each cup.

GINGER: Ginger tea is a cold remedy mentioned in the folk literature of New England, Appalachia, North Carolina, Indiana, and even China. Ginger induces sweating, which helps to cool the body during fever. Ginger contains 12 different aromatic anti-inflammatory compounds, including some with aspirin-like effects. Its other proven actions result from its antinauseant and antivertigo properties. Ginger also has carminative (gas relieving), diaphoretic (sweat inducing), and antispasmodic activities.

☞ Directions: Cut a fresh ginger root (about the size of your thumb) into thin slices. Place the slices in 1 quart of water. Bring to a boil. Cover the pot and simmer on the lowest possible heat for thirty minutes. Let cool for thirty minutes more. Strain and drink ½ to 1 cup three to five times a day. Sweeten with honey, as desired.

PEPPERMINT: Peppermint *(Mentha piperita)* is a folk remedy used in Indiana to treat colds. Cornmint *(Mentha arvensis),* a close relative of the plant, is used in China for the same purpose. Both plants, when taken as a hot tea, induce sweating and help to cool a fever. Also, the essential oils in the plants, including menthol, act as decongestants when drunk as a tea or inhaled. Peppermint also has antispasmodic and carminative properties.

☞ Directions: Place ½ ounce of peppermint leaves in a 1-quart jar. Fill the jar with boiling water and cover tightly. Let steep twenty minutes. Strain the liquid and drink 2 or 3 cups a day. Wrap yourself in blankets and rest in bed after each cup.

THYME: Thyme tea *(Thymus vulgaris)* is recommended as a treatment for cold or flu in the folk medicine of Indiana and China. Thyme taken in the form of a hot tea also induces sweating and helps to cool a fever. In addition, its constituent oil, thymol, is a powerful expectorant and antiseptic. The constituent readily disperses in the steam of a hot tea. Inhaling the steam may effectively spread the thymol throughout the mucous membranes of the upper respiratory tract and bronchial tree. Thus, thymol may help inhibit bacteria, viruses, or fungi from infecting the membranes. Thyme also has mild analgesic and antipyretic (fever reducing) properties.

This remedy from Indiana suggests sipping the tea slowly while inhaling its fragrance. In China, the same method is used as a preventive—for when colds or flu are "going around."

☞ Directions: Put 1 teaspoon of dried thyme leaves in a cup and fill with boiling water. Let steep for five minutes while inhaling the fumes through both the nose and mouth. Then, strain the tea, sweeten with honey, and sip slowly. Go to bed and bundle up warmly in blankets.

HORSEMINT AND BEEBALM: Two closely related species, horsemint *(Monarda punctata)* and beebalm *(Monarda menthaefolia, M. didyma)*, are used in folk medicine similarly to the way thyme is used. (Horsemint is native to the eastern United States; beebalm to the Rocky Mountains.) Both plants, like thyme, contain high amounts of the constituent thymol, which acts as an expectorant and antiseptic (see "Thyme," left). Both plants also induce sweating and can help cool a fever.

☞ Directions: Put 1 teaspoon of dried leaves of either plant in a cup and fill with boiling water. Let steep for five minutes while inhaling the fumes through both the nose and mouth. Strain, sweeten with honey, and sip the tea slowly. Do this three to five times a day.

LEMON BALM: Several Indiana residents responding to a poll of folk remedies in the 1980s recommended lemon balm *(Melissa officinalis)* tea for cold and flu. The plant, which is native to southern Europe and northern Africa, now grows throughout North America as well. Lemon balm has long been used as a relaxing and sweat-inducing herb. The 12th century German mystic and healer Hildegarde von Bingen stated, "Lemon balm contains within it the virtues of a dozen other plants."

Lemon balm is approved today by the German government as a medicine for digestive complaints and sleeping disorders, though it is not recommended specifically for colds or flu. Its aromatic oils contain antiviral compounds that may help disinfect the mucous membranes, however. Of the sweat-inducing herbs included in this section, lemon balm is probably the mildest and the most suitable for use in children. Lemon balm is also a mild sedative and can help relax a restless patient suffering from cold or flu.

☞ Directions: Place 1 teaspoon of the dried herb in a cup and fill with boiling water. Let steep for ten minutes. Inhale the steam from the cup. Strain and drink up to 4 cups a day. Sweeten with honey as desired.

GARLIC: The recommendation to take garlic for colds comes from New England, the American Southwest, and all the way from China. Garlic has been used for colds, bronchial problems, and fevers in cultures throughout the world since the dawn of written medical history—even the ancient Egyptians used it to treat cough and fever.

Garlic's constituents are antibacterial, antiviral, and antifungal. Garlic also stimulates the immune system, increasing the body's resistance to invaders. In addition, garlic is an expectorant and induces sweating, helping to reduce fever. Garlic has been approved as a medicine for colds and coughs and a variety of other illnesses by the pharmaceutical regulatory commission of the European Union, a confederation of modern European nations that has dropped trade barriers and is working toward economic regulation and a common currency. Garlic can also lower cholesterol and thin the blood. Note that garlic taken in high doses can irritate the stomach.

☞ Directions: Blend 3 cloves of garlic in a blender with a little water. (A clove must be cut or crushed in order to release its constituents.) If you want, add half a lemon, skin and all, to the garlic. Put the contents in a cup and fill the cup with boiling water. Let steep for five minutes, inhaling the fragrance. Strain, add honey, and drink the entire cup in sips. Do this two to three times a day while you have a cold or flu or once a day to prevent infection during epidemics.

Alternately, peel and chop 3 whole garlic bulbs and soak them in 1 pint of wine (red or white) in a closed container for a month. Shake the jar once a day. Then, strain and take 1 tablespoon of the wine each day as a preventive measure.

ONIONS: Onions are used to treat colds in virtually every folk tradition in North America—whether eaten raw, roasted, or boiled; taken in the form of teas, milk, or wine; worn in a sock or in a bag around the neck; or applied to the chest as a poultice. Wild onions have been used for the same purpose by American Indian tribes in every region of the country. Using onions to treat colds continues today in the folk medicine of New England, upstate

continued on page 129

American Indian Healing

American Indian tribes lived in many environments and had many different cultural and belief systems. All native peoples' beliefs about health and healing, including the use of natural materials such as plants, were based in their religions. Today all American Indian groups have been influenced by modern medicine, though many individuals still hold traditional beliefs and use traditional American Indian medical practices. For many indigenous peoples, there is no contradiction in using both their own remedies and "white" medicine. It should be kept in mind, however, that the following descriptions about the beliefs of different American Indian tribes do not apply to all members of each tribe.

For North American tribes east of the Rocky Mountains, diseases were traditionally things that entered the body to do harm. Thus, the cure was to remove them. For example, the Cheyenne have held the belief that a person can become seriously ill when a foreign object such as a ball of hair, a feather, or a thorn enters the body. The cure is a ritual that is performed by the tribal medicine man or healer and a woman, often his wife. Once the offending object is located, the healer sucks on the spot until the object is dislodged and removed. Similar treatments by "sucking doctors" are found in many parts of the world.

For tribes west of the Rockies, most illnesses (and all misfortune) were explained by the disruption of balance or harmony in nature. Disruption in relationships among humans, and in relationships between humans and the supernatural, could also bring on illness. These tribes believe that all living and non-living things had a life force or divinity; therefore, conflicts or behavior that went against community values could cause soul loss, which resulted in disease. Disease could also be caused by supernatural beings who were displeased in some way with human behavior.

PLANT MEDICINES: American Indian knowledge of curing plants is extensive, and for ordinary health problems, such as dysentery, menstrual problems, bladder infection, warts, and burns, healers use a wide variety of plant medicines. Of all the plants Indians used for food, healing, and ritual purposes, corn, or maize, is probably the most prevalent. The Hopi used corn- meal for every ceremony. They believed that corn was a divinely created spirit, referred to as the corn mother. The Spanish were impressed by the Inca's use of corn to treat kidney and bladder problems. The Aztec used a decoction of ground corn in water for treating heart problems and dysentery and to promote lactation in nursing mothers.

Among the Pueblo, blue cornmeal mixed with water was used to treat heart pain. The Chickasaw cured itchy skin by holding the affected area over smoke released from burning dry corncobs.

Following the arrival of Europeans in the Americas, whites adopted many of the cures taught to them by the native people. For example, Indians taught white settlers how to make maple sugar and syrup and how to use it for curing. Physicians of the time, too, recommended its use for both nutrition and healing. (It was said to relieve stomach problems, colds, coughs, and rheumatism.) Many medicinal plants used by American Indian tribes have even been added to the medical pharmacopoeia. For example, cinchona bark was the source for quinine. Corn smut, a corn fungus, used for food and healing by some Indian tribes, was used by the Zuni to increase the progression of labor. It was accepted by U.S. physicians to help in childbirth and was put into the *United States Pharmacopoeia* in 1882. Cornsilk was another food as well as medicine for some Indian groups. It was recognized as a diuretic by the *United States Pharmacopoeia* and by the National Formulary in the early 20th century. One of the most widely used plant medicines among the Indians is now considered a public health scourge: tobacco!

MYSTICAL MEDICINE: For most American Indians, medicine isn't simply a remedy or a treatment. It is mysterious, magical, and supernatural, and it signifies power. For instance, before planting, the Iroquois soaked seed corn in a boiled mixture of herbs. They called this mixture "corn medicine," and it was said to protect the corn from parasites and ensure its health and a good harvest.

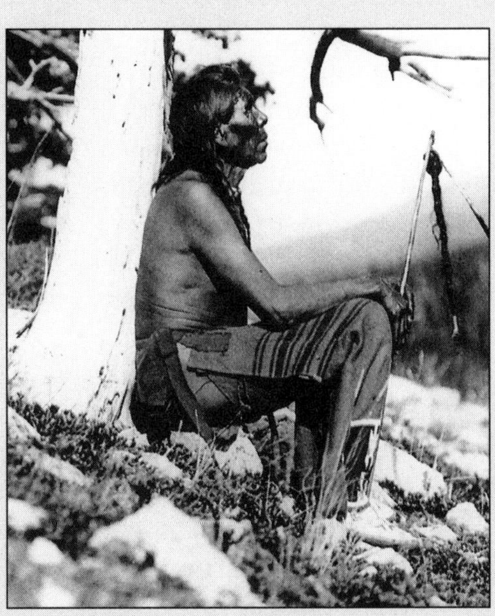

Beliefs about health were based in religion.

For prolonged and serious illnesses or severe injuries, American Indians called on their tribal medicine man, diviner, or shaman. Shamans are religious individuals who operate between the material and the supernatural worlds. Through mystical techniques, they learn procedures for diagnosis and healing. They also communicate with the spirit world to get supernatural help, learn about the universe, and receive guidance on proper behavior in the world. Serving as healers and philosophers, shamans often play a very influential role in a tribe's political, economic, and religious decisions.

During public performances, a shaman will induce himself into a trance and then use supernatural means to diagnose and cure. A trance can be induced by a variety of methods, including smoking tobacco, ingesting drugs, beating on a drum, dancing, and meditation. The most common form of trance was believed to be brought on by possession by a spirit. While experiencing the trance, the shaman acts as a medium, relaying mes-

American Indian Healing

sages from ancestors. With the help of good spirits, the shaman can identify the causes of illness and prescribe cures. While trance is a common part of shamanic practice in many American Indian tribes, it is not universal. Many cultures have part-time specialists who do not use trance but who diagnose and cure disease as well as perform other functions for their people. In the past, women were usually excluded from the sacred realm and thus were not allowed to become shamans, although they could often take on the role of lesser specialists, such as an herbalist or midwife.

WARFARE MEDICINE: American Indian tribes, especially those who engaged in warfare, had extensive knowledge of wound treatment and broken bones. Their healers, who were often more able than the white 18th century physicians, knew how to set badly broken bones in rawhide casts, remove embedded arrowheads, stop bleeding with astringents, and reduce inflammation. They also used steam baths and massage for a variety of ailments. For instance, many tribes used massage to relieve pain in the abdomen no matter the root cause.

VISION QUESTS: Even where shamans are common, tribal members may choose to conduct a religious ceremony individually. One of the most common is the vision quest, practiced by certain North American tribes and Eskimos. An individual's vision quest usually occurs at puberty when he ventures into the wilderness alone to receive a name and a totem (a spirit guardian).

A vision quest refers to power, protection, or guidance acquired during a hallucinatory experience when a person has direct and personal contact with the supernatural. This visionary experience was mandatory for every warrior who sought immunity and success in battle and personal power for healing. The Guardian Spirit, or totem, comes during the vision quest and adopts and aids the individual during his lifetime. Among the Cheyenne, if a spirit comes during the vision quest, it gives a blessing with instructions on how to prepare amulets and paint the body and which songs to sing to evoke power.

Until recently, many North American tribes did not induce visions through drugs like peyote but instead through self-inflicted pain. The Crow, for example, traveled alone into the wilderness, stripped off their clothes, fasted, and if this was not enough to induce a vision, resorted to severing a portion of the fourth finger on the left hand.

In the United States today, American Indians as well as whites are increasingly interested in American Indian philosophies and healing approaches. Sweat lodges, something like an Indian sauna but with more specific spiritual elements, are undergoing a resurgence of use among Indians, but they are also being tried by whites, too. It seems the native shaman has become somewhat of a cultural hero, symbolizing the precious knowledge of his people's past.

New York, North Carolina, Appalachia, Indiana, and within Chinese cultures throughout North America.

The constituents in onions—the same that cause onion's volatile vapors to burn the eyes—are antimicrobial. Onions also have expectorant qualities, which induce the flow of healthy cleansing mucous. Onions induce sweating as well, helping to cool a fever.

☞ Directions: Cut up 1 whole large onion and simmer in a covered pot for twenty minutes. Strain if desired to remove pulp. Drink a cup of the tea three to four times daily when you have a cold or flu.

Alternately, try chewing raw onions—but don't swallow until the onions are thoroughly chewed. Note: Chewing too many onions can cause stomach irritation.

To make an onion poultice for chest colds, slice 3 large onions, discarding the outer paper-like skin. Cover with water and simmer for twenty minutes. Strain. Layer the cooked onions between two cloths. Apply to the chest for twenty to thirty minutes.

Beware of Alcohol

Several folk traditions from the eastern United States suggest taking alcohol to treat a cold. In fact, a recommendation from a collection of Indiana folklore suggests hanging your hat on a bed post and drinking whiskey until you see two hats!

Getting drunk may well help you to forget the misery of a cold, but, from a medical standpoint, it is not such a good idea. Drinking to the point of intoxication depresses the immune system. Alcohol reduces the rate at which white blood cells engulf invading organisms; it also depresses antibody production. Thus, the duration and severity of a cold can only be made worse by alcohol consumption during the infection. Alcohol can also make your cold worse if you are exposed to cold air. The alcohol dilates the blood vessels near the surface of the skin, which promotes loss of body heat. The body then has to work even harder to maintain its normal temperature or a healthy fever.

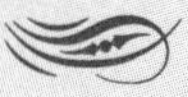

SAGE: Some residents of New England, North Carolina, and Indiana recommend hot sage tea to "break up" a cold. Sage *(Salvia officinalis)* contains volatile oils, which have been shown to kill viruses in laboratory studies. It specifically kills the rhinovirus, the virus most often responsible for causing colds. Also, because of sage's astringent qualities, it traditionally was used to treat sore throats. So, if you are suffering a sore throat with your cold, hot sage tea may be just the remedy for you. Other documented properties of sage include mild hypotensive effects, anti-inflammatory properties, and analgesic and anticonvulsant effects.

☞ Directions: Place 1 teaspoon of sage in a cup and fill with boiling water. Cover and let steep for ten minutes. Strain, add a little lemon and honey, and drink.

Repeat three to four times a day for as long as you have a cold.

LEMON: The contemporary folk traditions of New England and Indiana call for drinking "hot lemonade" during a cold or flu. The practice is at least as old as the ancient Romans.

Lemon juice, like vinegar, is acidic. Drinking it helps to acidify the mucous membranes, making the membranes inhospitable to bacteria or viruses. Lemon oil, which gives the juice its fragrance, is like a pharmacy in itself—it contains antibacterial, antiviral, antifungal, and anti-inflammatory constituents. Five of the constituents are specifically active against the influenza virus. Lemon oil is also an expectorant, increasing the flow of healthy mucous. And lemon is very tasty—its flavor is used to promote compliance in taking cold and flu products.

☞ Directions: Place 1 chopped whole lemon—skin, pulp, and all—in a pot and add 1 cup of boiling water. While letting the mixture steep for five minutes, inhale the fumes. Then, strain and drink. Do this at the onset of a cold, and repeat three to four times a day for the duration of the cold.

VINEGAR: A cold remedy from Indiana calls for inhaling the fumes of vinegar. This remedy is as old as ancient Greece—the Greek physician Hippocrates recommended the treatment for coughs and respiratory infections. Vinegar is a weak acid. Inhaling its fumes changes the acidity of the mucous membranes in the upper respiratory tract, making the membranes inhospitable to viruses. Due to its acidic nature, avoid splashing vinegar into the eyes or onto cuts.

☞ Directions: In a jar, pour ½ cup of boiling water over ½ cup of vinegar. Gently inhale the steam. Be careful not to burn yourself.

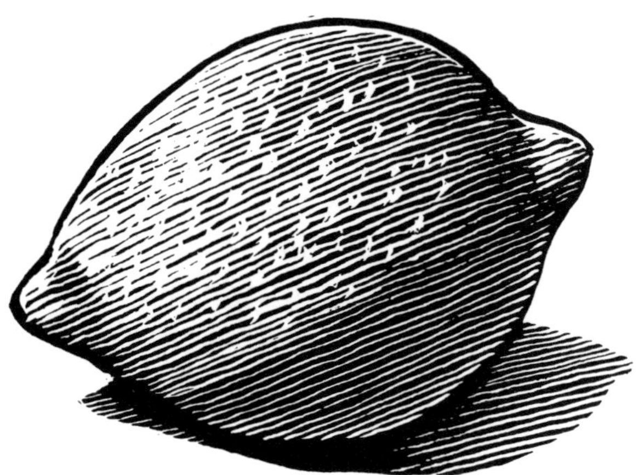

MUSTARD PLASTER: The mustard plaster has been used medicinally in Europe at least since the time of the ancient Romans. The contemporary Amish still recommend it for treating chest colds and bronchitis. It works mainly by increasing circulation, perspiration, and heat in the afflicted area. In addition, when its irritant antimicrobial and anti-inflammatory volatile substances are inhaled, mustard may also have a medicinal effect on the mucous membranes of the upper respiratory tract. The active principle is allylisothiocyanate, which is also present in horseradish and watercress.

☞ Directions: Mix ½ cup mustard with 1 cup flour. Stir warm water into the mustard and flour mixture until a paste is formed. This allows for the active principle to be released. Spread the mixture on a piece of cotton or muslin that has been soaked in hot water. Cover with a second piece of dry material. Lay the moist side of the poultice across the person's chest or back. Leave the poultice on for fifteen to thirty minutes. Remove promptly if the person experiences any discomfort. (Be careful not to blister or burn the skin. You may want to lift the cloth every five minutes or so to see how red the skin is.)

Chicken Soup

Chicken soup is a universal remedy for colds. It is mentioned in the folk literature of New England and in the traditions of Jewish immigrants. Research articles on the medicinal properties of chicken soup have appeared in the scientific literature in the past ten years. Because no specific medicinal properties have been found in the chicken, scientists suspect the "active constituents" in chicken soup may be the garlic and/or onions that are commonly added.

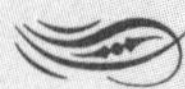

VAPORIZE IT: The contemporary Amish suggest using a vaporizer and adding essential oils to the water, such as pine, cedar, or mint. Many of the aromatic constituents of these plants have antimicrobial properties. If you can smell the aroma, then at least a small amount of the constituent has reached your mucous membranes and may assist in killing viruses there. Peppermint oil also contains menthol, which acts as a decongestant. Excessive inhalation can be hazardous to sensitive or allergic young children, however.

☞ Directions: Add a few drops of essential oils to the water of a commercial vaporizer. If you've purchased concentrated essential oils, be sure to dilute them with at least five parts of a carrier oil (such as almond oil) before adding them to the water. Place the vaporizer next to the sick bed and keep it running around the clock.

SALT WATER: According to New England and Indiana folk medicine, a good remedy for treating a head cold is sniffing warm salt water. The salt itself is antimicrobial, and the heat from the warm water kills the viruses that attack the mucous membranes (see sidebar, "Hot Water Treatments," page 123).

☞ Directions: Put ¼ teaspoon of salt in a glass of hot or warm water. Sniff some of the water. Do this after being exposed to someone with a cold or flu or at the first sign of infection. Repeat every three to four hours while suffering from a cold.

WATER TREATMENTS: The Seventh Day Adventists suggest a variety of water treatments for curing a cold.

☞ Directions: At the first sign of a cold, put your feet in hot water. Keep the water hot for twenty minutes. Then run cold water over your feet and dry them. Cover your feet well or go to bed for half an hour.

Also, you can try drawing hot water up into the nasal passages and then blowing the water back out. Just make sure the water isn't too hot. This action lubricates the passages and helps expel phlegm.

Gargle hot water four times daily for ten minutes if a sore throat or earache accompanies your cold.

For general muscle and joint aches, take a fifteen minute hot hip bath (see "Cold Hip Bath," page 262). Follow with a brief cold shower and rapid, vigorous drying with a rough towel.

To treat a sore throat, soak a cotton cloth in cold water. Wring the cloth out and wrap it around the neck. Place a warm wool scarf over the cold cloth. Keep the cloths in place until the body has warmed up the cold cloth.

BUTTER: An old New England remedy for treating colds is to eat butter, either straight or melted in a cup of hot water or milk. Adding butter to hot tea is a remedy used as a cold preventive in the high altitudes of Nepal and Tibet. Cough syrups made with butter are also popular remedies in folk medicine.

Butter contains about 15 percent short- and medium-chain fatty acids, which, in laboratory tests, exhibit antibacterial, antifungal, and immune-stimulating properties. A single tablespoon of butter also contains more than 400 IU of vitamin A, about half the minimum daily requirement. Vitamin A also helps to maintain the health of the mucous membranes of the respiratory tract.

☞ Directions: Eat 1 tablespoon of butter three or four times a day. Alternately, add 1 tablespoon of butter to 1 cup of hot tea. Let the butter melt so that it forms a thin layer across the top of the tea. Stir and drink.

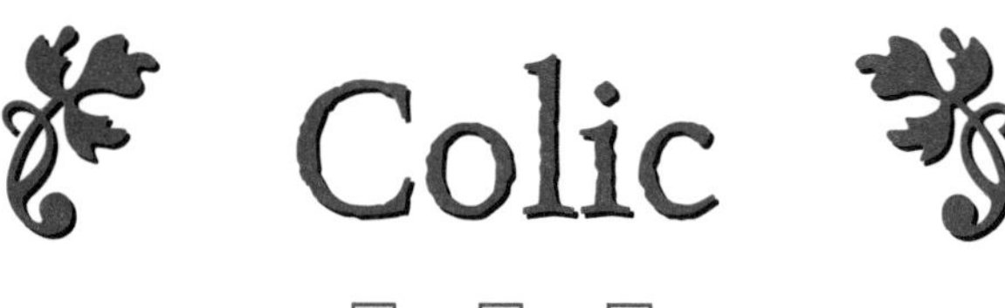

Colic

If your infant's colic is keeping you and your baby up at night, try one of the folk remedies below—and you'll both be sleeping a little easier

A wailing, colicky baby is perhaps the most familiar trial of a new parent's patience. We have included plenty of folk remedies for treating colic, developed no doubt by parents of the past who were very familiar with the condition. Colic is a common condition in babies under four months of age. It is characterized by intense crying, apparent abdominal pain, and irritability. One of the many causes of colic is that a baby's intestines are not fully mature, and sometimes normal foods, even the constituents in breast milk, are irritating. (An infant's intestines are not fully formed until about seven months of age. Giving an infant cow's milk, the soy protein in formulas, or solid foods before this time may stimulate the spasms of colic.)

Both conventional physicians and midwives recommend that a nursing mother avoid eating foods known to cause colic in infants, including garlic, onions, beans, cabbage, chocolate, excessive amounts of exotic or seasonal fruits, melons, rhubarb, peaches, or even tomato juice. If colic persists, the nursing mother might experiment by removing specific foods from her menu. Food sensitivities may cause colic in some infants.

In bottle-fed babies, allergies to cow's milk and soy formulas have been suspect. Cow's milk is much less suitable for the baby than mother's milk. Cow's milk has much higher levels of hard-to-digest casein protein and much lower levels of the beneficial milk sugar lactose. (Goat's milk is closer in composition to human milk, with lower amounts of casein and more lactose.) Breast feeding has advantages for the baby besides reducing colic, however. When a woman breast-feeds her baby, much of the immunity she has developed passes on to her infant through the antibodies present in her breast milk. Many studies show that breast-fed babies have fewer and milder illnesses and fewer hospitalizations.

Parents shouldn't allow the condition to interfere with the relationship they're developing with their child. It is perfectly natural to feel some resentment, confusion, and even anger when all your best efforts at comforting a colicky baby meet with no success. But be reassured the colic will end soon, and no physical or emotional problems have been found to result from it.

Most of the folk remedies for colic are herbs classified as carminatives. These are plants that, when taken as teas, may help reduce intestinal spasms or expel gas. Most are common kitchen spices that are used in contemporary professional medical herbalism in Europe and North America for treating indigestion in adults and children.

Spice It Up

Besides adding a little flavor to some of our blander dishes, many common kitchen spices also improve our digestion. That's because they possess antispasmodic properties. These properties help to reduce cramping and tension in the digestive tract. Perhaps this is why we enjoy on occasion a dash of this or a dash of that!

Most of the herbs listed in this section contain a dozen or more different volatile constituents. Some typical examples include caffeic acid, eugenol, and limonene. Many have antispasmodic (reducing the tendency of smooth muscle to cramp) and sedative (relaxing to the nervous system) actions.

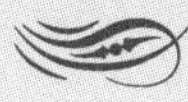

Remedies

CATNIP: Catnip *(Napeta cataria)* tea has been a popular sedative and sleep aid throughout American history. The plant arrived with the first European immigrants and became rapidly naturalized here. Indian tribes, such as the Onondaga and Cayuga, used it for sleepless and peevish children.

Catnip is also a well-known folk remedy for colic—it is mentioned in the folkloric lit-

continued on page 135

Remedying Colic

Because there are few experiences more frustrating for parents than to have their new baby cry inconsolably, treatments for colic are featured in many folk medical traditions. Colic has often been called "three-month colic" because it usually extends from shortly after birth until three months of age (though occasionally twice that long). Its cause is not known, but true colic does involve signs of intestinal gas, and it has long been assumed that the crying is caused by abdominal pain.

This theory has resulted in such common colic cures as massaging the baby's stomach. The massage sometimes used castor oil as a lubricant and was followed by warm cloths. Warm water or various warm herbal teas were given, especially those teas believed to have a sedative effect, such as catnip, or a carminative effect—that is, helping to expel gas.

Asafetida, a foul smelling plant resin, was placed around the neck as an amulet to treat colic. (Asafetida was used similarly in treating numerous other childhood diseases.) Asafetida actually is a carminative, but, of course, for the real relief of gas, a carminative needs to be swallowed not worn!

Other colic cures have a less obvious logic. For instance, giving a baby two spoonfuls of cold water as soon as possible after birth was a common colic preventive. Another cure involving water, this one from Indiana, recommends whiskey (never acceptable for children!) and sugar in warm water. Fortunately the remedy was used to treat "colic" in adults!

There were religious approaches as well. One was to have the baby swallow some of the baptismal water from his own Christening. From the Ozarks come directions to walk backwards without speaking for three steps (a common magic number in Christian culture) while holding the baby in an upright position. Then the baby should be given a drink of water from a brass thimble. Whether or not this remedy worked, such a routine might at least distract the suffering infant!

Some remedies were somewhat dangerous. In the Ozarks, folklorists collected numerous colic cures involving the use of tobacco smoke. The most innocuous was to blow tobacco smoke on the baby's stomach or under the baby's clothing. Similar uses of tobacco smoke turn up in other treatments for children, such as blowing smoke into the ear to cure earache. More drastic is the recommendation to blow tobacco smoke through a reed into the baby's bottle. Then the milk in which nicotine has dissolved is given to the baby.

The use of bees, with their powerful venom, turn up in folk medicine as well. This recipe for treating colic comes from the Ozarks: Roast nine live honeybees in a can in the oven, pulverize the dried bees into a fine powder, and give the powder (mixed in syrup) to the baby.

Conventional German Medicine

Medical herbalism is not an alternative practice in Germany; instead, both physicians and pharmacists are required to study the subject. The German equivalent of the U.S. Food and Drug Administration has a special branch that evaluates herbal medicines. That government agency has approved peppermint, fennel, and chamomile, all described in this section, as treatments for colic.

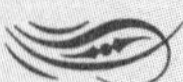

erature of North America more than any other remedy for that condition. It has been used to treat colic by residents of New England, Appalachia, North Carolina, Indiana, and New Mexico and by blacks throughout the deep South and by Hispanics in the Los Angeles area. It was an official medicine in the *United States Pharmacopoeia* from 1840 until 1870. Like many herbs in this section, catnip combines both carminative and sedative properties, with seven antispasmodic and five sedative constituents.

☞ Directions: Place 1 teaspoon of the dried herb in a cup and fill with boiling water. Let stand (covered) for ten minutes. Strain and, while warm, give to the infant in a bottle. If nursing, the mother may also drink the tea.

MINTS: Several types of mints are recommended for treating colic in North American folk literature, most commonly peppermint *(Mentha piperita)* and spearmint *(Mentha spicata)*. Peppermint seems to be the favorite in contemporary Indiana folklore and spearmint is favored in other areas, including New York, New Mexico, and California. Both species contain antispasmodic constituents, many of which may help reduce the intestinal spasms in colic. Due to their carminative and antispasmodic properties, a contemporary German medical text called *Lehrbuch der Phytotherapie (Herbal Medicine)* by R.F. Weiss recommends taking the mints as digestive aids. Peppermint is, in fact, an official digestive aid in Germany.

☞ Directions: Place 1 teaspoon of the dried herb in a cup and fill with boiling water. Let stand for ten minutes. Strain well and, while warm, give to the infant in a bottle. If nursing, the mother may also drink the tea.

FENNEL: In the folk medicine of both New England and China, a tea of fennel seeds *(Foeniculum vulgare)* is used to calm a colicky baby. In fact, according to medical herbalism, fennel seed tea is probably the most commonly prescribed tea for treating adults with abdominal cramping and gas in contemporary Great Britain, Canada, and the United States. It is an approved medicine in Germany for treating mild gastrointestinal complaints. Animal studies have shown that at least 16 chemical constituents in fennel have antispasmodic qualities.

☞ Directions: Place 1 teaspoon of the seeds in a cup and fill with boiling water. Cover and let stand for ten minutes. Strain well, and, while warm or at room temperature, give it to the infant in a bottle. If nursing, the mother may also

drink the tea. (A New England recipe suggests mixing the fennel seeds half-and-half with dried catnip leaves.)

DILL: Dill *(Anethum graveolens)* is used by the residents of the Appalachian mountains to treat infant colic; it is also used by residents in rural China for the same purpose. Dill, which was used as a digestive aid by the ancient Egyptians, came to North America with the European colonists and remains primarily a garden herb rather than a wild plant. The name dill comes from the Norse *dylla*, meaning "to soothe." Of the herbs in this section, dill contains more antispasmodic constituents than any other—more than 20, in fact. Dill seed has been approved by the German government as a medicine for digestive complaints.

☞ Directions: Place 1 teaspoon of the seeds in a cup and fill with boiling water. Cover and let stand for ten minutes. Strain well, and, while warm or at room temperature, give it to the infant in a bottle. If nursing, the mother may also drink the tea.

GERMAN CHAMOMILE: Chamomile *(Matricaria recutita)*, like catnip, combines both antispasmodic and sedative properties and may thus relieve intestinal cramping and induce relaxation at the same time. The herb is recommended for infant colic in the folk traditions of both New England and the American Southwest. Chamomile contains at least 19 different antispasmodic constituents, as well as five sedative ones. A 1993 clinical trial showed that chamomile was effective in relieving infant colic. The plant is approved by the German government as a medicine for gastrointestinal complaints.

What's Your Position?

Conventional medical texts suggest putting a colicky infant on his stomach, tightly swaddled with a sheet. The same recommendation appears in a variety of folk traditions, with some variations. One suggestion from North Carolina is to place the baby on his stomach and rub his back. Another common recommendation is to hold the baby upside down: An Appalachian source says to hold "the victim" by the feet and let his head hang down. A variation of this remedy from African-American folk medicine of Louisiana is to say prayers three times an hour while holding the baby "head down and heels up." Another African-American tradition, one recommended for preventing colic, advises against feeding an infant when the child is lying down. If you have questions about the best way to treat or prevent colic, speak with your doctor.

☞ Directions: Place 1 teaspoon of chamomile flowers in a cup and fill with boiling water. Cover and let stand for ten minutes. Strain well, and, while warm or at room temperature, give it to the infant in a bottle. If nursing, the mother may also drink the tea.

ANISE SEED: Another kitchen spice used in the folk medicine of New England and by Hispanics of the American Southwest is anise seed *(Pimpinella anisum)*. Anise seed contains ten antispasmodic constituents. Its constituent eugenol, which is common in many plants used to treat digestive cramping and pain, has carminative properties.

Blowing Smoke

Several folk traditions recommend blowing tobacco smoke on a colicky baby, or at least onto the child's food. Such traditions, however, even if they actually work, ignore the negative effects of secondhand smoke on a baby's health. Passive tobacco smoke increases the frequency of upper respiratory infections and ear infections in babies and young children. These effects, only demonstrated scientifically in the last decade, were unknown to American pioneers and others who used the smoke remedy.

A carminative helps to expel gas and relax intestinal muscle. (Purified eugenol is used in dentistry as a pain reliever.)

☞ Directions: Place 1 teaspoon of the seeds in a cup and fill with boiling water. Cover and let stand for ten minutes. Strain well, and, while warm or at room temperature, give it to the infant in a bottle. Add honey if desired. If nursing, the mother may also drink the tea.

LEMON BALM: "Lemon balm contains within it the virtues of a dozen other plants," said Hildegarde von Bingen of Germany, a 12th century mystic and healer. One reason for lemon balm's *(Melissa officinalis)* reputation is that, like chamomile and catnip, it is thus antispasmodic and sedative and will benefit any condition related to spasm and tension, including infant colic. Lemon balm contains nine constituents with antispasmodic properties and seven with sedative effects. It is approved by the German government as a medicine for digestive complaints or sleeping disorders.

☞ Directions: Place 1 teaspoon of the dried herb in a cup and fill with boiling water. Cover and let stand for ten minutes. Strain well, and, while warm or at room temperature, give it to the infant in a bottle. If nursing, the mother may also drink the tea.

ASAFOETIDA: Asafoetida, a pungent kitchen spice with a flavor similar to garlic, is used in Appalachia to treat infant colic; it is also used by some blacks in Louisiana for the same purpose. The herb is even used today as a treatment for colic in Ayurveda, the traditional medicine of India. Asafoetida is used in a variety of folk remedies both as a sedative and a carminative for digestive com-

continued on page 140

Illnesses Unique to Folk Medicine

The most obvious difference between folk medicine and modern medicine is the existence of entirely different kinds of sicknesses. Often called "folk illnesses," some of the best known examples of such illnesses in the United States are found among Latino ethnic groups. But all cultures have traditions about certain sicknesses. Some of these traditions vary from modern medicine only in the way that the illnesses are diagnosed and explained. For example, in some traditions, folk healers will diagnose cancer as being caused by a curse.

Other folk illnesses are more difficult to equate with a recognized medical condition. This is especially true in the case of psychiatric illnesses. For example, among the Hopi Indians, there exists an illness that is called "heart broken," but can also be translated as "heart is dying" or "spiritual death." The symptoms of the illness seem mostly physical (and include loss of appetite and difficulty sleeping) and are caused by the loss of an important relationship. Psychiatrists have identified this condition as one of five different kinds of emotional problems that can be equated with what mainstream medicine terms as depression.

Other folk illnesses seem to have no equivalent at all in Western society. These illnesses are called "culture-bound syndromes," and some anthropologists and psychiatrists believe that they are actually produced by the culture in which they are found.

CULTURE-BOUND SYNDROMES

One of the best examples of a culture-bound syndrome is *latah.* Latah is an Indonesian word that refers to a person who behaves in some very specific and bizarre ways when startled. The person who is latah will briefly obey commands—even ridiculous ones, repeat anything shouted at them, and often say dirty or blasphemous words. At one time scholars believed that this condition was caused by Indonesian child-rearing practices. But, as it turns out, the same condition is found in many cultures, just under different names. For instance, among French-Canadians living in New England, people who respond this way when startled are called "jumpers." Recently a psychiatrist named Ronald Simons, M.D., studied latah closely and showed that it is caused by being especially sensitive to being startled—and such people are found in every society. People in some cultures, like Indonesia, have traditional knowledge of this condition while others, like most of American society, do not. This suggests that culture does not so much cause these conditions as it shapes the way that they are experienced and understood.

SPIRITUAL MEANS

Folk illnesses usually have a prominent spiritual element, and they are typically treated by spiritual means. This spiritual element is one factor that differentiates certain folk illnesses from Western medical diagnoses, since Western medicine has excluded spiritual explanations and diagnoses for centuries.

Soul loss illnesses, such as Mexican *susto,* make up a kind of folk illness where folk tradition's knowledge may be beyond the learning of scientific medicine. Susto may actually be based on local knowledge of near-death experiences and the emotional changes that can follow these events, something that psychiatrists are only beginning to investigate and understand. Susto, which means "fright," is one of the best known of the Latino folk illnesses. It is caused by severe fright or emotional shock. It is believed that this shock may cause a person's soul to be separated from his body. If the soul cannot return, the person will begin to feel depressed and disinterested in life, he will lose sleep and his appetite and become nervous or anxious at small things.

In addition to experiencing the loss of your soul, you could also suffer from any of the folk illnesses thought to be caused by spirits. An example of a spirit-caused illness is *ghost sickness,* which is found among a number of American Indian tribes. This illness involves a preoccupation with the dead, feelings of suffocation, and, sometimes, even a loss of consciousness.

THE PHYSICAL ELEMENT

Some folk illnesses seem very physical, but they differ from sicknesses described by modern medicine. An example is *áwachse,* or "liver grown" (the common English translation). This ailment is best known in the United States among the Pennsylvania Germans. It is also known in Germany, England, and the American South. Áwachse means "to grow together." It is believed that the disorder is caused by the liver becoming attached to the ribs or other parts of the body cavity. The condition is believed to be most common in young children, especially after they have been exposed to strong wind, kept outside too long, or been "shaken up" in travel.

In the American South, the most common symptom of liver grown is a child's failure to thrive. The treatments for this condition include magical remedies as well as the act of stretching the arms and legs behind the child's back to loosen the liver. Among the Pennsylvania Germans, a definite diagnosis comes from feeling the lower chest. If the child has áwachse the healer will feel the flesh pulled inward, leaving both the ribs and abdomen with a raised appearance. For the Pennsylvania Germans, most treatments for this disorder involve passing the child under or through something: beneath a bramble bush or through a warm horse collar.

Some researchers have suggested that similar culture-bound disorders may be found in modern, Western culture. Thus, it is important for doctors and nurses to be aware of the existence of folk illnesses. When health care providers do not recognize or understand folk illnesses, several things can happen. Patient mistrust of the physician can develop. Also, a physician may misdiagnose a patient as mentally ill, even if the patient's symptoms are an appropriate response to stress and distress in his own culture. When there is understanding between patient and physician, however, it is possible to incorporate culturally sanctioned healing (as in rituals by a community healer) into medical treatment, yielding more effective and humane care. In addition, these folk illnesses are useful to us: They represent bodies of knowledge that Western medicine has yet to recognize.

plaints. Modern science supports its virtues as an intestinal disinfectant (kills bacteria in the intestines), but its other properties have not been formally studied. Asafoetida contains the antispasmodic aromatic oils alpha-pinene and ferulic acid. Eclectic physicians of the past century prescribed the spice as a sedative.

☞ Directions: Place ⅛ teaspoon of asafoetida spice in ½ cup of hot water. Stir and let stand for ten minutes. Strain and give warm to the infant.

SALT WATER: In his collection of remedies called *American Folk Medicine*, folklorist Clarence Meyer suggests giving a colicky baby a few drops of warm salt water. The practice survives in the contemporary folk medicine of Indiana.

☞ Directions: Dissolve 1 teaspoon of salt in a glass of warm water. Using your finger or an eyedropper, give the baby a few drops as needed. (If the baby doesn't like it, you'll know soon enough!)

BASIL: Another colic remedy from the kitchen is basil *(Ocimum bascilicum)*, recommended in the folk medicine of Mexico and the American Southwest. Basil is a European plant; it came to North America with the colonists, often those arriving from Mediterranean countries. The herb is steeped in sweetened water before it is given to an infant in the contemporary folk medicine of the Hispanics of New Mexico.

Basil contains large amounts of eugenol. Eugenol, which is used in a purified form in dentistry as a local anesthetic, has antispasmodic, sedative, and carminative properties. Eugenol is also present in several of the

Castor Oil

A suggestion from the folk medicine of contemporary Indiana is to rub warm castor oil on a colicky baby's stomach and keep the baby covered with warm clothes. (Castor oil taken internally is a strong laxative, and it should never be given to a baby or a child.) The *external* use of castor oil for digestive pain and complaints gained great popularity in North American folk traditions in the second half of the 20th century, thanks to the teachings of mystic Edgar Cayce. (Cayce, an American Christian, was known for giving medical advice, often while in a trance-like state. His books remain popular today.) Cayce claimed that castor oil improved the functioning of the gut's immune system. No scientific evidence exists to support the claim, but the practice continues and appears to be harmless.

other plants in this section, including peppermint, spearmint, dill, anise, and lemon balm.

☞ Directions: Place 1 teaspoon of dried basil leaves in a cup and fill with boiling water. Cover and let stand for ten minutes. Strain well, and, while warm or at room temperature, give it to the infant in a bottle. If nursing, the mother may also drink the tea.

Constipation

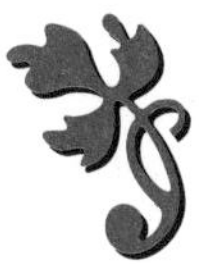

Regularity is actually a relative term. What matters is not the frequency of your bowel movements, but whether your normal routine alters

Constipation can mean either difficult or infrequent passage of the feces. Normal healthy bowels will produce between one and three bowel movements a day. Not an illness in itself, constipation, whether chronic or acute, can be the symptom of anything from a low-fiber diet to more serious illnesses. A medical checkup is warranted in any case of severe or persistent constipation. Constipation accompanied by nausea, vomiting, abdominal pain, or rectal bleeding or in the presence of any inflammatory bowel disease should never be treated with laxatives.

The most common cause of constipation in modern society is the modern diet. Constipation is classified by medical anthropologists H.C. Trowell and D.P. Burkitt as a "Western" condition, meaning that the condition does not appear in primitive people eating traditional diets—that is, until Western foods, such as sugar, white flour, and canned goods, are added.

Conventional physicians, alternative doctors, and folk healers alike all warn against the use of strong laxatives to force a bowel movement. From a medical point of view, if the constipation is due to a serious underlying disease, the laxative can cause injury and make that condition worse. Chronic use of strong laxatives also creates "laxative dependence"—a condition in which the bowels become so exhausted that they can no longer provide a normal bowel movement without the stimulation of more laxatives. Laxative dependence can also cause electrolyte (such as sodium and potassium) imbalances.

Conventional treatment for constipation, after a thorough investigation of the cause, is to increase fiber and liquids in the diet and to administer bulk laxatives (also called stool softeners) such as psyllium husks. An increase in fruits and vegetables in the diet is also encouraged. Eat six or more servings of vegetables each day.

Many of the folk remedies for treating constipation include herbs that act as strong laxatives, but their use for more than seven to ten days is not warranted. Anything stronger than a bulk laxative is contraindicated in pregnancy, however, because the same constituents that make the colon wall contract to produce a bowel movement can make the uterus contract as well. Stimulating laxatives are also contraindicated for use in children under 12 years of age.

The Wisdom of Father Kneipp

During the late 1800s and early 1900s, German immigrants to New York and to other eastern states arrived with the book *My Water Cure* (English translation) written by Bavarian peasant priest and healer Father Sebastian Kneipp. Within thirty years of the book's arrival to this country, Kneipp's recommendations for diet, herbs, and water treatments were widespread. There was a monthly magazine promoting this opinions, and tens of thousands of medical professionals and lay people practicing his advice. Said Father Kneipp about laxative herbs and chemicals: "It will be noticed that I have not given the well-known and generally used laxatives, such as rhubarb, senna, epsom-salt, etc. And the reason? These in themselves harmless remedies are nevertheless too strong for me; help can be obtained by milder means. No one would chase a gnat or a flea with a gun." Simply increasing the amount of water we drink each day may help many disorders of the gastrointestinal tract.

Remedies

SENNA: Well-known as a laxative, senna leaves *(Cassia senna),* most of which are imported from India, were brought to this country by European colonists. A North American variety of senna was used in the same way by Indians in eastern parts of the United States. Senna leaves have been used as a laxative by the Amish. Senna has been used for the same purpose in the folk medicine of New England, Appalachia, and the Southwest. Senna is also a component of some over-the-counter laxatives in North America and Europe. Senna is contraindicated in children, during pregnancy, and for more than ten days at a time.

☞ Directions: Do not use excessive amounts of senna. Place ¼ to ½ teaspoon of the dried crushed leaves or powder in a cup and fill with boiling water. Let steep seven to ten minutes. (A full teaspoon in a cup of tea is strong enough to produce abdominal cramping.)

CASCARA SAGRADA: At least 14 western Indian tribes have used cascara sagrada, or "sacred bark" *(Rhamnus purshiana),* as a laxative. Colonists learned its laxative effects from American Indian tribes in the

Pacific Northwest. Its use spread to the folk medicine of the Southwest, New England, and Appalachia. Cascara sagrada is a common component of many of today's over-the-counter laxatives in North America.

Cascara sagrada bark must be aged for more than a year before it is used, or else it can induce vomiting. Usually the bark you buy in herb shops has been properly aged, though in rare instances, you might inadvertently purchase young bark. If the cascara leaves you feeling at all sick to your stomach, return it for a refund and shop somewhere else. The use of cascara sagrada is contraindicated in children, during pregnancy, and for more than ten days at a time. Do not use cascara sagrada in herbal formulas intended to help you lose weight.

☞ Directions: Place 1 rounded teaspoon of the bark powder in a cup and fill with boiling water. Let steep until room temperature. Drinking a cup before bedtime will usually produce a bowel movement in the morning.

Alternately, place 1 ounce of aged cascara sagrada bark in a 1-quart jar, fill with boiling water, and let stand. The dose is 1 teaspoon in the morning and evening.

Appalachian Wisdom

Like Father Sebastian Kneipp (see sidebar, "The Wisdom of Father Kneipp," page 142), traditional Appalachian herbalist Tommie Bass cautioned against the habitual use of strong laxatives. Rather than avoid them, however, Bass recommended that a laxative be taken in small doses—doses that would soften the stool but not produce strong bowel movements. He cautioned that the use of low-dose laxatives was only for short term use, however.

Bass, who died in 1997, formulated and sold a herbal laxative mixture through his herb shop that combined small amounts of the stronger laxatives (senna and cascara sagrada) with more than a dozen other herbs. It was an herbal formula that seemed to work; users also noted improved overall digestion and liver function.

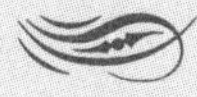

EPSOM SALTS: Epsom salts are composed of magnesium sulfate. The salt was first prepared from the waters of mineral springs in Epsom, England, where it was discovered in 1695. Their use as a commercial laxative spread quickly in the medicine of Europe; the salts remain popular there today. Epsom salts are now produced industrially and not from the springs in Epsom. The salts act as a laxative by drawing water out of the body and into the intestine. Epsom salts are listed in the folk medicine of New England and are widely used throughout North America as an over-the-counter laxative. Habitual use can cause dehydration and laxative dependence, however, so don't use Epsom salts for more than seven days.

☞ Directions: Place 2 or 3 teaspoons of Epsom salts in a glass of warm water and drink. Do this once a day.

continued on page 146

Asian-American Folk Medicine

Asia is a vast continent composed of many cultures and belief systems. Asian immigrants to the United States in the 19th century were primarily from China. More recent immigrants come from Japan, Korea, India, the Philippines, Laos, Vietnam, and Thailand.

Many Asian societies have been complex civilizations since ancient times. These highly developed societies generated great wealth, so they had the economic resources needed to support specialization in various fields of medicine. The medical systems of these societies, often called "great traditions" in contrast to local folk traditions, have been based on a written body of text from before the time of Christ. The physicians in these systems were high-ranking specialists who were often associated with the religious and political elite. These official healing systems occupied the same place of prestige and power that Western medicine holds in our culture today. And like America today, each of these "great" healing traditions was accompanied by folk medical traditions as well.

The oldest traditions based on ancient writings originated in the areas surrounding the Mediterranean and in what is now present-day India and China. Through cultural contact, the ancient Asian healing systems spread outward from their place of origin. The various systems have influenced and borrowed from each other as well as from other local folk medicine traditions. Although each of the great traditions and folk traditions of Asian medicine differs from the others in details of theory and practice, they all share certain broad similarities. For example, rather than focusing on the anatomical parts of the body, all of these traditions look at the body's functions. Physiological processes, as well as the development and treatment of disease, are explained in terms of oppositions such as hot and cold, wet and dry, light and dark. These contrasting qualities are applied to the physical parts of the body, emotional states, and the environment. For instance, in Chinese medicine, the whole universe is divided according to the qualities found in heaven and earth. These qualities are called *yin* and *yang*. The idea of yin and yang, and the processes they represent, are found in many Asian folk medical beliefs. The simplest way of characterizing yin and yang is to call them female and male. Yin, considered feminine, is dark, heavy, and passive (earth). Yang is masculine and bright, light, and active (the heavens). All people, men and women, are assumed to have and need both yin and yang, and health is found in a balance of the two, as illustrated by the yin-yang symbol. In the symbol, a bit of darkness shows up in the light half (yang), and a bit of light appears in the dark half (yin), and all combine to make a perfect circle. The yin and yang forces are said to constantly interact. And although they are, in a sense, in opposition to each other, their natural state is one of balance.

The body and mind and the physical environment are all seen as interrelated and reflective of one another. In their natural state, the relationship among the organs of the body, the thoughts of the mind, and the features of environment are one of balance. Imbalances can occur for a number of reasons, but it is when harmony is disrupted that disease can occur. The local folk traditions in Asian cultures added to these ideas of harmony and balance the practices of shamanism, astrology, and faith healing. Today, Asians and Asian Americans often integrate various practices (including Western medicine). Some practices may be alternatives to each other, but many are used as complementary strategies for coping with an illness.

The Hmong people provide an example of the diversity of belief systems that characterize Asia. The Hmong are an ethnically distinct group who lived in the mountains of Laos and Vietnam. Beginning in 1976, many Hmong resettled in the United States with government support because of displacement during the Vietnam War. The Hmong religion has a long history, but unlike the "great tradition" systems, Hmong medicine is not standardized. (The practices are similar from one healer to another, but they do not follow a single, written formal doctrine the way that a practitioner of Chinese medicine in "the great tradition" would.) Similar to many other farming peoples, their religious beliefs are inseparable from other aspects of everyday life. They are animists, meaning they believe that spirits reside in nature in both animals and inanimate objects. They also practice ancestor worship. They believe that spirits in nature may cause illness if they have been angered either intentionally or unintentionally. Since life and death are viewed as complementary, they believe that the needs of life on earth are the same after death. Therefore, ancestors, especially the recently dead, who lack food or money may indicate their need by causing sickness or misfortune to their living relatives. The proper response includes burning paper money or putting out food on a home altar for the ancestors to use.

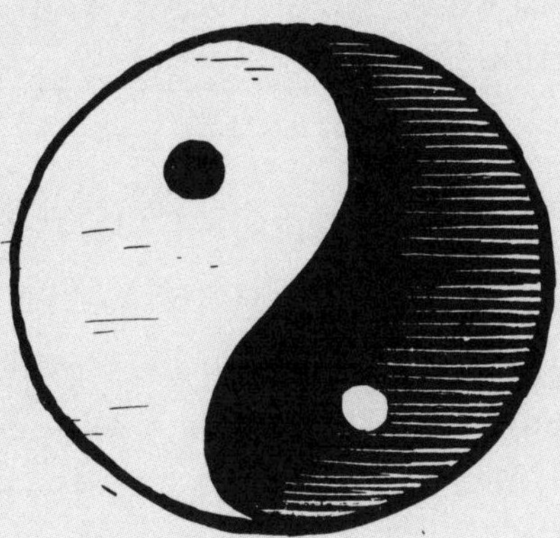

A healthy balance: the traditional yin-yang symbol

The Hmong believe that people have more than one soul, and that losing one or more of these souls is one of the main causes of illness. Souls are thought to be loosely attached to their material bodies, so that souls can separate from their bodies for any number of reasons, including sudden fright or because of a curse. The Hmong also believe in reincarnation and that how long one will live in a particular incarnation is predetermined. (A fatal illness is therefore understood to be the time that death was scheduled to arrive.) Although a Hmong shaman may try to bargain with the spirits for an additional bit of time, if the request is rejected, then the person's fate is sealed and death occurs.

Asian medical traditions, both great and small, have very much influenced American folk medicine. This is largely due to the impact of literature and film about such practices as acupuncture. It is also the result of the Asian peoples, who through immigration, have proudly brought their traditions with them.

FLAX SEED: Flax seed *(Linum usitatissimum)* is a New England folk remedy for treating constipation. The remedy is also used among the Amish and by some Gypsies. Flax is a bulk laxative, meaning that its fiber absorbs water, expands, and provides bulk for bowel movements. Flax seed also contains high amounts of essential fatty acids. Flax seed works in the same way as psyllium seed, the chief component of the commercial bulk laxative Metamucil.

☞ Directions: Take 2 teaspoons of flax seeds. Grind them in a coffee grinder and add to an 8-ounce glass of water. Let stand for half an hour and drink, seeds and all.

A GYPSY FORMULA: The following formula, related by a Spanish Gypsy in Wanja von Hausen's *Gypsy Folk Medicine,* combines several laxative substances with herbs to reduce tension and improve digestion. Note the absence of any strong laxatives, making it a safe formula for regular use.

☞ Directions: Mix a half-handful of rosemary blossoms or leaves and a handful of black elderberries in a pint of extra-virgin olive oil. Shake well and store for three days in a cool, dark place.

Crush 1 tablespoon of flax seeds in a coffee grinder or with a mortar and pestle. Place the crushed seeds in a bowl, adding the olive oil and herb mixture. Crush 2 tablespoons of valerian root and add to the mixture as well. Place the entire mixture in a jar, shake well, and store for seven days, shaking it once or twice a day. Strain the oil through cheesecloth or gauze, and store in a cool, dark place. Take 1 tablespoon first thing in the morning on an empty stomach. If needed, take a second tablespoon in the evening before dinner. Keep taking the oil until your bowel movements are regular.

BONESET: In colonial days, boneset *(Eupatorium perfoliatum)* was one of the most often used medicinal herbs in North America. Ethnobotanical sources say that it was found hanging in the houses or barns of every "well regulated" household in the

Prunes vs. the FDA

In both New England and Appalachia, prunes or prune juice are recommended for treating constipation. Nineteenth century German immigrants also stood by the remedy. In fact, anyone who has had the misfortune of drinking too much prune juice can attest to the remedy's effectiveness!

The U.S. Food and Drug Administration (FDA) recently ordered American food companies to halt claims that their prune juice products acted as laxatives, however, because that effect had never been proven in clinical trials. This incident illustrates a common dilemma with many effective folk remedies in the United States—they remain outside the fold of official medicine because they have never been formally tested in a university, laboratory, or hospital setting.

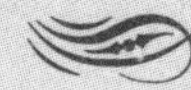

Enemas

The use of enemas is occasionally mentioned as a treatment for constipation in the literature of folk medicine. It was a widespread practice among American Indians and persists today among the Seventh Day Adventists. Overuse of enemas can be injurious to the bowels, however, because the enemas wash away normal protective mucus, deplete the body of electrolyte salts, and possibly introduce foreign or irritating matter into the bowels.

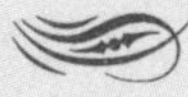

colonies. Hot boneset tea was taken to treat fevers, colds, and flu. Cold boneset tea was taken as a digestive tonic, and, sometimes, as a mild laxative.

The use of boneset as a laxative was recorded among the Mohawk Indians and persists today in the folk medicine of Appalachia. When using boneset, always use the dried leaves, however, because fresh boneset contains mildly toxic substances. And don't exceed the recommended amounts, because larger amounts can cause nausea or induce vomiting, one of its older medical uses.

☞ Directions: Place 1 teaspoon of dried boneset leaves in a cup and fill with boiling water. Cover and let stand until cooled to room temperature. Drink ¼ cup three times a day for up to five days.

SESAME SEEDS: According to the Amish, sesame seeds have a laxative effect. Chinese folk medicine claims the same. The seeds are nutritious and also contain about 55 percent oil, which helps to moisten the intestines in those suffering from dry constipation.

☞ Directions: Eat up to ½ ounce of sesame seeds a day. Grind them fresh in a coffee grinder and sprinkle on food like a condiment.

HOT WATER: A remedy from New England also mentioned by the Amish is to drink a cup of hot water in the morning. Similar practices, slightly modified, appear throughout the world. In the folk medicine of India, the prescription is to drink a quart of room temperature water in the morning. German followers of the water cures of Father Sebastian Kneipp (see sidebar, "The Wisdom of Father Kneipp," page 142) take the water hot in 1-tablespoon doses every half hour all day.

Drinking water in the morning to produce a bowel movement has a solid physiological basis. An internal digestive reflex causes the bowels to contract and move the stool in the direction of the anus in response to stretching of the stomach. The stretch reflex can be triggered most easily in the morning, when the stomach is most contracted. Drinking water can trigger this stretch reflex.

☞ Directions: Drink 1 to 3 cups of hot water first thing in the morning on an empty stomach.

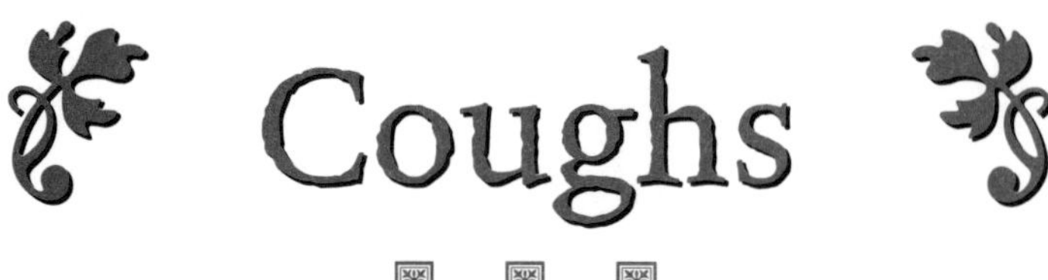

Coughs

Coughing is more than an annoyance—it's a reflex that protects your breathing passages (including your lungs) from secretions that can clog them and hinder your intake of oxygen

Coughing can result from inhaling dust, dirt, or irritating fumes; from breathing icy air; or from mistakenly drawing food into the airways. It can also be caused by mucus and other secretions from such respiratory disorders as the common cold, influenza, pneumonia, or tuberculosis.

The respiratory passages in the throat and lungs are constantly kept moist by a layer of mucus. This mucus traps small particles, viruses, bacteria, dust, pollen, or other materials. The surfaces of these passageways are so sensitive to touch that any irritation there will cause a cough reflex—a reflex that expels the irritating matter at velocities as high as 100 miles an hour. This reflex usually removes any loose mucus or other matter. A cough is thus a healthy healing mechanism, necessary to remove allergens, viruses, bacteria, or foreign matter from the respiratory tract.

Both pharmaceutical drugs and folk remedies aid coughs in several ways. Some folk remedies, like the herbs licorice or marshmallow, are demulcents; they moisten and soothe the throat and bronchial tract, reducing the cough reflex by reducing irritation of the tissues. Others, such as garlic or honey, are expectorants and work by promoting the secretion of fresh mucus, which aids the body in washing out irritants. Finally, cherry bark and the over-the-counter drug dextromethorphan, are respiratory sedatives. They act on the nervous system to reduce the cough reflex. Such a reduction is appropriate for short-term use when an unproductive cough interferes with sleep or is overly-exhausting. Sedatives are not appropriate for productive coughs with a lot of mucus, however, because the cough is necessary to clear the lungs of mucus.

According to the Public Citizen Health Research Group, dextromethorphan is the best cough suppressant to use. It is a component of many over-the-counter cough remedies and syrups. The Public Citizen Health Research Group recommends purchasing generic dextromethorphan at a pharmacy or taking a product containing only dextromethorphan, which will suppress a cough for about twelve hours and allow a good night's sleep.

The actions of cough remedies, even the over-the-counter pharmaceutical types, are difficult to prove. There is no scientific evidence supporting that these herbs effectively treat coughs, probably due to the difficulty in accurately measuring expectoration.

Remedies

WILD CHERRY BARK: The use of wild cherry bark *(Prunus serotina)* to treat coughs was taught to the British colonists by the Cherokee and the Iroquois eastern Indian tribes. Other tribes throughout North America have used various wild cherry species in the same way. Use of the bark became very popular throughout the United States in the 19th century. Wild cherry bark is still used as a cough remedy in the folk medicine of the Amish, New Englanders, and residents of the Southwest. It is also used in contemporary North American and European medical herbalism. "Wild cherry" cough drops are available in stores today, although they are now made with artificial flavors instead of actual wild cherry bark.

The bark's constituent prunasin reduces the cough reflex, so wild cherry is classified as a cough suppressant. Thus, it requires the same cautions as the over-the-counter medication dextromethorphan. Prunasin is a potentially toxic compound. But, if taken as a tea in the correct quantities, adults are safe using it. All cases of toxicity from wild cherry have occurred in children eating the fruit—called "choke cherries"—along with the toxic pits, which contain large amounts of prunasin and related compounds.

Wild cherry has expectorant and demulcent properties, too, so this herb is like a complete cough formula all rolled up in one. Wild cherry bark is especially suited to dry, irritating coughs. Combining it with another demulcent will further improve its effects.

☞ Directions: Place 1 tablespoon of wild cherry bark and an equal part of licorice root in 1 pint of water. Boil for five minutes, remove from heat, sweeten with ½ cup of honey. Let stand until the mixture cools to room temperature. The dose is ¼ cup, no more than five times a day. To remain on the side of caution, don't give cherry bark to children under the age of twelve. Adults shouldn't take cherry bark for more than three consecutive days. Women should avoid cherry bark altogether if they are pregnant or nursing.

FLAX SEEDS: New Englanders and residents of other eastern states use boiled flax seeds *(Linum usitatissimum)* to

continued on page 151

Pass the Honey

Honey has been used in traditional Chinese medicine for more than 2,000 years. It is used for conditions ranging from asthma, cough, and chronic bronchitis to stomachache, constipation, chronic sinus congestion, canker sores, and burns. A folk remedy from China for treating coughs calls for a tablespoon of honey in hot water. Expectorant syrups made from honey are widespread throughout the folk traditions of the world, and appear in the folk medicine of every region in the United States. Honey is a natural expectorant, promoting the flow of mucus.

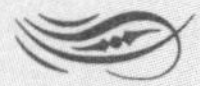

Worms Be Gone!

In folk medicine, from aloe to yucca root, the catalog of plant-based remedies for worms is long. The most widely used medicine in the country for a century and a half was the Cherokee recipe for pulverized root of pinkroot. Plant-based teas used across the country included pumpkin seed, horsemint, peach leaf, and butternut bark.

Garlic was a mainstay, usually eaten but sometimes worn on a string around the neck. (Some mothers put raw cloves on the ground for crawling babies to pop into their mouths—along with the nastier things they might eat.) Recommended foods included burnt toast, sauerkraut, and raw potatoes.

If these remedies didn't work, people could always try patent medicines, whose makers were quick to exploit the grotesque potential of worms. *Dr. Jayne's Medical Almanac* of the 1800s was decorated with a huge staring tapeworm. Medicine-show men would display roundworms in glass jars for their customers' contemplation.

The ancient theory that something repulsive must be driven out by something even worse is evident in worm remedies with appalling ingredients, such as tea of earthworm, sulphur, or kerosene. One of the most common "cures" was also the most dangerous: turpentine.

Perhaps it was a good thing that there were magical cures as well. Some charms addressed the worms themselves. One from 13th century England begins, "I adjure you, worms, in the name. . . . " It may be compared with one recorded in Pennsylvania six hundred years later: "Worm, I conjure thee by the living God that thou avoid this flesh and blood."

The belief that a tapeworm eats the "host's" food inspired the Scottish cure whereby the sufferer chews bread, spits it out, then drinks some whiskey. The worms smell the bread, open their mouths, and are choked by the alcohol.

No longer an everyday worry, worms still wiggle into our folklore.

Legendary Creatures

In many places around the world, people avoid drinking from open water lest they ingest eggs that can hatch and grow in the stomach. According to legend, this happened once to a Newfoundland man, who at first didn't realize the cause of his swollen belly. An old woman told him to fast for a day, then eat something salty and lie down by the brook he had drunk from. He did, and out of his mouth crawled a thirsty little waterwolf in search of a drink.

In the southern United States, such legendary creatures as waterwolfs are called "springkeepers," in Ireland "mankeepers." The luring-out cure is sometimes advised for the lowlier tapeworm, too, who is said to be especially fond of milk.

treat coughs. Boiled flax seeds make a thick demulcent that is soothing to the throat and bronchial tract.

☞ Directions: Boil 2 or 3 tablespoons of flax seeds in 1 cup of water for a few minutes, until the water becomes gooey. Strain. Add equal parts of honey and lemon juice. For a dry irritable cough that's not producing much mucus, take 1-tablespoon doses as needed.

BLACK PEPPER: A remedy for coughs from New England, which also appears in Chinese folk medicine, is black pepper *(Piper nigrum).* The irritating properties of black pepper stimulate circulation and the flow of mucus. Black pepper works best on coughs producing a thick mucus; it is inappropriate for a dry, irritable cough with little expectoration.

☞ Directions: Place 1 teaspoon of black pepper and 1 tablespoon of honey in a cup and fill with boiling water. Let steep for ten to fifteen minutes. Take small sips as needed.

Coughs, Dry and Wet

A cough is a healthy healing mechanism, necessary to remove allergens, viruses, or bacteria from the respiratory tract. Mucus traps these invading and irritating substances. The secretion of the mucus and its expulsion from your body when you cough is part of the body's healing process.

With some coughs—such as "wet" coughs—plenty of mucus is present, but the mucus is thick, gummy, and hard to expel. Acrid, irritating, and stimulating herbs are helpful for treating these types of coughs because they stimulate the flow of new clean mucus, which helps expel the old.

"Dry" coughs typically accompany the flu. Acrid and stimulating herbs only irritate dry coughs further because there is little mucus to expel. To treat a dry cough, try a soothing herb such as slippery elm, mallow, or licorice.

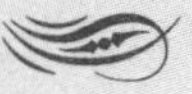

MUSTARD SEED: An old New England cough remedy calls for mustard seed. Mustard is also used for treating coughs in the folk medicine of China. Mustard has irritating sulfur-containing compounds that stimulate the flow of mucus. Like pepper, above, it is only appropriate for congested productive coughs with plenty of mucus present. It will irritate a dry cough and make it worse.

☞ Directions: Crush 1 teaspoon of mustard seeds or grind them in a coffee grinder. Place the seeds in a cup and fill with warm water. Steep for fifteen minutes. (The expectorant compounds are not released until the mustard seeds are crushed or broken and allowed to sit in water or some other medium for about fifteen minutes.) Take in ¼-cup doses throughout the day.

GARLIC: Early medical records from all over the globe show that garlic *(Allium sativum)* was used as a treatment for coughs and bronchial conditions. Garlic-honey syrups are standard cough treatments in the folk medicine of the Southwest today.

Garlic was acknowledged as an expectorant in the National Formulary of the United States from 1916 until 1936. Garlic is not appropriate for treating dry, unproductive coughs, however. It is best for treating coughs that are producing mucus.

☞ Directions: Put 1 pound of sliced garlic in 1 quart of boiling water; let it soak for ten to twelve minutes, keeping the water warm (but not boiling). Strain and add 4 pounds of honey. Strain and bottle the syrup. When you feel congested, take 1 teaspoonful.

ONION SYRUP: In *American Folk Medicine,* folklorist Clarence Meyer suggests taking a honey-and-onion syrup for treating coughs. Onions have anti-inflammatory properties that may reduce throat irritation, and honey is a natural expectorant, promoting the free flow of mucus. Onions also contain the antiviral constituent protocatechuic acid, which attacks viruses, including the one that may be causing the cough.

Formulas for Coughs

The practice of giving cough remedies as formulas rather than as single herbs is universal in contemporary North American and British professional medical herbalism. For an effective cough syrup, use expectorant, demulcent, and respiratory sedative plants with the natural expectorant honey. Single-herb formulas don't work as well. Here are two remedies you can try:

DRY COUGH, FORMULA #1: Here is a formula from the contemporary southern Appalachians for soothing dry, irritable coughs.

☞ Directions: Stir ½ ounce of slippery elm bark powder, ¼ ounce of sage leaves, and 3 tablespoons of honey into 1 pint of boiling water. Let stand for half an hour. Strain and take 1-tablespoon doses as desired.

DRY COUGH, FORMULA #2: Another Appalachian formula for treating dry coughs uses wild cherry bark, which may help suppress a cough that is keeping you up at night.

☞ Directions: Boil ½ cup slippery elm bark powder, ½ cup wild cherry bark, and ½ cup mullein leaves in 1 gallon of water. Simmer for half an hour. Add 4 pounds of sugar or honey to the hot water, strain, and drink as desired. Wild cherry bark is not appropriate for consumption by children under the age of 12 or by pregnant or nursing women.

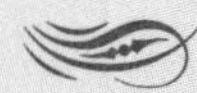

☞ Directions: Chop 5 or 6 white onions and place them in a double boiler. Add ½ cup of honey and the juice of 1 lemon and cook at lowest heat possible for several hours. Strain the mixture and take by the tablespoon as needed—from every half an hour to every few hours.

HOREHOUND: A folk remedy for coughs from contemporary New Mexico is horehound *(Marrubium vulgare),* a European plant that arrived in North America with both the Spanish and northern European colonists. Horehound has been used to treat coughs in European folk medicine since the time of the ancient Greeks. It was an official cough remedy in the *United States Pharmacopoeia* between 1840 and 1910, and it remains an approved medicine for coughs by the German government today.

Horehound stimulates the flow of mucus, and is indicated for use in moist unproductive coughs. It can be irritating and increase the discomfort of dry coughs, however.

☞ Directions: Place 1 tablespoon of dried horehound in a cup and fill with boiling water. Cover and let steep for fifteen minutes. Sweeten with honey. Drink in ½-cup doses as often as desired.

OSHA SYRUP: Osha *(Ligusticum porteri)* was a medicinal plant popular among American Indians and settlers residing in the higher elevations of the Rocky Mountains. Osha has a hot acrid taste, and its constituents possesses both expectorant and antiviral properties. American Indians of the area believed that osha has the power to repel evil spirits.

☞ Directions: Grind 1 ounce of osha root in a coffee grinder. Heat 1 pint of honey in a pot, and add the osha root. Simmer slowly until the honey becomes thick. Leave the root in the honey and let cool to room temperature. Do not strain. Take 1-tablespoon doses of the syrup four to six times a day as desired.

That's Pine

Pine bark or pine pitch (congealed pine sap) was a commonly used American Indian cough treatment. The practice also dates back to the ancient Greeks. Colonists in the eastern states, whether they brought the practice with them from Europe or learned it from the American Indians, used pine pitch and pine bark as well—often adding it to their cough formulas or syrups. One simple syrup from folklorist Clarence Meyer's *American Folk Medicine* calls for a tea of the inner bark of pine, sweetened with honey and made into a syrup. Pine oils are extremely stimulating, however, and the bark or sap should never be used on dry, irritable coughs.

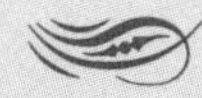

MULLEIN: Did you know you can make a cough syrup with the leaves of the mullein plant? Mullein *(Verbascum thapsus)* came to North America with the European colonists and is now naturalized throughout the United States and Canada. Its use as a

continued on page 157

Herbalism

Humans have used plants as medicine for longer than recorded history. An ancient Egyptian papyrus, from the 16th century B.C., describes more than 800 plant medicines, including castor oil, mandrake, and opium. An ancient Chinese botanical text, thought to be from about 1600 A.D., includes more than 1,000 medicines, many of which are plant medicines. Today, some of these medicines, such as camphor and ephedra, are currently recognized and used by Western medicine. Marijuana was used in ancient China, India, and Greece. Today, conventional medicine is investigating its use as a treatment for relieving nausea in cancer patients.

During the Middle Ages, the Crusaders brought new herbal lore back from the Holy Land. The constant mixing of traditional plant knowledge has enriched cultures all over the world. But where did this plant knowledge come from? It is, of course, impossible to know for certain, but herbalists have always suggested that observations of nature may be a major source. For example, when an animal is sick, it may eat a certain plant to heal itself. From this behavior, an herbalist may learn of a plant's healing capabilities.

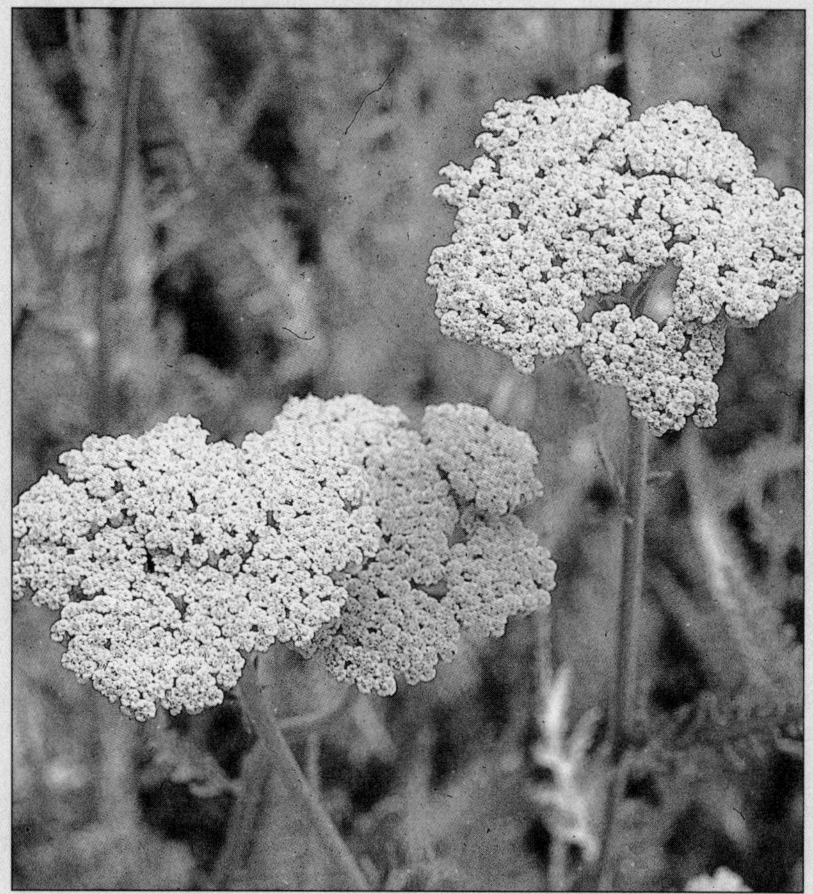

Yarrow has been used to treat wounds and burns.

What's more, efforts to find edible plants, especially during times of scarcity, forced many people to taste plants they would have previously avoided. Through this experimentation, it was also discovered that the difference between a poisonous plant and a medicinal plant is often just a matter of dosage. So, although such experimentation sometimes led to sickness or death, it also introduced new foods and new medicines, including stimulants, sedatives, laxatives, and diuretics, to the community. Of course, in every society, there have always been those daring naturalists who purposely experimented on themselves, including Samuel Hahnemann, who developed homeopathy. Those who survived these experiments added to their culture's store of herbal knowledge.

The testing of plants, however, has not always been a matter of chance or necessity. The search for cures has sometimes been based on theory. For example, in the Doctrine of Signatures, it is taught that a plant bears a visible sign, a "signature," of its medicinal purpose. Thus, herbalists tried red plants for treating blood problems, yellow plants for jaundice, and walnuts for brain disorders! Mandrake (*Mandragora officinarum*), a medicinal plant of the nightshade family, is famous as an aphrodisiac in folk medicine and it was consumed for this purpose. The root is often forked, giving the rough appearance of a human form with legs, and additional forks in the root can look like male genitals. Many times the Doctrine of Signatures must have mislead herbalists (for example, mandrake is a powerful sedative!), but it did provide a basis for experiment.

Just how knowledgeable were herbalists before modern botany? There is evidence they knew quite a great deal. In 1976, for example, two scientists published an important study. Plants used by herbalists around the world in the treatment of cancer were compared to a list of plants known to be effective against tumors. The list of plants recognized as effective came from the studies of the National Cancer Institute (NCI), where plants from all over the world are screened for anti-cancer effectiveness. The scientists discovered that the effective plants were identified by folk tradition about twice as often as were identified in the NCI screening program. Apparently, traditional herbalists had accumulated a lot of accurate knowledge of anti-cancer plants.

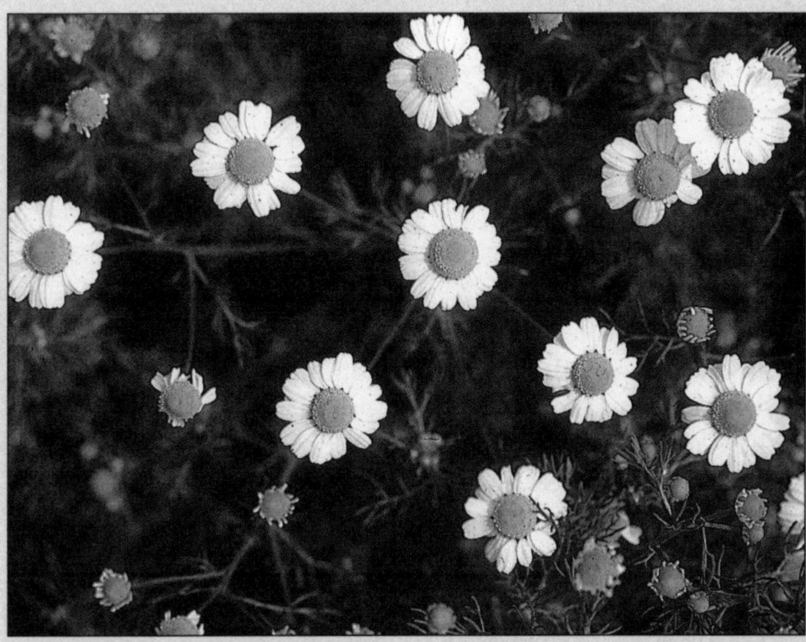

Chamomile can be used to improve digestion.

In the past, when scientists looked at folk medicine, they tended to separate "magico-religious" practices from "natural folk medicine," which includes herbalism, massage, and other physical remedies. But in folk tradition this distinction does not hold up. Folk herbalists consistently describe their beliefs and practices in a spiritual way. One very common belief among herbalists is that God has provided a natural treatment for each illness found in a specific region. For example, quinine, a treatment for malaria, is derived from the bark of cinchoma trees. The trees grow in South America in areas where malaria is found.

Also related in folk religion is the connection between the medicinal use of herbs with astrology and beliefs about phases of the moon. For instance, in the South, it is often said that herbs taken internally should generally be consumed during the "dark of the moon" (that is, when the moon is waning, and the visible part growing smaller). It is believed that, during this phase of the moon, it is the best time for making things get smaller or stop, just as the moon appears to be getting smaller during this period. For example, a salve made from boiled buckeyes mixed with lard, which is a Midwestern folk treatment for external cancers, would be applied to the cancer during the waning moon in order to increase the salve's effectiveness in making the cancer wane.

Related to spiritual ideas in herbalism is "vitalism," which is the idea that organic things are unique from nonliving material because they have a "life force." The idea of vitalism was widely accepted during most of human history. But this view changed in 1828 when a German pharmacist created urea—a component of the urine of mammals—in a laboratory experiment. Even though no kidney was used, this urea was indistinguishable from that found in the urine of mammals. The idea that artificially created substances—called "synthetic compounds"—were identical to those found in nature would have a tremendous effect in medicine. Earlier in the century, a German chemist had isolated morphine, the active ingredient of opium. These two developments, the ability to isolate active principles and then copy them, led to the creation of simple, synthetic drugs that could be readily standardized—and did not depend on locating particular plants in the wild.

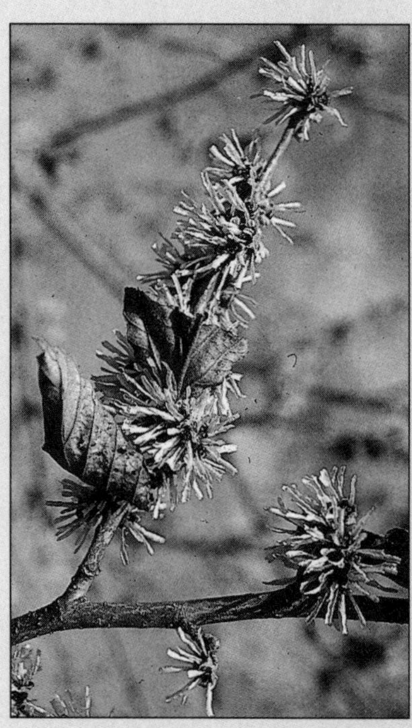

Witch hazel acts as an astringent.

After these discoveries, herbalism and medical science began to separate, and herbalism became more and more the property of folk tradition. Only in the latter part of the 20th century have the ecology movement and related developments in modern society begun to raise questions about the adequacy of synthetic materials and the possible value of a return to natural plant medicines. This return includes more gentle action on healing the body, fewer side effects, and less negative impact on the environment. As a result, folk herbalism, much like the rest of folk medicine, is increasingly joining the rest of alternative medicine to change modern ideas about health and medicine.

cough medicine was quickly adopted by several American Indian tribes, including the Mohegan, Delaware, Cherokee, Creek, and Navaho. It appears today in the folk medicine of Appalachia and the Southwest. Mullein was an official cough medicine in the *United States Pharmacopoeia* from 1888 until 1936 and remains an approved medicine for cough in Germany. Recent research shows that mullein tea also may have an antiviral effect against the influenza virus.

☞ Directions: Place ½ pound of mullein leaves in a 1-quart jar. Fill with boiling water and let cool to room temperature. Strain and add honey until the mixture has the consistency of a syrup. The dose is 1 tablespoon as needed.

Great Expectoration

For a dry cough or one accompanied by thick (rather than watery) mucous secretions, be sure to drink enough liquids. Water is a natural expectorant, so drink plenty of it—whether in the form of water, soups, or teas. A Seventh Day Adventist treatment calls for taking a sip of water every time you cough.

You can also moisten the respiratory tract with steam from a vaporizer or a hot shower or simply by inhaling steam from hot water running in the sink.

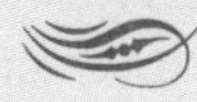

SLIPPERY ELM: Slippery elm bark *(Ulmus fulva)* has a slimy mucilaginous texture that is soothing to inflamed tissues in the mouth and throat. It is ideally suited to treat a cough that accompanies a sore throat. Slippery elm cough lozenges have been sold in the United States since the late 1800s. It was an official cough remedy in the *United States Pharmacopoeia* from 1820 until 1930. It is used to treat coughs in Appalachia today.

☞ Directions: Stir 1 ounce of slippery elm bark powder and 3 tablespoons of honey into 1 pint of boiling water. Let stand for half an hour. Strain and take 1-tablespoon doses as desired.

MALLOW: For a dry or inflamed cough high in the respiratory tract that's accompanied by a sore throat, a tea made from marshmallow *(Althea officinalis)* or hollyhock *(Althea rosea)* and honey may bring relief. Both plants have been used in traditional European herbalism at least since the time of the ancient Greeks. The plants came to North America as garden plants and are still used today to treat coughs in professional medical herbalism.

Dried marshmallow root contains up to one-third mucilage. Marshmallow is also expectorant, so the double action of the plant mucilage and its ability to increase natural mucus will help soothe the inflamed membranes of the throat.

Hollyhock flowers may be used instead of marshmallow root. Says the 19th century German herbal *My Water Cure* (English translation), a popular book among German immigrants in the United States, "Among the flowers in the garden, hollyhock must not be missing. When the good creator painted its blossoms, so pleasing to the eye, he poured a drop of medicinal sap into the paint for every petal."

☞ Directions: Cover 1 ounce of chopped marshmallow root with 1 pint of boiling water and let steep until cool. Add 2 tablespoons of honey to a cup of the tea and sip as often as desired throughout the day. Also, try placing a handful of hollyhock flowers and a handful of dried mullein leaves in a 1-pint canning jar. Fill with boiling water, cover, and let stand overnight. Strain, and sweeten with honey. Take ¼-cup doses as desired.

LICORICE: Licorice root *(Glycyrrhiza glabra)* has been used to treat coughs and bronchial problems in many traditions throughout the world. It is listed in several 19th century folk remedy collections from the eastern United States. It was an official medicine in the *United States Pharmacopoeia* from 1820 until 1975; it was recommended as a flavoring agent and a demulcent and expectorant for cough syrups. (Most licorice candy in the United States is really flavored with anise oil.)

☞ Directions: Cut 1 ounce of licorice sticks into slices, and add to 1 quart of boiling water. Steep for twenty-four hours. Drink throughout the day, adding honey to taste.

GINGER: Several North American Indian tribes, including the Allegheny and Montagnais, used wild North American ginger *(Asarum canadensis)* for treating coughs. Cultivated ginger *(Zingiber officinale)* is mentioned for the same purpose in a collection of American remedies called *American Folk Medicine* by folklorist Clarence Meyer. Ginger is commonly used today in Chinese folk medicine. Ginger contains both anti-inflammatory and antispasmodic chemical constituents.

☞ Directions: Thinly slice a fresh ginger root (about the size of your thumb). Place in 1 quart of water. Bring to a boil and then simmer in a covered pot on the lowest possible heat for thirty minutes. Let cool for thirty minutes more. Strain and drink ½ to 1 cup, sweetened with honey, as often as desired. Ginger can be irritating to hot, dry, unproductive coughs and should thus be avoided when such a cough is present.

COMBINATION TREATMENT: Folklorist Clarence Meyer's *American Folk Medicine* suggests the following combination of herbs and spices when making a cough remedy. (The formula was first published in 1931; it has been slightly adapted to include modern ingredients and measurements.) This remedy is appropriate for treating either dry or wet coughs.

☞ Directions: Take ¼ pound of horehound, 3 tablespoons of flax seeds, and 3 tablespoons of powdered ginger. Bring to a boil and simmer on low heat for one hour in a covered pot. Add 1 pound of honey. Simmer, stirring often, until the mixture is reduced to a quart and a half of syrup. Strain and store. The dose is 1 or 2 teaspoons four to six times a day.

MULLEIN AND HOREHOUND: This formula from *American*

Folk Medicine is appropriate for treating either dry or wet coughs.

☞ Directions: Place 1 ounce of mullein leaves and ½ ounce of horehound leaves in 1 quart of water. Bring to a boil, and simmer for forty minutes. Strain and add 1 pint of molasses. The dose is 1 or 2 tablespoons three times a day.

ELECAMPANE: Elecampane *(Inula helenium),* has been used to treat coughs and bronchitis since the time of the ancient Greeks. (Its Latin name, *helenium,* comes from Helen of Troy, who supposedly was holding the plant as she left her home for Troy.) A native plant of southeastern Europe, elecampane came to North America with the European colonists. Its use for coughs was quickly adopted by the American Indians, and it is still included today as a cough medicine in the folklore of the Iroquois. It is also used in contemporary Chinese medicine for the same purposes. Elecampane is a mild expectorant, so it may be irritating to a dry cough.

☞ Directions: Place 1 tablespoon of dried elecampane root in 2 cups of water and simmer for twenty minutes in a well-covered pot. Drink 2 to 3 cups a day.

BUTTERY SYRUPS: Adding butter to a hot cough syrup is common throughout North American folklore, especially in the eastern and northeastern states. Butter may be soothing to the tissues because of its texture, but some of its constituents may also be beneficial. Butter contains vitamin A, which helps to regenerate mucous membranes. It also contains short- and medium-chain fatty acids, which possess antimicrobial properties. It may thus help kill germs in the mouth and throat that may be responsible for causing the cough in the first place. The recipe below is from *American Folk Medicine.* (It has been adapted to substitute honey for sugar.)

☞ Directions: Mix equal parts of butter, vinegar, honey, and hot water. Add a pinch of cinnamon. Simmer for thirty to forty minutes to make a thick syrup.

HYDROTHERAPY: Hydrotherapy has its roots in the German tradition of naturopathy; it was brought to North America by immigrants near the turn of the 20th century. Here's a hydrotherapy treatment from New England for treating coughs.

☞ Directions: Soak a cotton cloth in cold water. Wring it out and wrap it around the front of the neck below the ears, carefully avoiding contact with the back of the neck. Wrap a warm wool scarf around the wet cloth and lie down. The cold cloth will attract circulation to the area, soothing the cough and promoting healing.

 Depression 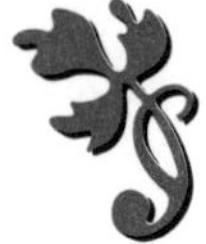

If you suffer from sadness that is intense and severe, it may not simply be the blues. You could be suffering from depression

Depression is a psychological condition characterized by prolonged sadness, combined with other symptoms, including persistent low, anxious, or "empty" feelings, decreased energy, loss of interest or pleasure in usual activities, sleep disturbances, and feelings of hopelessness. Depression may be due to an imbalance or lack of certain necessary brain chemicals.

Some types of depression run in families, indicating that a biological vulnerability to the condition can be inherited. Psychological makeup also plays a role in vulnerability to depression. People who have low self-esteem, who consistently view themselves and the world with pessimism, or who are readily overwhelmed by stress are prone to depression. A serious loss, chronic illness, difficult relationship, financial problem, or unwelcome change in life patterns can also trigger a depressive episode.

Depression can occur because of normal chemical changes in the body. Two examples are premenstrual depression and postpartum depression, both thought to be linked to female hormonal activities. In addition, certain drugs, including oral contraceptives, alcohol, and some sedatives, may cause a side effect of depression in some people. Certain infections (including influenza) can depress a person's mood, as can over- or underproduction of hormones by the outer layer of the adrenal gland, or a deficiency of vitamin B_{12}. Scientific evidence has also linked some forms of depression to deficiencies of the vitamins biotin, folic acid, pantothenic acid, pyridoxine, riboflavin, thiamine, vitamin C, and vitamin E. Deficiencies in the minerals calcium, copper, iron, magnesium, potassium, and zinc can also cause depression. (In fact, deficiencies of magnesium and zinc alone can cause symptoms that can lead to a diagnosis of depression. According to the U.S. Department of Agriculture, the average American does not consume the minimum daily requirement of either mineral.) So, before taking antidepressant drugs, patients with mild depression would be wise to undergo a thorough screening of their nutritional status.

Traditional societies are less likely than we are to report depression in their literature because they are more likely to consume a whole-food, nutrient-dense diet and to get sufficient exercise. Weston Price, a nutritional anthropologist who studied traditional societies around the world in the 1930s, found that primitive people consuming a traditional diet take in from three to ten times the vitamin and mineral content found in modern diets.

Very few folk remedies appear for depression in folk literature; the word itself is a 20th century medical term. Older texts are more likely to refer to depression as melancholy (depressive mood), neurasthenia (nervous exhaustion), malaise (profound fatigue), possession, or witchcraft.

Depression can be very serious. Depression with thoughts of suicide requires immediate medical attention. Conventional treatment for depression includes taking an antidepressant and, sometimes, participating in psychotherapy.

Remedies

ST. JOHN'S WORT: St. John's wort is a common meadowland plant that has been used as a medicine for centuries. (It is mentioned in early European and Slavic herbals.) The genus name *Hypericum* is from the Latin *hyper,* meaning above, and *icon*, meaning "spirit." The herb was hung over doorways to ward off evil spirits or burned to protect and sanctify an area. German immigrants to the United States at the turn of the century used it as a digestive herb for "melancholy."

St. John's wort is reported to relieve anxiety and tension and to act as an antidepressant. The herb is an approved medicine in Germany. With long-term use, hypericin, one of the constituents, may make the skin of a few individuals more sensitive to sunlight, however.

☞ Directions: Purchase St. John's wort from a health food store, herb shop, or pharmacy. Take as directed. Alternately, you can purchase a St. John's wort tincture at a health food store or herb shop.

continued on page 164

The Sluggish Liver

Sluggish liver function has little meaning in North American conventional medicine. But "bile deficiency," the physiological equivalent of sluggish liver function, is commonly treated in both French and German contemporary medicine. Contemporary French physicians attribute conditions such as fatigue, physical sluggishness, and headache to this low-grade liver dysfunction.

In traditional Western medicine, melancholy, an older term for depression, was associated with sluggish liver function. The connection between liver function and depression is also seen in contemporary Chinese medicine. In fact, Chinese herbs, foods, and formulas designed to stimulate the liver are frequently prescribed for treating depression. Several of the remedies in this section are traditional treatments for sluggish liver, including St. John's wort, wormwood, boneset, dandelion, and increased exercise.

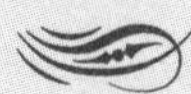

Prayer vs. Magic

According to research, the great majority of Americans pray for health and healing for themselves and loved ones. Prayer is, of course, an ancient way of enlisting supernatural powers to fight disease. The word "prayer" is usually used to refer to religious practices and it comes from the Latin word *precari,* to entreat or plead.

Some scholars find it useful to classify worship of supernatural persons as religious prayer, and to reserve the term "magic" for techniques that are supposed to force spirits to do one's bidding. But the following Pennsylvania "charm" for stopping blood, when the patient is not present, seems magical. To perform the charm, you must first pronounce the bleeding person's name correctly, then state from which side the person is bleeding, and then say:

On Christ's grave grows three roses;
The first is kind,
The second is valued among rulers,
The third stops blood.

According to tradition, the blood will then stop. This charm is very formal and must be stated in exactly the right way. If it is, the result is certain.

There does not seem to be any communication between the healer or the patient and God—or anyone else, for that matter! It is as though the words are commanding a mysterious force and not pleading for a favor from God. But the attitude and belief of the practitioner has to be considered. Many folk healers consider their work a religious vocation, and their charms are recited with the same heart-felt supplication to God as the most sincere prayer said in church. Thus, the magic-prayer distinction is not as clear as it may at first seem!

The tendency to insult the religion of others as "mere magical thinking" reflects the modern history of religion in western Europe and North America. In the Middle Ages, Christians believed strongly in miraculous answers to prayer. They also believed in the power of the saints and the souls in Purgatory to intercede with God. In short, they believed in a very complex kind of activity back and forth between the material world and the supernatural world. This belief included a great many ideas about health and healing, ranging from miracles obtained by prayers to the saints to the use of holy water and blessed oils as medicines. The Protestant Reformation, beginning in the 1500s, started out as an effort to reform certain practices of church officials that were felt to be excessive and to go against basic Christian belief. But by the time Protestantism had given rise to the major new denominations of Christianity, many Protestants had rejected far more tradition than the original reformers had targeted. Some (Calvinists, for example) dismissed the entire idea that miraculous events could burst into the everyday world on a regular basis. The idea of frequent answers to prayer and miracles reported from holy places were rejected as mere tricks of clergy used to impress the faithful.

This put folk tradition in a peculiar position. Folk

tradition, like Medieval Christianity, has always relied heavily on extraordinary and mysterious experiences and on the idea of a close social relationship between humans and spirits—God, angels, demons, and saints. So, while folk tradition and Christian religion had freely mixed in Medieval times, in Protestant lands, starting in the 16th century, most of folk belief was condemned as ignorant and "Popish," a term of insult for Catholic ideas and practice. Folk practices could lead to charges of heresy, and this led to the suppression of folk medicine, loaded as it was with ritual and stories of miraculous cures. It was preached against in churches and it was condemned in the schools as backward and foolish. As a result, folk medicine in much of the United States went underground.

During the past century, ideas about the supernatural underwent still more changes. In the 19th century, the supernatural ideas of folk tradition became associated with several newly developing religious groups such as Mormonism. In the early 20th century, the nondenominational "healing revival" sprang up in Protestantism, especially in the South. Preachers like Oral Roberts traveled around the country holding large meetings in tents. (After attending his meetings, many people said they were healed.) At the same time, among Catholic Americans, folk practices popular in the Middle Ages, such as promising to make a pilgrimage to a saint's shrine in return for healing, continued with little notoriety. The desire for healing and miraculous answers to prayer continued. Then, in the 1960s, the Charismatic Movement emerged. It was based on the belief that prayers continue to be answered miraculously even at the present time, and miraculous healing returned to a place of prominence in modern society.

Today, all sorts of ideas about prayer for healing have become popular again, and healing rituals from the religions of the world have a positive reputation. People from all educational backgrounds study shamanism and read about American Indian religions. Most Christian churches now offer healing services. Similar developments have occurred in Judaism and Islam and in other religions of the world. Not all of these modern spiritual healing practices are related to "folk medicine" by any stretch of the imagination. But folk medical prayer now has far more in common with institutional religion than it did a hundred years ago, and the need for embarrassed secrecy is greatly reduced. Today, the Pennsylvania German powwow or Mexican-American curandera is more likely to be consulted by college-educated patients than to be condemned by ministers and teachers in the community.

Even in medicine there is a new openness to the idea that prayer can make a difference. In 1988, Randolph Byrd, M.D., a cardiologist, published a double-blind, controlled, scientific trial of prayer aimed at a large group of heart attack patients. His study found a strong, statistically significant effect of prayer. Those hospitalized patients who were prayed for by strangers who volunteered for the trial recovered with fewer complications—even though they didn't know that they were being prayed for! As a result of these types of studies, the folk medical use of prayer—once viewed as a remnant of premodern, magical ideas—has returned to an honored position in our society.

A good quality tincture will be dark red in color.

For a more traditional formula, try this Gypsy "soul-refreshing tonic": Gather properly identified wild St. John's wort leaves and flowers, enough to fill a loosely packed pint or quart jar. To follow ancient traditions, harvest them on St. John's day, the day after the summer solstice. (You can do this in most parts of the country, but at higher elevations the flowers will not yet be in bloom, so you'll have to wait a little longer to try this remedy.) Cover the leaves and flowers with 90 proof liquor. Let stand for one cycle of the moon, shaking the bottle daily. Strain and rebottle. Take 10 to 20 drops daily.

How Depressing

Many people with borderline depression turn to alcohol or recreational drugs to lift their mood. But alcohol is a "pick-me-up" that might just "bring you down."

Alcohol, the most popular drug of choice in modern society, is a depressant. Alcohol dulls the brain and the nervous system, slowing reactions and making drinkers feel relaxed and tranquilized. It can also lower inhibitions and make a person aggressive or hostile. In higher doses, it may block memory and impair concentration, judgement, coordination, and emotional reactions.

The liver is one of the primary targets of chronic alcohol abuse. In alcoholic hepatitis, liver cells are damaged or destroyed as a result of recent heavy drinking. Prolonged excessive drinking can lead to alcoholic cirrhosis, a condition in which large areas of the liver are destroyed or scarred. Liver damage is extremely serious and may be life threatening.

Chronic depression and anxiety are common in habitual drinkers. In fact, one or two glasses of alcohol a day may cause or contribute to depression in some individuals.

CALIFORNIA POPPY: California poppy *(Eschscholtzia californica)* was used as a treatment of the nervous system by the Costanoan Indians. California poppy eventually made its way into European medicine, and today pharmaceutical preparations of the herb are prescribed by physicians in Germany for nervous disorders, including mild depression. The Germans consider the herb to be so gentle that it is sometimes prescribed for treating mild emotional disorders in children. (Although it bears the name "poppy," the herb is not a narcotic and contains no morphine or codeine-type alkaloids.)

California poppy is not readily available in the herb trade, but it grows freely in the western United States and is a common garden plant in other areas. Do not use during pregnancy or while nursing.

☞ Directions: Pick some California poppies, using the stems, leaves, and flowers of the plant. Let them dry in a warm place, out of direct sunlight. Place 1 teaspoon of the dried herb in a cup and fill the cup with boiling water. Cover and let steep for twenty minutes. Strain and drink 1 to 3 cups a day, as desired.

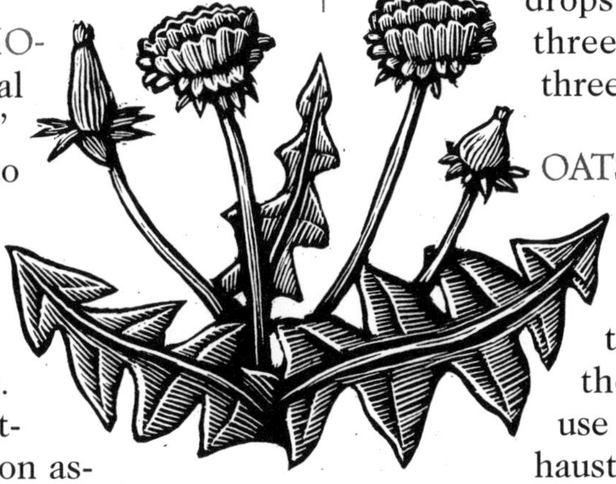

DANDELION AND MOLASSES: A traditional treatment for "bilious" depression, according to folklorist Clarence Meyer in his book *American Folk Medicine,* combines dandelion root with molasses. This "double-duty" treatment may help depression associated with a sluggish liver while, at the same time, restore mineral deficiencies that contribute to fatigue and low energy. Blackstrap molasses contains high amounts of essential minerals—a tablespoon contains more than 15 percent of the daily requirement of calcium, magnesium, iron, potassium, copper, and manganese.

☞ Directions: Simmer 4 ounces of dandelion root in 2 quarts of water until half of the water is gone. Strain and add a cup of molasses. Take 1 tablespoon three to four times a day, twenty minutes before meals. Try the treatment for three weeks, then take a break for a week or two.

WORMWOOD: Wormwood *(Artemisia absinthum)* has been widely used to treat "melancholy" in European medicine. Also, at least seven North American Indian tribes used it as "witchcraft medicine"—the symptoms of possession and depression may have been similarly interpreted.

In addition to its mild antidepressant effects, wormwood increases the secretion of bile in the liver and has anti-inflammatory properties. Wormwood may be toxic, however, if taken for long periods of time.

☞ Directions: Purchase a wormwood tincture at a health food store or herb shop. Using a dropper, take 15 drops of the tincture two or three times a day for two to three weeks.

OATS: Oats *(Avena sativa)* are a folk remedy for neurasthenia, or "nervous exhaustion," which is an old term for the condition. At the turn of the century, the use of oats to treat nervous exhaustion was widespread among the Eclectic physicians, a school of physicians who used herbal remedies.

Oats are highly nutritious. In fact, one cup of oats contains 26 grams of protein, 4 grams of essential fatty acids, 7.4 milligrams of iron, 276 milligrams of magnesium, 0.5 milligrams of copper, 6 milligrams of zinc, 7.1 milligrams of manganese, and 97 micrograms of folic acid—values that are more than half the recommended dietary allowance for each of these nutrients. Clinical research has demonstrated that oats may also aid in withdrawal from addictions.

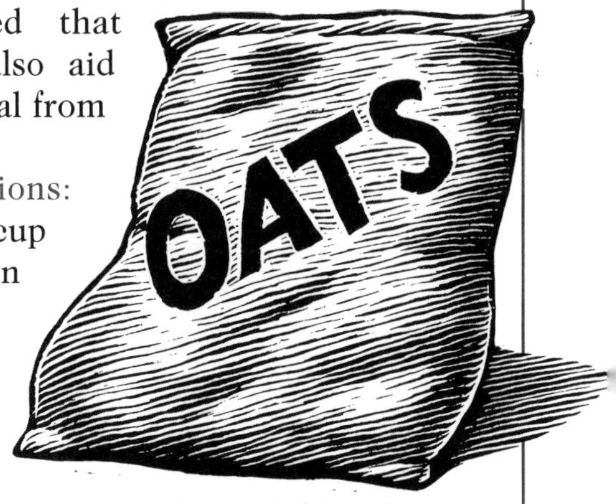

☞ Directions: Place 1 cup of oats in 3 cups of water and simmer for forty minutes in a covered pot. Add molasses

continued on page 168

Aphrodisiacs and Love Potions

Few aspects of folk medicine attract more interest than traditional aphrodisiacs. Most people are familiar with the belief that oysters increase sexual desire, and many more have heard of Spanish fly—without knowing exactly what it is. All species, including humans, are driven to reproduce, and the influence of this instinctual drive constantly permeates our thoughts and actions. The word "aphrodisiac" comes from the Greek name for the goddess of love and beauty, Aphrodite. In folk traditions, aphrodisiacs come in many different forms. There are remedies for sexual dysfunctions such as impotence and foods like oysters that serve both as a symbolic communication of amour and a hoped-for physical boost. There are also a variety of recipes that are intended either to arouse sexual desire in another (sometimes without their knowing) or to destroy someone's sexuality.

Over the centuries many foods and drugs have had a reputation for exciting sexual desire or increasing sexual capacity. Oysters are probably the best known aphrodisiac food, and their reputation seems to come from their resemblance to testicles. This illustrates the "doctrine of signatures," a very old idea that was accepted by physicians in the days when astrology and magical ideas were a part of science. According to this doctrine, medicinal substances in nature were thought to be marked by a visual indication of their proper use. This mark was their medicinal "signature." Medicines for the blood were often red, and beans were believed to be beneficial for the kidneys because of their kidney-like shape. Besides oysters, the tubers of some orchids have also been considered aphrodisiacs because their shape resembles testicles—in fact, the source of the word "orchid" is the Greek word for testicle, orkhis. One final example of the doctrine of signatures is the folk use of pickled cucumbers as a love charm—the phallic shape of cucumbers has always been a part of their lore.

After oysters, onions and garlic are probably the best known "love foods" in folk tradition, but there are others. Cayenne pepper, in various combinations, is believed to be a powerful stimulant and effective for rousing passion because it is "hot." Summer savory *(Satureja hortensis)* has been prized for centuries both as a seasoning and as a means to increase sexual desire. Winter savory *(Satureja montana),* on the other hand, was considered to be an anaphrodisiac—a substance that decreases sexual desire—and was less popular!

The very well-known aphrodisiac Spanish fly deserves mention as well. Spanish fly is a toxic substance prepared from the dried and crushed bodies of dried beetles. This preparation causes irritation of the genito-urinary tract and increases blood flow to the area. It has never been shown scientifically to produce sexual excitement, however, and it is poisonous. There have been several cases of death due to its ingestion.

Mandrake *(Mandragora officinarum)* is a medicinal plant of the nightshade family that has a dramatic sexual reputation in folk medicine. The mandrake root is often forked, giving the rough appearance of a human form with legs. Additional forks in the root sometimes look like male genitals, and these particular roots are especially prized. Mandrake growing beneath a gallows was believed to be particularly powerful. Some even believed that the mandrake grew there from the semen of hanged criminals, increasing the sexual connection. The effects of mandrake that have been identified are sedative and anesthetic, however, so it seems very unlikely that it actually is a sexual stimulant!

American ginseng *(Panax quinquefolium)* is another herb with a powerful reputation as an aphrodisiac. Ginseng root comes originally from Asian medicine traditions. It is very difficult to cultivate, so naturally occurring ginseng is very valuable. By the 19th century, the root, often called "sang" by its Appalachian gatherers, was being exported from America to Asia in large quantities. Then, as the influence of Chinese medicine increased in the United States, ginseng became a very popular herb in American folk medicine. Like mandrake, the ginseng root sometimes has a human-like appearance. Recent investigations of ginseng credit it as an adaptogen, a substance that aids the body in adapting to stress. If there is any truth to the folk medical idea that ginseng is a sexual tonic, especially for older men, it may lie in this sort of tonic property.

Many folk aphrodisiacs seem magical, especially those love potions intended to arouse overwhelming attraction and desire in a particular person. For example, from North Carolina comes the statement that a woman can compel a man to love her by making a powder from dried leaves shaped like hearts and sprinkling it on her intended's clothing. A more dramatic recipe from North Carolina calls for moss from the skull of a murder victim that must be taken during a full moon in a cemetery. The moss is then worn around the neck as a sort of amorous amulet. Tradition also says that if you think constantly of the one you love, she will love you back!

Love Blood

Most magical love potions involve the use of blood. For example, from the southern United States comes the idea that if a man can secretly place some frog's blood on the woman he loves, she will be forced to fall in love with him. The most common use of blood in love potions, however, requires that a woman place a small amount of her menstrual blood in a man's food. If he consumes it, he will be powerfully attracted to her—regardless of other competitors. This use of menstrual blood is believed to bind a woman's lover or husband to her in an overpowering way—so much so that some women say their husbands will not eat their cooking during the period of menstruation! This belief continues in many communities in the United States. And though it may sound bizarre and grotesque to our modern ears, folk traditions all over the world also consider menstrual blood to be extremely powerful for many purposes.

Adaptogens: Asian Remedies for Depression

Adaptogens are plants that help the body respond to sources of stress, including such things as overwork, lack of sleep, and overexposure to the elements. Three of the key symptoms of depression are fatigue, appetite loss, and lowering of sexual libido, and adaptogens are used in the traditional medicine of Asia (and in Chinatowns throughout North America) to treat all three of these symptoms. The two most famous of the Asian adaptogens are Asian ginseng *(Panax ginseng)* and Siberian ginseng *(Eleutherococcus senticosus)*. A wide array of products containing the plants are available in health foods stores, herb shops, pharmacies, supermarkets, and Asian groceries.

Asian ginseng can be overstimulating, however. The symptoms of overstimulation include a stiff neck and headache. If these symptoms occur while taking Asian ginseng, stop taking it, and try a different remedy.

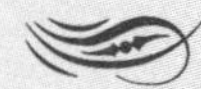

or honey to taste. Pour off the liquid and save—you can drink it during the day. Eat the remaining gruel.

WATER TREATMENT: A hydrotherapy treatment for depression that was popular among German immigrants at the turn of the century, and remains in use by the Seventh Day Adventists today, is the neutral bath. In a neutral bath, the patient relaxes in water that is kept within a degree or two above body temperature for twenty to forty minutes. Water immersion has been shown in clinical trials to lower the circulating levels of stress hormones in the body. The treatment itself may be as old as the ancient Romans, who used hot, cold, or neutral water to treat medical conditions.

☞ Directions: Run a tub of bathwater at 96–98°F. Soak in the bath for twenty to forty minutes. Repeat most days as part of your daily routine for three to six weeks.

WORK ON YOURSELF: If you are depressed, the Amish suggest you should "work on yourself." The same advice is recorded in the folk literature of the southern Appalachians.

A modern version of this view is psychotherapy. Fortunately, in the last two decades, some of the stigma of "seeing a therapist" has fallen away, and most people today view participating in therapy as a sign of healthy growth rather than an indication of mental illness. If you decide to participate in therapy, it's important that you find a counselor who's right for you. In a counseling situation, you should feel safe—physically and emotionally. Keep in mind you are investing your money, time, and effort, and no therapist, no matter how skilled, works well with all clients. The goal is to find the right fit between your personality and problems and the therapist's personality and expertise.

Many personal emotional problems can be greatly improved or even permanently overcome within six visits to a psychotherapist. The therapist often then becomes an ally that the individual can visit occasionally during crises or periods of change in life circumstances.

☞ Directions: Ask a friend for a referral, or consult a directory of local therapists. Talk to a few therapists on the phone or in person before making a selection. Explain what you need help with and ask candidates if they've had any experience in this area. Try to determine which therapist you feel a "chemistry" with. Also, ask about the therapist's training and qualifications.

Beating Depression

According to *Herbal Medicine Past and Present* (Volume I), by John K. Crellin and Jane Philpott, there is plenty of non-herbal advice for the depressed patient. Suggested methods for overcoming depression include paying attention to diet, spending time in the fresh air, exercising, taking a break in routine, getting away from it all, engaging in amusements, being in nature, and working on discovering why you're depressed.

BLACK COHOSH: The American Indians used black cohosh *(Cimicifuga racemosa)* to treat menstrual complaints. Later, the Eclectic physicians adopted the plant, and it soon became one of the most commonly prescribed herbs for treating depression, especially depression associated with the menstrual cycle. Today, black cohosh is an approved antidepressant in Germany.

☞ Directions: Purchase a tincture of black cohosh in a health food store or herb shop. Take 1 dropperful three times a day for up to three months, taking breaks during the menstrual period. Also, you can purchase a standardized extract of black cohosh at a health food store and take it as directed.

BONESET: Boneset *(Eupatorium perfoliatum)*, taken as a cold tea, was a famous remedy for sluggish liver (see sidebar, "The Sluggish Liver," page 161) and melancholy in the colonies before American independence. Previously, boneset was used as a witchcraft medicine by the Iroquois Indians. Cold boneset tea is bitter, which stimulates digestive secretions and bile production by the liver.

☞ Directions: Put 1 teaspoon of dried boneset leaves in a cup. Fill the cup with boiling water, and let stand until the water reaches room temperature. Drink one third of the cup before meals, three times a day, for a week or two.

 Diarrhea 

Whether it's the flu or something you ate, if you're like the average American, you'll suffer once or twice this year from diarrhea

Diarrhea is abnormally frequent and excessively liquid bowel movements. This is often the body's defensive attempt to rid itself of irritating or toxic substances. It is a symptom that accompanies many disorders, both mild and serious.

There are two basic types of diarrhea: acute (or short-term) diarrhea, the more common form, which comes on quickly and usually lasts no more than two or three days, although it can last as long as two weeks; and chronic (or long-term) diarrhea, which may also appear suddenly but lingers for many weeks or months, with symptoms either constantly present or appearing and disappearing.

Both acute and chronic diarrhea can become a serious problem because of the excessive loss of body fluids (called *dehydration)* and the loss of the nutrients sodium, potassium, and chloride. Simply drinking more water is not sufficient to replace these losses. Minerals as well as glucose must be replaced in severe diarrhea. Electrolyte replacement drinks for infants are readily available in grocery stores. Use of such replacement liquids has revolutionized diarrhea care for infants throughout the Third World in the last ten years, where diarrhea is a leading cause of infant death. The accompanying sidebar shows the composition of electrolyte replacement formulas (see sidebar, "Electrolyte Replacement Therapy," page 172).

In an infection, the intestines may pour out massive quantities of fluids and salts in response to a bacterial toxin (poison) or other irritant. Viruses may cause minor epidemics of diarrhea, usually referred to as "intestinal flu." (The influenza virus is actually not involved.) In inflammatory bowel disease (also known as *colitis),* protein, blood, and mucus are lost through the inflamed lining of the colon; large quantities of water are also lost. Other disorders speed up the normal movement of the colon, thereby not allowing time for absorption of fluids. Yet another type of diarrhea is caused by poor absorption of a type of sugar (called *lactose)* that draws fluid out of the colon. Other causes of diarrhea include changes in the diet, certain medications, stress, and food allergies. Diarrhea is a symptom and not a disease, and conventional treatment for diarrhea varies widely depending on the cause. Most important is the replacement of fluids and electrolytes if diarrhea is severe. Constipating drugs or bulk fiber may also be given. Common medical wisdom, both conventional and alternative, is to let normal mild diarrhea run its course because it is a natural defense mechanism that washes infectious bacteria, viruses, or toxins out of the body. Diarrhea may be suppressed with constipating astringents, whether herbal or over-the-counter, but that may make you sicker. According to *My Water Cure,* by Father Sebastian Kneipp, a 19th century German peasant priest and folk healer: "Sudden stopping of diarrhea is never to be recommended: the foul matters should be gradually removed. . . ."

The folk remedies below focus on removing or correcting the cause of the condition.

Kitchen Spices for Diarrhea

Many folk remedies for diarrhea use simple kitchen spices. These spices are probably most appropriate for treating simple diarrhea that results from poor digestion and malabsorption, not severe diarrhea that's caused by an infectious agent. The volatile oils in the spices may also be effective against mild intestinal "flu." The oils act as digestive stimulants, increasing the natural digestive secretions of the stomach, intestines, and gallbladder. Because the stomach acid and digestive enzymes can destroy some invading organisms, the oils may have an indirect effect against infectious organisms. The kitchen spices basil, cinnamon, clove, ginger, nutmeg, black pepper, cayenne pepper, and thyme have all been mentioned in North American folk tradition as treatments for diarrhea.

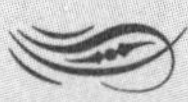

Remedies

BLACKBERRY ROOT: Perhaps the most commonly recommended remedy for diarrhea in North American folklore is blackberry root tea. Blackberry roots *(Rubus hispidus)* are not usually available in the commercial herb trade, but, if you are willing to brave the thorns, then start picking—the plant grows throughout most of the United States.

Taking blackberry root was a popular remedy in the United States during the 1800s. A listing in the 1849 book *The Family Physician* states that blackberry root "often provides a sovereign remedy [for diarrhea] when all other remedies fail." The text states that, during a dysentery epidemic, none of the local Indians using blackberry root died, while many of their white neighbors did. The root was used to treat diarrhea by the Oneida, Rappahannock, and Shinnecock Indians. It was likely that the whites died of mercury poisoning—mercury was what the white physicians used to treat diarrhea at the time.

The use of blackberry root for treating diarrhea survives today in the folk medicine of New England, Indiana, Appalachia, and among the Amish in the eastern states. The roots contain astringent tannins, which dry up the watery secretions of the intestines. The following suggestion comes from the folk traditions of New England.

☞ Directions: Simmer a handful of the roots in 1 pint of water until the liquid turns dark. Drink 1 cup. Wait a few hours and, if necessary, drink another. Don't take more than 2 cups a day. Gather the roots in the fall.

WORMWOOD: German immigrants at the turn of the century used wormwood tincture *(Artemisia absinthium)* to treat diarrhea. They arrived in this country carrying with them a popular health book called *My Water Cure* (English translation) by Father Sebastian Kneipp. The book warned against taking the remedy for a prolonged period of time or at high doses.

In the past, Europeans who consumed large amounts of wormwood, via an alcoholic drink called "absinthe," developed a form of insanity. The artist Vincent Van Gogh probably suffered from this mental illness, which may account for his progressive insanity and the increasing hallucinatory quality of his paintings at the end of his life.

A related plant from New Mexico, estafiate *(Artemisa ludoviciana),* is used identically in the folk medicine there. New Mexican folklorist Michael Moore suggests that wormwood treats minor diarrhea by restoring normal secretions of the stomach acid and bile.

☞ Directions: Purchase a tincture of wormwood in a health food store. Take a dropperful three times a day for no more than two days for treating simple diarrhea.

CHARCOAL: The use of charcoal for treating diarrhea in North America was well

continued on page 174

Electrolyte Replacement Therapy

The World Health Organization recommends the following formula for electrolyte replacement after excessive diarrhea or vomiting:

3.5 grams sodium chloride (table salt)

2.5 grams sodium bicarbonate (baking soda)

1.5 grams potassium chloride (available at a pharmacy)

20 grams of glucose (available at a pharmacy)

Add the ingredients to a liter (1 quart, 2 ounces) of water and drink.

For electrolyte replacement, you can also try the formula below. This remedy, taken from a German medical text, includes peppermint, which is a traditional folk treatment for diarrhea.

☞ Directions: Make a tea by simmering 1 tablespoon each of peppermint leaves and fennel seed in 1 quart of water for fifteen minutes in a covered pot. Strain and allow to cool to room temperature. Add ½ teaspoon salt, ¼ teaspoon baking soda, ¼ teaspoon potassium chloride, and 2 tablespoons glucose. Drink freely.

Finding the Balance

Many cultures around the world define health as a condition of balance. There are many factors, both internal and external, that may be involved in this complex balance. One factor that is found in many cultures is the balance between hot and cold. This balance of hot and cold principles is found in many Asian, Arabic, European, and Latino cultures. For example, the well-known yin and yang principles of Chinese medicine correspond (among other things) to the balance of hot and cold.

Interestingly, the terms hot and cold do not refer to actual temperatures, but to actual qualities or characteristics of symptoms and conditions; states of the body; foods and beverages; and medicines. (Temperature does play some part in treatment, however. Patients may need to be kept warm or cool as part of their recuperation. Also, temperature may be responsible for causing illness; exposure to cold air or drafts is believed to cause sickness, for example.) The ideal of health in a hot-cold system usually requires a state very near to neutral, sometimes with a preference for being just slightly on the warm side.

As a rule of thumb, "hot" conditions and symptoms usually involve blood or a hot substance. These hot conditions tend to be very outward in their manifestations and they may cause gnawing pain. Some examples of hot conditions include pregnancy, skin rashes and eruptions, diarrhea, stomach ulcers, and anything causing reddening of the skin or sweating without chills.

"Cold" conditions and symptoms involve phlegm or a cold substance. These conditions are usually very inward in their expression and can cause aching pain or stiffness. Some examples of cold conditions include colds and other upper respiratory infections, arthritis and rheumatism, flu, and anything causing pallor or chills.

Foods, beverages, and medicines of all types (including folk remedies, vitamins, and prescription drugs) are classified according to the kinds of effects they have and symptoms or side effects they produce. Acidic foods, such as oranges and other citrus fruits, tend to be classified as cold because they have a contracting effect and they may stimulate production of mucus, or phlegm. Alcoholic drinks, because they cause reddening of the face and induce sweating, are considered hot (even if served chilled!).

The basic principle of therapy in a hot-cold system is to move the patient's inner state back to a neutral center, using foods, beverages, and medicines. Cold conditions are treated with hot substances; hot conditions with "cool" ones. (Cold substances are not used.)

Although the idea of a hot-cold balance may sound strange to some, consider your own beliefs. Do you believe that a hot breakfast is important for health in the winter time? Do you worry about the effect of going from air conditioned surroundings out into a hot summer day? All such ideas are descended from the ancient idea of the importance of balancing hot and cold.

under way before the arrival of the European colonists. The Kwakiutl tribe from the Pacific Northwest would burn the bark of a fir tree, pulverize the coals, add the ash to water (sometimes with other herbs), and drink the mixture to end diarrhea. The use of "hardwood ashes" in water to treat diarrhea is also recorded by folklorist Clarence Meyer in his folk collection *American Folk Medicine.* Today, the use of charcoal to treat diarrhea is used by the Amish and Seventh Day Adventists.

Charcoal is absorbent, meaning that toxic substances attach to it and are tightly bound. It is used in emergency medicine to treat some types of poisoning. Be sure to use activated charcoal, which is very finely powdered and treated to be free of contaminants and gases.

☞ Directions: Purchase charcoal capsules from a pharmacy. Take 4 to 8 capsules three to four times a day.

ORANGE PEEL TEA: In reference to orange peel, a 9th century medical text from Baghdad, Iraq, says that "candied skin" is good for the stomach. Orange peel teas were used to treat digestive problems in Arabic medicine and European medicine during the Middle Ages, until the 1600s. The peels of related citrus fruits are still used for treating digestive complaints in China and India today. The practice also survives in the folklore of Indiana.

The oils in the peels stimulate digestion. (Today, dyes and pesticides are used on oranges, so if you want to try this remedy, you'll have to obtain organic oranges.) An Indiana remedy says to drink freely of orange peel tea sweetened with sugar.

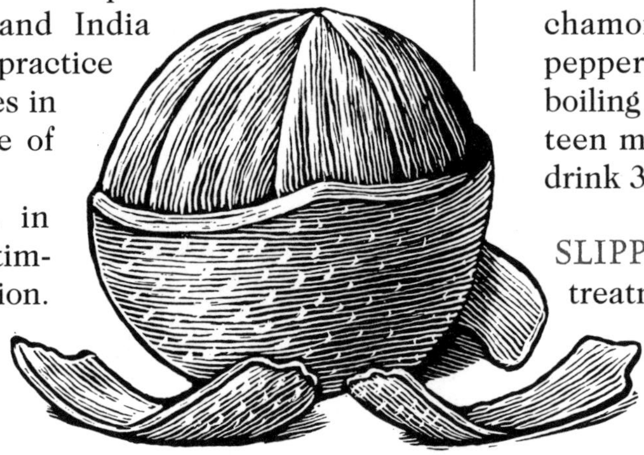

☞ Directions: Peel 1 organic orange and chop the skin into small pieces. Place the skin in a pot and cover with 1 pint of boiling water. Cover well and let stand until the water reaches room temperature. Sweeten with sugar or honey and drink freely.

CHAMOMILE (GERMAN): German immigrants to the United States used German chamomile *(Matricaria recutita)* to treat diarrhea. Chamomile is also mentioned as a treatment for diarrhea in Gypsy folklore.

Chamomile contains strong anti-inflammatory oils as well as other active principles. It may be best used in treating diarrhea caused by intestinal inflammation. Modern studies show it has antispasmodic properties as well. One German source suggests combining the tea half-and-half with peppermint. A Gypsy treatment calls for adding 25 blueberries to the tea. Thus, chamomile is probably viewed in folk medicine as a supportive treatment rather than a singular one. The following suggestion offers contemporary German advice.

☞ Directions: Place 1 teaspoon of chamomile flowers and 1 teaspoon of peppermint leaves in a cup. Fill with boiling water. Let steep, covered, for fifteen minutes. Sweeten, if desired, and drink 3 cups a day.

SLIPPERY ELM: An American Indian treatment for diarrhea is slippery elm bark *(Ulmus fulva).* Slippery elm bark is soothing and demulcent to inflamed tissues and may be best suited to treating diarrhea caused by intestinal inflammation.

☞ Directions: Place 1 tablespoon of powdered slippery elm bark in a cup. Fill with boiling water. Let steep ten minutes. Stir, without straining, and drink the whole cup.

BLACK TEA: Simple black or green tea *(Camellia sinensis)* is suggested as a treatment for diarrhea in the folk medicine of New England. One collection of remedies called *American Folk Medicine* by Clarence Meyer recommends taking the tea with no milk and very little sugar.

The tea contains astringent tannins, which help "dry up" the watery secretions of the intestines. In addition, the leaves contain at least 16 different antiviral constituents, which may be helpful for treating intestinal "flu."

☞ Directions: Make a tea using a black or green tea bag or with 1 teaspoon of tea leaves per cup of boiling water. Drink 2 to 4 cups a day, unsweetened and without milk.

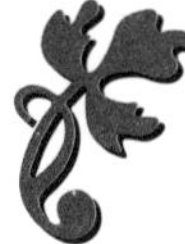

Digestion

According to traditional medical systems of Greece, India, and China, the digestive tract is the root of the tree of good health. Modern physiologists would agree

If the digestive tract is healthy and digestion and absorption of the nutrients are efficient, then the entire body will be well-nourished and will function optimally. Any irregularity in digestion, however, can cause or contribute to disease anywhere in the body.

Below are some common signs of a poorly functioning digestive system:

- flatulence or belching
- nausea
- pain anywhere in the digestive tract
- undigested food in the stool
- offensive breath
- constipation (less than one bowel movement per day)
- lethargy or depression after meals
- food cravings other than normal hunger
- lack of satisfaction after meals
- lack of hunger for breakfast

These symptoms—all considered to be serious signs that require treatment in traditional medical systems—are often left untreated by conventional physicians in North America. This is not so in the modern medicine of Germany and France, however, where symptoms such as "biliousness" (sluggish liver function), poor appetite, gas, and bloating or feelings of fullness after meals are routinely treated by doctors, often with herbal medicines from the European folk tradition.

According to folk medicine throughout the world, which offers many remedies for weak and sluggish digestion, healthy digestion requires:

- a balance of fats, proteins, and starches in the diet, and adequate fiber from sources such as grains, beans, fruits, and vegetables.
- food intake in moderate quantities. Overeating strains the capacity of the digestive system to process the consumed food, and undigested or partially digested remnants can cause inflammation and other problems in the digestive tract and elsewhere in the body.
- a relaxed state during meals. For the stomach and intestines to function normally, and for digestive secretions to be adequate, the body cannot be in a state of stress during meals.
- a healthy number of normal bacteria in the gut. The "garden" of friendly bacteria in the intestines acts as a defense against harmful bacteria, yeasts, molds, and other microorganisms by competing with them for food. (As the friendly bacteria proliferate, the nutrients they consume deprive the harmful microorganisms of their food supply.) Some of these friendly bacteria manufacture essential vitamins. The good bacteria can be disrupted by courses of such drugs as birth control pills, steroids, and antibiotics, however, leading to poor digestion and inflammation and infection of the intestinal wall. This in turn can cause inflammatory diseases in other parts of the body as the intestinal contents leak through the inflamed gut wall and overwhelm the immune system.

Folk remedies may improve digestion by stimulating the secretion of more stomach acid, digestive enzymes, and bile (a digestive secretion of the liver) from the liver. The remedies may also improve the absorption of nutrients by increasing blood flow to the mucous membranes of the intestines. Finally, antispasmodic constituents in folk remedies may prevent spasms in intestinal wall muscles that often accompanies gas and bloating.

Any severe or persistent digestive tract symptoms merit a visit to your doctor, however.

Remedies

GINGER: Ginger *(Zingiber officinale)* is a folk remedy for treating gas or nausea in the folk traditions of both New England and the southern Appalachians. It is used the same way in the traditional medicine of India, China, and Arabia. Ginger contains at least 13 antispasmodic constituents, which may help reduce spasms and tension in the digestive tract muscles. Also, circulatory stimulants in ginger increase circulation to the mucous membrane lining of the digestive tract, which in turn increases digestive secretions and absorption of nutrients. What's more, in clinical trials, ginger has shown to be effective in soothing some kinds of nausea and vertigo. Avoid excessive doses of ginger if you're taking drugs for heart or blood conditions or diabetes.

> ☞ Directions: Stir ½ teaspoon of ground ginger into a cup of hot water. Let stand two to three minutes. Strain and drink.

MINTS: Different types of mints are recommended for treating indigestion in North American folk literature, most commonly peppermint *(Mentha piperita)* and spearmint *(Mentha spicata).* Mints appear in the folk medicine of New England, New York, Indiana, Appalachia, New Mexico, and California. Mints have also been used as carminatives (see sidebar, page 180) by members of the Cherokee, Chippewa, Dakota, Omaha, Pawnee, Ponca, and Winnebago American Indian tribes. Mint species contain the antispasmodic constituents carvacrol, eugenol, limonene, and thymol, which may help reduce intestinal spasms. A contemporary German medical text, *Lehrbuch der Phytotherapie* by R.F. Weiss, M.D. (in translation: *Herbal Medicine*), recommends the mints as digestive aids for their carminative and antispasmodic properties. Peppermint is used as an official digestive aid in Germany.

☞ Directions: Place 1 teaspoon of the dried herb in a cup and add boiling water. Cover and let stand for ten minutes. Strain well and drink the tea warm three times a day on an empty stomach. Don't take peppermint if you are experiencing heartburn or painful belching.

FENNEL: A tea of fennel seeds *(Foeniculum vulgare)* is used for treating sluggish digestion or gas in the folk medicine of both New England and China. It is also the most often prescribed tea for abdominal cramping and gas in adults in the medical herbalism of contemporary Great Britain, Canada, and the United States. It is an approved medicine in Germany for mild gastrointestinal complaints. At least 16 chemical constituents in fennel have demonstrated antispasmodic effects in animal trials.

☞ Directions: Place 1 teaspoon of the seeds in a cup and add boiling water. Cover and let stand for ten minutes. Strain well and drink three cups of warm tea a day on an empty stomach until digestion improves.

CARAWAY SEEDS: Caraway seeds *(Carum carvi),* with a flavor and a medicinal action similar to that of fennel are recommended for gas and poor digestion in Appalachia and in the folk medicine of Indiana. Their medicinal use originated in Arab culture. Their use for poor digestion spread to ancient Rome, and from there to European folk medicine. Caraway seeds are approved for medical use for weak digestion by the German government.

☞ Directions: In a cup, pour boiling water over 1 teaspoon of the crushed seeds. Cover and let stand for ten minutes. Strain well and drink three cups of warm tea a day on an empty stomach.

Alternately, you can chew on the seeds. A common practice in households in India and the Middle East is to pass a small bowl of caraway, fennel, or anise seeds for nibbling after meals.

AMERICAN GINSENG: American ginseng *(Panax quinquefolium)* is used as a digestive tonic throughout the Appalachian mountain chain where it grows. A related species of ginseng *(Panax ginseng),* known as Asian ginseng, is perhaps the most famous tonic herb in China. (American ginseng, however, is also exported to China in large quantities.)

Even though both species are called "ginseng," the Chinese use the two plants for entirely different purposes. Asian ginseng is

continued on page 179

Medicinal Teas

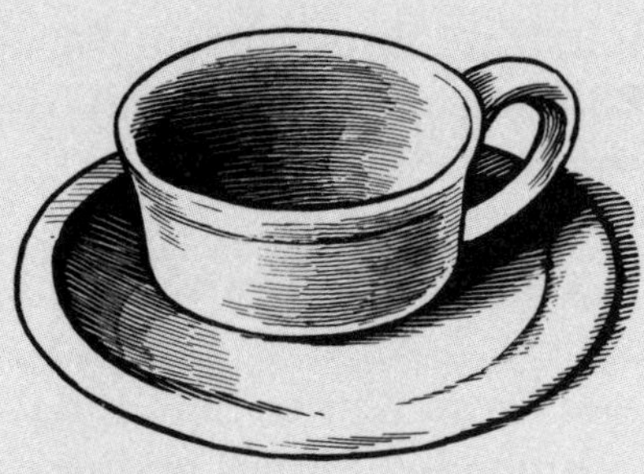

Teas from almost every conceivable plant are a mainstay of the traditional pharmacy. These teas, often referred to as infusions, can be taken as tonics, sedatives, stimulants, inhalants, emetics (to cause vomiting), and laxatives. Some teas were made on a seasonal basis, like sassafras (which is no longer used because of carcinogenic constituents) or dandelion in the spring; some were made specifically to serve a need, like alfalfa for arthritis, boneset for migraine, or pennyroyal to induce a missing menstrual period. Other teas were meant to be drunk regularly to maintain health. Teas could also be applied externally, like burdock root tea for acne or walnut hulls for hair growth.

The earliest noted folk medicine of North America may be a recipe for tea given to Jacques Cartier in the winter of 1535 by the native people of Quebec. The infusion of white cedar bark cured his crew of scurvy as well as some other longer-standing diseases. North America's earliest medical book was an herbal, written in the year 1552 in the Nuahuatl Aztec language by the Aztec physician Martin de la Cruz.

The vast catalogue of medicinal teas is representative of the traditional healer's intimate knowledge of the environment. In addition to identifying plants, the healer might also have to know the time of year, time of day, or phase of moon when it was best to gather the plants, as well as the proper methods of preparation and storage. Unfortunately, many of the healers' cures were ultimately lost when the plants disappeared due to overharvesting or the vernacular names for them were no longer recognized as languages changed overtime.

Of course tea can be made from things other than plants, but these kinds of teas are not as common—and it is easy to see why. One formula for treating a "run-down condition" called for a mix of horses' hooves, eggshells, and banana stalk. A Louisiana drink to stop vomiting in children was made from boiled flies. Sheep dropping tea was used in many places for measles. After these, the spearmint or peppermint teas advised for bad breath sound all too sweet!

Chamomile: A Chameleon

"One table-spoon to be taken at bed-time." When Peter Rabbit's mother put him to bed with chamomile tea after his fright in Mr. MacGregor's garden, she was using a well-known brew. An Old World plant imported to the New, chamomile tea has been employed not only to calm the stomach and nerves, but as an eyewash, tonic, laxative, and hair rinse.

Bitter Tonics

In folk medicine and traditional herbalism, bitter tonics are one of the most often prescribed categories of herbs and foods. In fact, a 1994 poll of the most-often prescribed medicinal herbs by North American professional herbalists showed that half of the top ten herbs had important bitter constituents.

The key indication for bitter tonics is poor appetite. The bitter constituents in the plants stimulate the secretion of stomach acid and liver bile, thereby improving digestion and nourishment. Because they stimulate these secretions, however, they are contraindicated if you have heartburn or other kinds of digestive pain.

Bitter tonics in this section include wormwood, chamomile, goldenseal, Oregon grape root, gentian, and boneset. Bitter tonics are often combined with carminative herbs in simple formulas (see sidebar, "Carminatives," page 180).

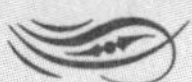

considered to be stimulating; in fact, it is sometimes used in large doses as a stimulant in Chinese hospital emergency rooms. American ginseng, however, is used as a sedative for individuals who are tense and nervous from prolonged stress or illness.

American ginseng earned the attention of the turn-of-the-century medical doctor Arthur Harding, M.D., who, out of disillusionment with the conventional medicines of his day, abandoned his regular medical practice in order to investigate folk remedies. He said in his book *Ginseng and Other Medicinal Plants*, published in 1909: "If the people of the United States were educated as to its use, our supply of ginseng would be consumed in our own country and it would be a hard blow to the medical profession." In his book, Harding recounts case studies of patients whose generally deteriorated health improved only after a few weeks or months of treatment with ginseng. He attributes the plant's power to restore health to its ability to restore weak digestion.

Unlike Asian ginseng, very little scientific research has been performed on American ginseng. Thus, we have to rely on contemporary Chinese medicine or on the folk traditions of this country for guidance on its use.

☞ Directions: American ginseng can cost more than $200 a pound, and many adulterated or ineffective products are sold in health food stores. The most reliable way to use it is to make your own powder from whole roots with the fine rootlets attached.

Purchase the roots and grind them into powder in a coffee grinder. (Consume the powder from one root before grinding another, because the constituents are more likely to be preserved in the whole root than in the powder.) Stir ¼ to ½ teaspoon of the powder into 1 cup of warm water and drink one dose daily on any empty stomach before breakfast for two to three weeks. Then, repeat if desired after taking a break for one or two weeks.

CHAMOMILE (GERMAN): Chamomile *(Matricaria recutita)* is recommended for intestinal spasm or gas in the folk traditions of New England, Indiana, and the American Southwest. It combines both antispasmodic and sedative properties and may relieve intestinal cramping and induce relaxation at the same time. Chamomile contains at least 19 antispasmodic constituents, as well as five sedative ones. The plant is approved in Germany as a medicine for gastrointestinal complaints. In addition, a 1993 clinical trial in Germany showed that chamomile was effective in relieving infant colic.

☞ Directions: Pour boiling water over 1 tablespoon of chamomile flowers in a cup. Cover and let sit for ten minutes. Strain and drink warm three times a day on an empty stomach. Do this for two to three weeks. Taking one of the doses before bed may also work as a sleep aid. Avoid using if signs of allergy appear. Avoid excessive use during pregnancy and lactation.

WORMWOOD: Wormwood *(Artemisia absinthium, Artemisia spp.)* is described as a digestive stimulant in the Hispanic folk medicine of southern California. The active constituents of wormwood include bitter digestive stimulants and anti-inflammatory volatile oils including azulenes, constituents that are also present in chamomile. The European species of the plant is approved as a digestive stimulant by the German government.

Carminatives

Carminative herbs and spices are hot digestive stimulants that have traditionally been taken for indigestion accompanied by gas. Exactly how they work is not clear, but some scientific experiments give us a hint.

German researchers observed that carminative spices may reduce gas pressure in the stomach by promoting belching and the release of gas. Carminatives also increase circulation to the stomach wall, which reduces spasm and improves the absorption of nutrients.

In addition, according to a German textbook on medical herbalism called *Lehrbuch der Phytotherapie* by R.F. Weiss, M.D. (translation: *Herbal Medicine*), which is used in schools of medicine and pharmacy in Germany, carminatives improve the tone of the intestinal muscles and increase the secretion of digestive juices. These herbs and spices invariably contain antispasmodic substances as well, which is why a key indication for using carminatives is poor digestion accompanied by gas or spasm. Carminatives are often combined with bitter herbs in formulas.

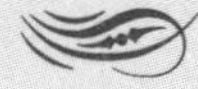

☞ Directions: Place 1 teaspoon of wormwood leaves in a cup of water and fill with boiling water. Cover well to prevent the escape of aromatic substances. Let cool to room temperature. Take ½ doses three or four times a day. Don't take wormwood for more than ten days at a time and take a ten-day break before starting the therapy again. Avoid excessive consumption of wormwood.

CINNAMON: Cinnamon *(Cinnamomum verum)* is used as a digestive stimulant in the folk medicine of New England and China. It is also used for this purpose in the Hispanic folk medicine of the Southwest. Cinnamon contains at least 16 different antispasmodic constituents, especially in its aromatic oils. It contains the antispasmodic and circulatory stimulant cinnamaldehyde in large quantities. Cinnamon is approved by the German government for treatment of poor digestion. It is contraindicated in medicinal quantities during pregnancy, however, because it can stimulate uterine contractions.

☞ Directions: Stir ¼ to ½ teaspoon of cinnamon powder into a cup of hot water. Let stand three to five minutes. Stir again and drink without straining.

GENTIAN: In this country, five of the six North American gentian species were used as digestive aids or bitter tonics by American Indians. Gentian *(Gentiana lutea)* is the most famous component of the pre-dinner "bitters" commonly consumed in European folk medicine. (Bitters are traditionally taken in many cultures ten to twenty minutes before meals to improve the appetite.) Experiments show that bitters increase the secretion of stomach acid, which helps the digestive system prepare for the meal.

The use of gentian also appears in the contemporary folk literature of British Columbia. Gentian is approved as a bitter tonic by the German government. Like other strong bitters, it is contraindicated if you are experiencing heartburn or other digestive pain or if you have an ulcer.

☞ Directions: Chop up three fresh lemon peels and place with 1 ounce of chopped gentian root in 1 quart of water. Bring to a boil and simmer on the lowest heat for ten minutes. Let stand until the tea reaches room temperature. Strain and store in the refrigerator. Take a teaspoon twenty minutes before meals. If the gentian causes heartburn, stop taking it. Avoid in pregnancy and lactation.

GENTIAN AND GINGER: In folk medicine, gentian is usually combined with other herbs or foods to make pre-dinner bitters (see "Gentian," above). Gentian is most commonly combined with a warming, spicy herb.

☞ Directions: Grind some gentian root in a coffee grinder to make a powder. Mix well with an equal amount of powdered ginger root. Stir ¼ to ½ teaspoon of the mixture into a cup of hot water. Let stand three to five minutes. Stir again and drink, without straining, twenty minutes before meals. If this remedy causes heartburn, try a different one.

GOLDENSEAL AND OREGON GRAPE ROOT: Goldenseal *(Hydrastis canadensis)* is the most famous bitter tonic in North American folk medicine. The colonists learned its use from the American Indians, and it entered into the folk medicine of New England in the 1700s. Goldenseal remained a common household remedy

continued on page 184

Soul Loss and Lost Souls

Soul loss. To many people in North America the loss of one's soul occurs at death. To others, soul loss is a crisis that leads to an illness that may ultimately result in debility or death. Medical anthropologists refer to soul loss as a "folk illness." Most of the illnesses treated in folk medicine are well known to doctors—from whooping cough to rabies, from burns to colds. From the medical viewpoint, some of the terms used in folk medicine to describe a condition are not quite right, even though the illnesses are recognizable. For example, in folk medicine, osteoarthritis and rheumatoid arthritis and a host of other achy, stiff conditions are all classified as rheumatism.

Some illnesses that are described in folk tradition are unknown to modern medicine. In fact, a case of soul loss may be mistaken for a contemporary disease, or doctors may believe that it is a sign of distress somehow caused by the culture in which the patient lives. However, it is always possible in such a case that folk knowledge may actually be ahead of medical knowledge, that a folk illness may be a real illness not yet recognized by medicine. This seems especially likely when the same illness is found in many different cultures—including some where it is not widely recognized. This is the case with soul loss.

In many cultures, it is believed that humans have more than one soul. In some cultures, it is believed that humans have many souls.

Although it is found in many cultural groups in America, probably the best known example of American soul loss is in the Latino culture, where soul loss is called "susto," meaning fright or trauma. The person suffering from susto is said to be restless in his sleep, and when he is awake he acts depressed, passive, or indifferent. Often the individual's grooming habits and cleanliness suffer. The illness is said to be caused by a sudden shock or fright that causes a person's soul to come loose and wander away or even be captured by a spirit. A typical situation leading to susto was described by a young Mexican woman who saw her father swept off his feet while fording a rapidly moving stream. He barely managed to save himself. Two weeks later she became ill and was diagnosed as suffering from susto.

In recent western European tradition, people are conceived of as having one soul. The soul is usually equated with consciousness. Therefore, many readers might expect a person whose soul has left them to appear unconscious. But, in many cultures, it is believed that humans have more than one soul. In such a tradition, one soul may be responsible for operating the basic functions of the body, such as breathing and heartbeat, and another for consciousness, since some activating principle obviously remains even when a person is unconscious. Still other cultures, for example the Hmong of southeast Asia, hold the belief that a body has many souls.

Although the majority of Americans believe that humans have souls, and that their soul departs at death, there really is no "scientific proof" that souls really exist. How, then, can we approach the question of whether soul loss may represent folk knowledge that is beyond medical understanding? Investigating the beliefs and experiences of those who believe in soul loss will not help, because their beliefs may actually be producing the events and behaviors that define soul loss. However, we can study the possibility that soul loss traditions are valid by looking at cultures that do not have beliefs about soul loss, and seeing whether the same experiences occur there. If the experiences do turn up in such nontraditional settings, then the idea of soul loss is valid.

Since Raymond Moody's book, *Life After Life,* appeared in 1974, the American public has shown a great deal of interest in one particular kind of "soul loss" experience, the near-death experience (NDE). In the classic NDE, as described by Moody and many others since 1974, the subject is unconscious while their conscious soul moves around the environment. But that is not the only way that people experience NDEs. Sometimes, after a classic NDE, when the person's viewpoint returns to normal and he can again speak and walk, something feels like it has remained outside the body. One woman, whose experience occurred as a result of a bad reaction to medicine, claimed it felt as though the "real" her remained up by the ceiling in the spot from where she had observed her resuscitation. The sensation of being separated continued for two weeks and only ended when she had a vision of deceased relatives and friends who asked her to choose between life and death. She chose to live because of unfinished personal business. This is a common scenario in NDEs.

The following morning when the woman awoke she said she felt as though her spirit, which had been trailing along behind her like a balloon on a string, was now back inside her. Before her spirit reentered her, she had been conscious but passive and indifferent to her surroundings. To others she had seemed depressed, though she did not recall feeling sad. She made a good recovery and returned to her daily activities. This woman's strange experience had been precipitated by a shock—a shock that occurred as a result of a reaction to medication. Her symptoms were the same as those reported from cultures where soul loss is recognized. Had she been in such a culture, she would have been diagnosed as susto.

There are several kinds of NDEs, although only a few are routinely publicized. It seems that people experience the sensation of self leaving the body in a variety of ways, and some of these are included in the folk illness category of "soul loss." This is an instance in which folk medical traditions may have knowledge of an important human state that is virtually unknown to modern biomedicine.

Anthropologists have found many cultures around the world where it is believed that a sudden shock can cause one's soul to be displaced, at least temporarily. Because of the connection to a sudden shock or fright, they have often called this type of soul loss "magical fright."

Fiber and Digestion

German naturopathic tradition, which arrived in this country with turn-of-the-century German immigrants, has long advocated a high fiber diet to improve poor digestion. In the last 20 years, conventional medicine has begun to recommend the same.

What is the single most important dietary change you can make to improve digestion? Eat more fiber, and not as fiber supplements, but in the form of whole foods—grains, beans, fruits, and vegetables. Fiber provides bulk for the stool, helping to maintain muscle tone in the intestinal walls. The result is faster passage of food through the intestines and less constipation. Fiber also feeds the friendly bacteria in the digestive tract, increasing their number and creating a defense against potentially harmful bacteria.

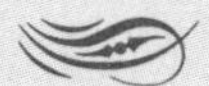

throughout the eastern states during the 1800s. It was also one of the most commonly prescribed herbs by doctors of the Eclectic and Physiomedicalist schools of medicine. Although goldenseal had several therapeutic uses, the physicians often prescribed it to restore the functioning of a "run-down" digestive system.

Today, goldenseal is an endangered species, so medical herbalists in North America frequently prescribe Oregon grape root *(Mahonia aquifolium, Berberis aquifolium)* as a substitute bitter tonic. (Because of its equivalent bitter effects, Eclectic physicians also prescribed Oregon grape root.) As with other strong bitters, don't take either of these herbs if you are experiencing digestive pain or if you have an ulcer.

☞ Directions: Grind Oregon grape root in a coffee grinder to make a powder. Stir ½ teaspoon into a cup of hot water. Allow to stand for three to five minutes. Don't strain, just stir. Drink the cup twenty minutes before meals for one to three weeks.

BONESET: Contemporary North Carolina folk traditions suggest taking a tea of boneset *(Eupatorium perfoliatum)* for weak digestion. Boneset was one of the most common folk remedies in the early American colonies, where it was considered to be a panacea. It was taken as a hot tea to treat colds, flu, and feverish diseases. As a cold tea, it was used as a bitter digestive tonic. Boneset is very bitter to the taste.

☞ Directions: Place 1 tablespoon of dried boneset leaves in a 1-pint jar and fill with boiling water. Cover and let cool to room temperature. Drink half of a cup twenty minutes before meals for one to three weeks.

CATNIP: Catnip *(Nepeta cataria)* tea, a sedative and indigestion remedy in European folk medicine, has been a popular remedy in this country since the arrival of the European immigrants. The plant rapidly became naturalized here, and American Indian tribes such as the Onondaga and Cayuga eventually used it for poor digestion as well, especially when treating children. It was an official medicine in the *United States Pharmacopoeia* from 1840 until 1870.

Catnip has been used in folk medicine to treat weak digestion, intestinal spasm, and gas by residents of New England, Appalachia, North Carolina, Indiana, and New Mexico and by Blacks throughout the deep South and by Chicanos in Los Angeles. Catnip combines both carminative and sedative properties, with seven antispasmodic and five sedative constituents.

☞ Directions: Pour boiling water over 1 teaspoon of the dried herb. Let sit covered for ten minutes. Strain and drink three cups a day, between meals on an empty stomach.

THYME: A digestive stimulant found in the folk traditions of both Indiana and China is thyme *(Thymus vulgaris)*. Thymol, the chief aromatic substances of thyme that gives it its fragrance, has antispasmodic and carminative properties. Animal research has shown that thymol relaxes the muscles of the intestinal tract, which relieves pressure from gas.

☞ Directions: Place 1 teaspoon of dried thyme leaves in a cup and fill with boiling water. Let stand, covered, for ten minutes. Strain and drink. Do this three times a day, before meals, on an empty stomach. Thyme oil is toxic and should only be used when highly diluted.

CHAMOMILE, PEPPERMINT, FENNEL, AND LICORICE: Jill Stansbury, N.D., who chairs the botanical medicine department at the National College of Naturopathic Medicine in Portland, Oregon, devised a formula for treating the digestive tract that combines three of the herbs in this chapter. Stansbury prescribes this remedy for a wide variety of digestive complaints.

☞ Directions: Place a handful each of chamomile flowers, peppermint leaves, fennel seeds, and licorice root in 1 quart of water. Bring to a boil and simmer on the lowest heat, covered, for twenty minutes. Strain and drink the quart in 3 or 4 doses throughout the day on an empty stomach at least twenty minutes before meals for three to six weeks.

WATER TREATMENT: A treatment for weak digestion, gas, and bloating from the Seventh Day Adventists tradition is to apply a heating pad or hot water bottle to the abdomen after meals. This presumably attracts circulation to the area, improving digestion. Relaxation during the period of application also promotes good digestion.

☞ Directions: Place a hot water bottle or heating pad over the abdomen and relax, lying down, for twenty minutes after meals.

CASTOR OIL: A suggestion for poor digestion, from the folk medicine of contemporary Indiana, is to apply a warm castor oil pack to the abdomen. Castor oil taken internally is a strong laxative. It does not have this effect with external applications, however.

The external use of castor oil for digestive pain and complaints gained popularity in North American folk traditions in the second half of the 20th century, thanks to the advice of mystic Edgar Cayce, who was known for giving medical advice while in a trance-like state. His books on health remain popular throughout the United States today.

Cayce claimed that castor oil packs improved the functioning of the gut's immune system. No scientific evidence exists to support this claim, although the practice appears to be harmless. Some benefits from the treatment may come from the relaxation and hot application involved. Castor oil packs for digestive problems are now a standard treatment in North American naturopathic medicine.

☞ Directions: Dip a cloth in castor oil and apply to the abdomen. Cover with plastic wrap and a second cloth, and finally with a heating pad on low heat. (The plastic wrap keeps the castor oil away from the heating pad.) Relax with the pad in place for forty to sixty minutes in the evening after dinner three nights a week. Do not used if appendicitis is suspected or during pregnancy.

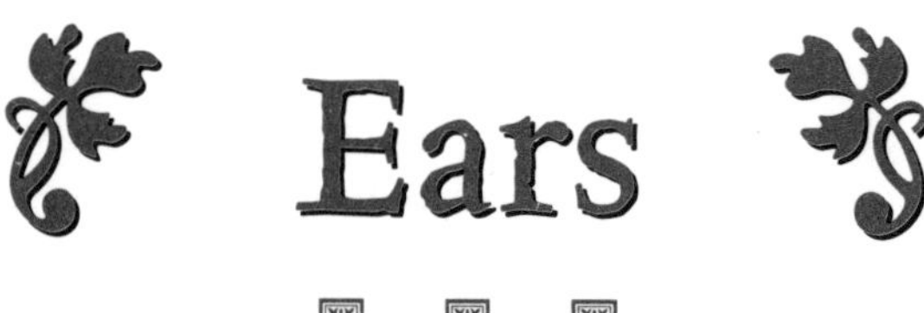

Ears

There are plenty of folk remedies available that can successfully soothe conditions of the ear

Today, ear infections are epidemic among toddlers in America. The incidence of the condition has risen dramatically in the last generation. One possible factor for the increase is the rise in attendance at day care centers, where increased exposure to infection is likely.

The ear can become infected in any one of its three parts—the inner ear, the middle ear, and the outer ear. However, infections most commonly occur in the middle and outer ear.

Middle ear infections develop when viruses or bacteria in the nose or throat travel to the ear through the eustachian tube, which connects the middle ear to the nose and throat. The middle ear also can become infected when infection spreads from a severe outer ear infection or injury. Allergic reactions or obstruction of the eustachian tube can also lead to ear infections. Ear infections are much more likely to affect children than adults; children are most susceptible between the ages of six months and six years.

Infection of the outer ear, sometimes called "swimmer's ear," is more common among adults. Water in the ears after swimming can create a warm humid environment that is congenial to bacteria, viruses, molds, or fungi. Personal hygiene is important to prevent outer ear infections. To prevent swimmer's ear, wet outer ears should be thoroughly dried with a soft towel. Blowing the ear dry with a hair dryer can also get the job done.

Middle ear infections are usually quickly eliminated by treatment with an antibiotic. (If a viral infection is present, however, antibiotics are not used, because viruses do not respond to antibiotics.) Conventional antibiotic therapy is controversial, however, because the antibiotics can have severe side effects. Also controversial is surgery to implant ear tubes into the ear drum. The procedure is designed to allow the middle ear to drain outward, instead of down the eustachian tube. When treating an ear infection, some conventional physicians advocate doing nothing more than keeping the child comfortable by giving simple decongestants to clear the eustachian tube.

Natural treatments for middle ear infections include screening for allergies and increasing the body's natural resistance to infection with nutritional, herbal, or homeopathic remedies. Ear tube surgery can frequently be avoided with such methods. John Collins, N.D., a naturopathic physician of the National College of Naturopathic Medicine, stated in a 1991 issue of *East West: A Journal of Natural Health and Living* that he has seen more than a hundred children who had been recommended for the surgery, but after using simple natural methods and screening for allergies, he only had to refer one child for the procedure.

Folk remedies occasionally appear for deafness. These types of remedies may also be effective in removing accumulations of ear wax, a common cause of hearing loss in the elderly. If you are experiencing hearing loss, we recommend visiting your doctor rather than experimenting with home remedies, however. Hearing loss can be a sign of serious underlying conditions.

Remedies

BASIL: Basil *(Ocimum basilicum)* is used in the American Southwest to treat earaches. The plant is used in Spanish-speaking areas of the United States (as well as in Mexico and Central America) for a variety of medicinal purposes.

Basil leaves contain high amounts of the essential oil eugenol, which has anti-inflammatory, anesthetic, and antiseptic properties. Research of the plant in India has shown its anti-inflammatory and fever-reducing effects. Applications to the outer ear may kill bacteria or other infecting agents and help reduce pain and inflammation in the outer and middle ear.

☞ Directions: Place 1 ounce of the leaves in 1 pint of vegetable oil, cover tightly, and let sit in a warm place for two weeks, shaking the jar daily. Using a dropper, put 6 to 8 drops directly into the ear canal. Do this four times a day. Don't confuse this vegetable oil preparation with the essential oil of basil, which is concentrated and can burn the skin.

CLOVE: Another earache remedy used in the Southwest, especially in Colorado and New Mexico, is clove *(Eugenia caryophyllata)*. Originally grown in Indonesia, the plant was traded as a medicine throughout Asia. The first shipment arrived in Alexandria in North Africa in A.D. 176. Clove was then used as a multi-purpose medicine by

continued on page 190

The Calendar

Time is a critical element in many folk medical practices. Certain days, months, or seasons of the year were said to be the best—or worst—time to take or make medicine, to get sick, or to get well.

January will search,
February will try,
March will tell if you'll
live or die.

A spring tonic was taken to "clean the blood" after the long winter. The great variety of teas and formulas used for this purpose attest to the widespread desire to "open the system and clean it out" and "pep it up." An Ohio farmer in the 1950s said he sold thousands of bunches of red sassafras for tonic each spring. He dug up the plants in the dark of the moon in February when they were supposed to be "full of the vitamins and minerals for a healthy life."

Some calendrical ideas and practices have an obvious basis in fact, while others are based on outmoded ideas about nature or the body. Winter is, of course, the riskiest season for influenza and other diseases that spread in close quarters, so there is reason in the rhyme above. But the idea that the blood needs "purifying," or that this can be done with laxatives (which is what many "tonics" were) is rejected by medical science. Despite this, digging sassafras root in February might—or might not—be done because it is believed the active compounds are most concentrated then. Many medicinal plants are supposed to be harvested at certain times of the day or year in order to be effective as medicine, so they well may have the desired properties only at a certain season or state of maturity.

The most magical health customs are the once-a-year observances to insure health for the rest of the year.

Sometimes it seems easy to separate "magic" from "material" medicine: The leaves or bark of a tree to be used for an emetic (a vomit inducer), for instance, is supposed to be stripped upwards. If it is to be used for a laxative, it is stripped downwards. Because the direction in which the leaves are stripped could not really reverse their medicinal effect, this is a magical cure even though it uses plant medicine. But say an herb is to be picked only on Saint John's Day. This remedy sounds more like "magic," but perhaps midsummer is when the herb is actually the most potent, and fixing that day merely encoded that fact.

One of the major shapers of American folk medicine, the almanac, influenced many time-related beliefs. Throughout the 16th and 17th centuries, these how-to guides were the only book other than the Bible in many households. Almanacs contained thousands of "receipts," or recipes, for cures. A perennial feature of the earlier almanacs was the "Man of the Signs"—a human figure surrounded by astrological signs designating various parts of his anatomy. The reader consulted tables inside as to the best time for attention to these parts. Well into the 20th century people spoke of remedies to be undertaken (or avoided) when "the sign is in the head" or "in the knees." The almanacs also gave health hints for each month. The readers of *Poor Robin's Almanac* for 1728 were given this advice for November:

"The best Physick in this month is good Exercise, warmth, and wholesome Meat and Drink. Kill your swine in this Month, and after Pork and Pease be sure to break Wind."

Phases of the moon have been thought to affect the body, especially the full moon, which was supposed to make sick people sicker. People having surgery during a full moon would bleed more. Light shining on the face of a healthy person while he slept could drain him of his strength. On the other hand, medicine taken during this time was especially effective because the sickness would decrease along with the moon. The principle was similar to planting crops, brewing, or butchering by the moon: Waxing and fullness fostered growth; waning produced the opposite. You could thus plant potatoes by the full moon for a healthy family.

The most patently magical health customs are the once-a-year observances to insure health for the rest of the year: Walk barefoot in the first snow and wash in the first May rain. New Year's Day is naturally favored for the practicing of customs, so you should wipe down all the doorknobs at the stroke of twelve on this day for better health. Holidays are common occasions for such magical actions, and sometimes religious symbolism from the church is carried over into the home. Catholics would put blessed palms from Palm Sunday on the walls of their houses or hang bouquets blessed on the Assumption. Other symbolic rites had a completely secular, spell-like character. You could eat the first fresh fruit of the season and say, "First fruit into my stomach, illness to hell." You could throw an apple, cake, and salt into the well on Christmas Eve and say, "Cold water, I am giving you these gifts, now you give me health and happiness." The most common annual health-bringing act was merely to eat a special food on a special day, like goose for Christmas and hog's head on New Year's.

Marking the calendar with health-related customs affirmed the importance of health in the cycles of life.

Getting Lucky

Lucky and unlucky days for health abounded. Marry on Monday (but not in May) and cut your fingernails on Thursday. If you get sick on a Sunday you won't get better. If you get sick on Friday the 13th you'll have the same sickness for every Friday the 13th after that.

Good Friday was an especially auspicious day. Bread baked that day was said to have curative powers and might thus be kept in the cupboard all year for first aid. To insure health all year, one could rise and wash before sunrise. Some activities were taboo on Good Friday, however. Cutting wood or driving nails—acts symbolic of the crucifixion of Christ—could result in injury. But a child born on Good Friday was said to have the power to heal.

the Arabs. Its use eventually reached Spain with the Arab conquest of that country. The medicinal use of clove possibly came to the Spanish colonies with the many Spanish Arabs fleeing the Spanish Inquisition in the 16th century. Many fled to Mexico and later settled in the upper Rio Grande Valley, where some of their folk customs survive today.

Although clove is considered a cure-all throughout Asia, Arabia, and Latin America, it has hardly been used medicinally in parts of Europe (other than Spain), and it is rarely mentioned in the folk medicine of North America. Clove, like basil, contains large amounts of a volatile oil, made up largely of eugenol, which has a strong, spicy odor. Clove is both analgesic and antiseptic.

☞ Directions: Grind ½ ounce of clove in a coffee grinder and add to ½ pint of olive oil. Cover and keep in a warm place for 3 to 4 days, shaking the bottle each day. Strain well and put 6 to 8 drops in each ear. Don't confuse this preparation of cloves with the concentrated essential oil of cloves, which can burn the skin if applied directly to it.

MULLEIN: The herb mullein *(Verbascum thapsus)* was used in ancient Roman medicine. The plant came to North America with the European colonists and is now naturalized throughout the continent. The American Indians quickly adopted it as a medicine for coughs, colds, and other upper respiratory infections, just as the Europeans did before them. The Iroquois Indians used the leaves specifically to treat earache. The German government today has approved the use of the herb's flowers as a medicine for treating colds and coughs. Mullein ear oils, made from the plant's flowers, and sometimes mixed with garlic oil, are available in health foods stores and herb shops.

☞ Directions: Purchase a mullein or mullein-garlic oil in an herb shop or health food store. Apply to the ears as indicated on the label.

Garlic and Baby

Oils made from garlic and olive oil (sometimes with the herb mullein added) are available in health foods stores and herb shops. Caution must be used when using these oils to treat an ear infection in a child, however. The garlic can cause further irritation. Cold or even room-temperature oil acts as an astringent and, put in a child's ears, may tighten swollen and inflamed tissues, causing pain. If you are using a commercial ear oil for a child, use simple mullein oil rather than a mullein-garlic combination when treating ear infections.

This treatment is not recommended for children under the age of two or if discharge is coming from the ear. If you suspect your child has an ear infection, make sure to see your health care practitioner.

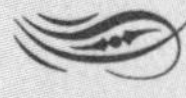

GARLIC, CRUSHED IN OLIVE OIL: Garlic was used to treat ear infections in the medicine of ancient India and Arabia. In this country, the Cherokee Indians used wild garlic as an ear medicine. Today, a traditional folk remedy of the southern Appalachians is to place garlic in the outer ear to cure ear infections or lessen ear wax. Garlic ear oils are also used by contemporary naturopathic physicians, called N.D.s, in the United States. (Naturopathic physicians, who are licensed to practice medicine in 13 states, primarily use natural remedies rather than pharmaceutical drugs or surgery.)

Garlic contains the powerful antibiotic allicin. After being aged in oil, the allicin breaks down into more than 30 medicinal constituents, including chemicals that inhibit bacteria, viruses, molds, and yeast. The allicin is only released when a clove is cut, crushed, or otherwise broken apart.

☞ Directions: Squeeze the juice from 3 cloves of garlic into a cup using a garlic press. Add 2 to 3 ounces of hot olive oil, and let the mixture stand until it reaches room temperature. Using a dropper, add 6 to 8 drops to the infected ear.

GOLDENSEAL: To treat earache, the Iroquois Indians applied drops of goldenseal tea in their ears. Goldenseal *(Hydrastis canadensis)* contains the alkaloidal constituents hydrastine and berberine, which may kill infecting organisms in the outer ear. Goldenseal is also soothing to inflamed, swollen tissues.

☞ Directions: Place 1 teaspoon of goldenseal root in a cup and add boiling water. Let steep until the water reaches room temperature. Using a dropper, add 6 to 8 drops to the infected ear. Do this four times a day.

YARROW: The Winnebago Indians used a tea of yarrow *(Achillea millefolium)* to treat earaches. The plant also was used as a universal remedy for infections among American Indian tribes throughout North America. Yarrow has been used in Europe as a disinfectant for wounds and other infections since the time of the ancient Greeks. Yarrow contains more

Blowing Smoke

Tobacco smoke, blown into the ear, was a widespread remedy for reducing the pain of earache among American Indians in the eastern United States. The practice subsequently entered into the folk medicine of New England, North Carolina, Indiana, and even northern New Mexico. (A contemporary method is to roll up a dollar bill to make a tube, and blow the hot smoke directly into the ear.) Herbs other than tobacco, such as mullein, are also sometimes used.

Using tobacco smoke is not an appropriate method for treating earache in children. Research shows that secondhand tobacco smoke increases the frequency of upper respiratory infections and ear infections in infants and young children.

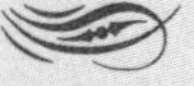

than a dozen constituents with antiviral, antibacterial, anti-inflammatory, and antiseptic properties.

☞ Directions: In a cup, pour 1 cup of boiling water over 1 teaspoon of crushed yarrow leaves. Let steep, well covered, until the mixture reaches room temperature. Strain and apply 6 to 8 drops to the infected ear. Do this four times a day.

URINE: In New England, Indiana, and the Southwest, urine is sometimes used as a remedy for ear infections. Urine therapy for cleansing wounds and treating a variety of infections has appeared in the ancient medical systems of Mexico, Egypt, Persia, India, and China, as well as in 17th and 18th century European medicine.

Modern science suggests reasons why urine may be an effective disinfectant. Urine from a healthy person is as sterile as boiled water, and thus is safe to apply to infected areas. Urine contains the substance urea, a disinfectant used today in pharmaceutical preparations to clean and disinfect burns and wounds. Urea also has strong drying properties and kills fungi, bacteria, and viruses by literally sucking the water right out of them. Also, urine was often the only sterile liquid available for cleaning wounds in earlier times before sanitation and purification.

New England tradition says that the urine used should be from a child under the age of ten. The reason: The urine needs to be free of sex hormones. These hormones are not found in young children because they have not yet experienced puberty.

☞ Directions: Allow about one third of the urine stream to pass. Catch the middle third in a cup or other container, and then let the last third pass as usual. The "middle catch" of urine is the most likely to be completely sterile. Place 6 to 8 drops in the infected ear. Repeat four times a day. (Generally, this procedure should only be preformed in emergency situations when proper antiseptic or clean liquids are not readily available.)

JUST PLAIN OIL: Several remedies in this section call for herb-infused oils to treat ear infections. Folk traditions from New England, North Carolina, southern Appalachia, and Indiana suggest using just plain oil, without the herbs. Types of oil range from skunk oil to butter, although olive oil is the most commonly mentioned. Olive oil is believed to work by creating an environment in the ear that is inhospitable to infection. The warmth of the oil may also help soothe the tissues. The following remedy comes from New England folk medicine.

☞ Directions: First warm a spoon in boiling water. Pour the oil onto the hot spoon, which will heat the oil. Place 6 to 8 drops in the infected ear. Plug the ear with cotton. Repeat 2 to 3 times a day until ear pain subsides.

BREAST MILK: New England tradition suggests putting breast milk in a baby's ear to treat an ear infection. Breast milk contains antibodies that may help disinfect the outer ear during an infection. Also, if the milk is warm, the warmth may also draw circulation to the area and soothe the pain.

☞ Directions: Using a dropper, add warm breast milk to the ear canal three times a day.

 Eczema 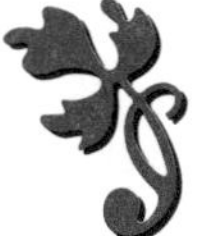

The cause of eczema is unknown, although allergies may play a role in triggering outbreaks. Find relief with a remedy below

Eczema is an inflammation of the skin and is most commonly equated with the medical term atopic dermatitis. It is characterized by red, oozing, and sometimes crusty lesions on the face, the scalp, the extremities, and the diaper area in infants. The lesions may also become infected with bacteria or other microorganisms, and infection with herpes virus can cause serious illness. Stress, food allergens, scratching, bathing, and sweating may also induce attacks.

Conventional treatment includes avoidance of triggers and administration of antihistamine topical steroid creams and antibiotics for infections of the eczema lesions. Alternative medical treatments include avoidance of triggers; optimizing vitamin, mineral, and essential fatty acid nutrition to reduce tendency to develop inflammation; internal or topical applications of anti-inflammatory or soothing herbs; and administration of bitter herbs to "stimulate the liver" and optimize digestion.

In alternative medicine, it is believed that to heal the skin, you must heal the digestive tract as well. Thus, a three-way link that exists between the liver, the digestive tract, and the skin is a key tenet of alternative medicine for treating allergic eczema and other skin inflammations. One physiological basis for this theory may be the detoxifying role of the liver. The liver normally transforms toxic substances so they can be excreted from the body either in the form of bile from the liver or as urine. If the liver is not doing its job, toxic substances may circulate freely in the body and irritate the skin "from the inside out."

The folk treatments below include bitter herbs to stimulate the liver and digestive tract, anti-inflammatory herbs for both internal and external use, astringent and disinfectant herbs for topical use, and treatments with water and clay.

Remedies

NETTLE AND DANDELION: A Gypsy folk remedy for eczema uses a combination of two "blood purifying" herbs (see "Blood Purifiers and Blood Builders," page 82) that are traditionally prescribed to treat skin conditions. Stinging nettle *(Urtica dioica, U. urens)* has been used by at least seven American Indian tribes—from the northeastern United States to the Pacific Northwest and down to Mexico—as an aid for healing skin conditions. Stinging nettle is used for the same purpose in traditional European herbalism. A recent clinical trial showed that nettle was effective for treating hay fever, and recent laboratory research has identified its anti-inflammatory and anti-allergic constituents.

Dandelion root is traditionally considered to be a "liver" herb—its use in this country is consistent with the traditional idea of treating skin ailments through the liver (see introduction to this section, above). It has been used to treat skin conditions by several American Indian tribes, including the Iroquois of the northeastern United States, the Aleuts of the Pacific Northwest, and the Tewa of the Southwest. The German government has approved the medicinal use of dandelion root as a "cholagogue," a medicine that increases the flow of bile from the liver. Constituents in dandelion have also been found to protect the liver and to enhance its detoxifying ability. Dandelion contains both antioxidant and anti-inflammatory constituents.

☞ Directions: Place 1 ounce of dandelion root and 1 ounce of nettle leaf in a pot, and cover with 3 pints of water. Bring to a boil and then simmer, covered, on low heat for forty minutes. Let cool to room temperature. Drink 3 cups a day. Do this for three weeks, and then take a break for seven to ten days before starting again.

BURDOCK ROOT: In the traditional herbalism of Europe and North America, burdock *(Arctium lappa, A. minus)* is probably the most well-known for treating skin complaints such as acne, boils, or eczema. It has been used to treat skin conditions by several American Indian tribes, including the Cherokee, Iroquois, Menominee, Micmac, Nanticoke, and Penobscot. Burdock is used today in folk medicine as a "blood purifier" among Pennsylvania Germans, the Amish, Indiana farmers, and throughout Appalachia. Burdock was an official medicine in the *United States Pharmacopoeia* from 1831 until 1842, and again from 1851 until 1916; it was prescribed as a diuretic, mild laxative, and treatment for skin ailments.

Modern scientific studies show that constituents in burdock root have anti-inflammatory properties. Its constituent polysaccharide inulin, which can make up 50 percent of the root by weight, provides food for the "friendly" strains of bacteria in the gut and may thus help reduce the toxic load on the liver and skin by reducing toxicity in the bowels.

For some individuals, however, burdock can worsen eczema. Perhaps this is because burdock promotes light sweating, and sweat can trigger eczema in some people. If you find that burdock makes your eczema worse, stop using it immediately and try a different remedy.

☞ Directions: Put 1 ounce of burdock root in 1 quart of water. Bring the water to a boil and simmer, covered, for forty minutes. Drink the quart throughout the day. Burdock is a mild herb and can be consumed this way for long periods of time.

YELLOW DOCK: Yellow dock *(Rumex crispus)*, like dandelion and burdock, is a traditional bitter, liver-stimulating herb. The Aleut, Cherokee, Cheyenne, Iroquois, Navaho, and Shoshone Indians, as well as other American Indian tribes, used it to treat skin ailments. It was a folk remedy for treating eczema of residents of the eastern states in the 1800s. It was listed in the *United States Pharmacopoeia* from 1860 until 1890; physicians of the last century used it to treat chronic skin ailments. It is still used today for this purpose in the Southwest.

☞ Directions: Make a tincture of yellow dock by placing 4 ounces of the dried root in a 1-quart jar and filling the jar with 100 proof vodka or gin. Let stand for three weeks, shaking the jar once a day. Strain and store in a cool dark place. The dose is 2 to 3 droppers twice a day, taken in a cup of warm water. Alternately, you can purchase a tincture of yellow dock at a health food or herb store.

BAKING SODA BATH: Contemporary Seventh Day Adventists recommend treating eczema by taking a baking soda bath. In New England, the same treatment is used for relieving hives and other skin conditions.

☞ Directions: Place a few handfuls of baking soda in warm bath water and take a long soak.

FRINGE TREE BARK: A contemporary Appalachian treatment for eczema is taking fringe tree bark *(Chionanthus virginicus)*. This bitter, liver-stimulating herb was one of the top ten most-often prescribed herbs by the Eclectic physicians in 1920; they used it to treat liver diseases in particular. American Indians used it externally on cuts, wounds, and skin inflammations. (Use external applications to treat eczema.)

Though fringe tree bark has been studied very little by modern scientists, its reputation persists thanks to its former popularity. Internal use requires a tincture. Use as a tea when applying as an external wash.

☞ Directions: Purchase a tincture of fringe tree bark at a health food store. Take a dropperful 3 times a day for seven to ten days. Discontinue if any digestive discomfort develops.

To apply as an external wash, simmer 1 tablespoon of the bark in a cup of boiling water for fifteen minutes. Strain and, using gauze, apply to the eczema.

OREGON GRAPE ROOT AND YELLOW DOCK: American Indian tribes in the North Central and Pacific Northwest states took Oregon grape internally to treat the digestive tract and applied it externally to treat skin conditions. The Cowlitz Indians applied it externally as a disinfectant; today, physicians in Germany use it in the same way for treating psoriasis.

The contemporary Amish use a combination of Oregon grape root *(Berberis aquifolium)* and yellow dock root *(Rumex crispus)* for treating eczema. Oregon grape, like yellow dock, is considered in contemporary British and North American herbalism to be a liver herb, and its constituents berberine, berbamine, and oxyacanthine all promote the flow of bile.

☞ Directions: Purchase a tincture of Oregon grape root and some capsules of powdered yellow dock root. Take 1 dropper of the Oregon grape tincture and 4 capsules of the yellow dock root three times a day until the eczema is relieved. In addition, dilute 1 ounce of the Oregon grape tincture with 5 ounces of water, and apply the diluted solution, using gauze or a clean cloth, to the eczema.

HONEY: Honey is a traditional remedy for infected eczema throughout Asia. Honey is also used by Chinese Americans. Honey is a powerful disinfectant and has been used by conventional physicians in both France and India as a disinfectant for burns.

☞ Directions: Cover gauze with a layer of honey, place over the eczema, and

continued on page 198

Witchcraft

There was once a child who was sick for weeks and who was becoming constantly weaker. His parents took him to doctors, but the experts could not diagnose his problem. Finally, a neighbor woman, one who was wise in spiritual matters, came to visit. She told the parents that, because the child had been bewitched by a woman in the neighborhood, the doctors wouldn't be able to help him. She told them to look inside the child's pillow. Some of the pillow's feathers, the parents found, had been woven together, forming nearly a complete wreath. According to the neighbor woman, the only reason the boy was still alive was because the wreath had not been completed. The family removed the feather wreath and pounded on it until it was in pieces. The next day, a woman in the neighborhood was found to have bruises all over her body—she was the one who had bewitched the boy. The boy recovered fully.

This story, told in similar forms in every region in the United States, illustrates many important points about witchcraft beliefs and folk medicine. Witchcraft is an explanation that is used when all else fails. Witchcraft comes to be suspected when a sickness does not respond to the doctor's medicines or common folk medicines. There is often some physical evidence of the witchcraft found near the sick person—in this case, the feather wreath. The treatment for the witch's spell often sends the spell back on the person who cast it, causing injury or death.

A witch is an individual who has supernatural powers. The belief in such people is found all over the world. There is a general agreement that their powers include predicting the future; changing their own form (or the forms of others), especially into animals; flying (either physically or by leaving the body behind); becoming invisible; and knowing the correct drugs and charms to use to make someone sick or well, to make others fall in love, and to create fertility or infertility. Some or all such powers have been attributed to medicine men, wise women, shamans, priests and priestesses of many religions, and all sorts of spiritually powerful individuals. Early Christianity, as it encountered other religions, taught that all such people and their practices were evil. By the Middle Ages, the idea had become firmly established that people who had such powers got them by bargaining with the Devil or other evil spirits. The person doing the bewitching was often, though not always, believed to be a woman. Midwives, in particular, were often accused.

The assistance of male physicians at births was not common until about 100 years ago. Prior to that time, and in most cultures, women were the birth attendants. Those who specialized in assisting other women in labor were called "midwives." (These women also offered a variety of other traditional women's health care, often providing help for the infertile as well as providing traditional methods for preventing conception and using both herbal and magical means to produce abortion.)

Birth is a very private time. It was also a very dangerous time in the years when infant and maternal mortality were high. The knowledge shared by the midwives and the other women (sisters, mothers, daughters, and neighbors) attending the births was unknown and mysterious to male members of society. This situation created great political tension in the societies dominated by men. Because midwifery, like the rest of folk medicine, included many charms and magical procedures, midwives were also viewed as particularly suspicious characters—especially by the Christian Church where the male ministers and priests were naturally excluded from attendance at births.

One of the most common magical practices for easing childbirth, found in the folk medical traditions of societies in many parts of the world, is the untying of all knots and opening of all doors and boxes in the vicinity of the laboring woman. This is an obvious kind of sympathetic magic. The Church condemned it as a diabolical practice and as typical of the kind of practices taught by midwives. As official medicine took over birth attendance through obstetrics, midwifery also experienced a great deal of legal pressure. Today, licensed nurse midwives practice legally in many parts of the United States, but there are also many non-licensed "lay" midwives, whose practices include a great deal of folk medicine. Even among licensed midwives, the use of herbs and other folk and alternative medical practices are much more common than in the labor and delivery rooms of hospitals! Although witch trials are no longer a threat for the midwife, religious as well as medical opposition to the practice continue in many places.

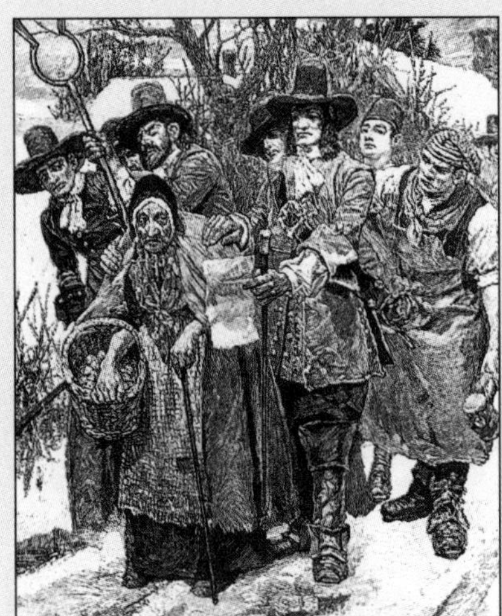

Healers and midwives were often accused of witchcraft.

Men have also been accused of witchcraft, especially men to whom extraordinary healing powers are attributed. It is widely believed that if a person can use supernatural power to heal, it would be easy to use the power to harm. Although there is no doubt there are individuals in most cultures who prefer to be feared, and who therefore encourage their reputation as evil sorcerers, many healers who are accused of witchcraft are only practicing their own religious views and trying to help their neighbors. Many people believe that this has always been true of witches, arguing that the idea of the "wicked witch" is a Christian invention used to suppress the pagan religions it encountered, especially when women were powerful figures in those religions. That is why today there are groups of modern witches who describe their tradition as part of "the old religion." These people, who often call their religion by the Old English word for witch—"wicca"—believe in spirits in nature and practice magic intended to promote healing and peace. They generally oppose any effort to employ magical or spiritual means to cause anyone harm. These "modern witches," though criticized in many ways by people who do not share their beliefs, are far from evil.

cover with tape or a bandage. Change the dressing every two hours until the infection is gone.

THYME: Another traditional Chinese folk remedy for treating eczema is to wash the affected area with a tea of thyme leaves *(Thymus vulgaris).* Thyme leaves contain about 2 percent thymol, a volatile constituent that has strong antiseptic and anti-inflammatory properties.

☞ Directions: Place 1 ounce of thyme leaves in a 1-quart canning jar and fill with boiling water. Cover tightly to prevent the thymol from escaping with the steam. Let cool to room temperature. Apply to eczema with gauze or a clean cloth three or four times a day. If you find the remedy irritating, dilute it in half and try again.

ECHINACEA: When applied externally, echinacea *(Echinacea angustifolia, E. purpurea)* has disinfectant, anti-inflammatory, and wound-healing properties. Taken internally, it increases natural resistance to both viral and bacterial infections. Subsequent research has shown that it has immune-stimulating properties. To the Plains Indians, echinacea was the panacea for all ills. Echinacea is now commonly prescribed by physicians in Europe for both internal and external uses.

☞ Directions: Make your own tincture of echinacea by purchasing 4 ounces of the root. Chop or grind the root in a coffee grinder and place it in a 1-quart jar. Cover with 100 proof vodka. Let stand for three weeks, turning the bottle each day. Then strain and store in a cool dark place. Dilute 1 ounce of the tincture with an equal amount of water and use as a wash on the eczema.

YARROW: Yarrow *(Achillea spp.)* is used as a universal treatment for skin ailments (including infected wounds) by the American Indians. In fact, a database of American Indian ethnobotany at the University of Michigan records the use of yarrow by 24 tribes for remedying skin conditions.

Yarrow contains the constituents azulene and chamazulene, both of which are antiallergic and anti-inflammatory. A strong tea of yarrow has been found to be more effective than steroid creams to suppress eczema. As with steroid creams, however, as soon as the treatment is stopped, the eczema returns. Thus, internal remedies as well as identification and removal of triggers are important for long-term healing.

☞ Directions: Place 1 ounce of yarrow leaves in a 1-quart canning jar and fill with boiling water. Cover tightly to prevent the active constituents from escaping with the steam. Let cool to room temperature. Apply with gauze to the eczema three or four times a day.

CHAMOMILE: Today, residents of Mexico and the American Southwest use a wash of chamomile tea *(Matricaria recutita)* to treat skin infections. The Cherokee Indians used chamomile to remedy afflictions of the skin as well.

For some individuals who are allergic to chamomile itself, however, chamomile can cause an allergic skin rash. If you are allergic to it, try using yarrow instead, which contains the same key constituents but belongs to another plant family and is not as likely to provoke an allergic response.

☞ Directions: Place 1 teaspoon of chamomile flowers in a cup and fill with boiling water. Cover and let stand for ten minutes. Strain well, cool, then apply several times a day.

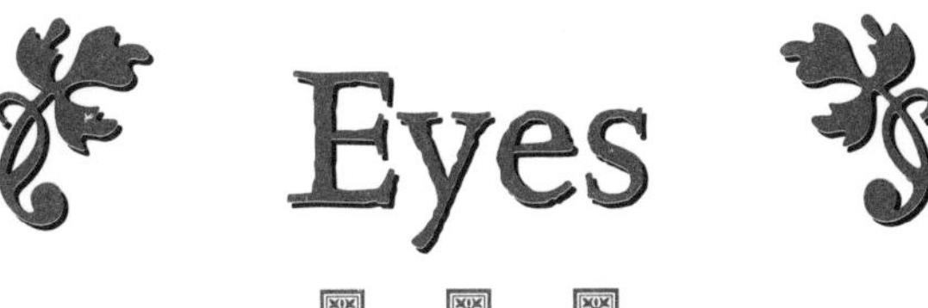

Eyes

The most common folk remedies for the eyes help to relieve soreness and infection. Soothe your eyes with one of the remedies below

Conjunctivitis, or pinkeye, is an inflammation of the conjunctiva. The conjunctiva is a delicate membrane that lines the inner surface of the eyelid and covers the exposed surface of the eye. Most cases of conjunctivitis result from disease-causing microorganisms such as bacteria, fungi, and viruses. Allergies, chemicals, dust, smoke, and foreign objects that irritate the conjunctiva may also lead to conjunctivitis. (Occasionally a sexually transmitted disease can cause pinkeye if the eyes are rubbed after touching infected genital organs. Herpes simplex keratitis is a painful viral infection of the cornea of the eye that can result in blindness if not treated.)

Most cases of conjunctivitis in North America are caused by viruses. In Asia and the Mediterranean region, however, eye infections are commonly caused by the organism *Chlamydia trachomatis.* Known as trachoma, this persistent infection can cause scarring and excessive drying of the membranes around the eyes and lead to blindness.

Conventional treatment depends upon the cause and resulting symptoms of the conjunctivitis. If the inflammation is environmentally caused, simply removing the irritant may be sufficient to eliminate the condition. For more difficult cases, a physician may prescribe antibiotics, steroids, or combination eyedrops to be used several times a day as directed.

A most important fact about conjunctivitis is that its infectious form is highly contagious. Individuals with infective conjunctivitis should not share handkerchiefs, towels, or washcloths. You should be careful to avoid touching the unaffected eye after touching or rubbing the infected eye because it can easily become infected as well.

The most common folk remedies for the eyes focus on relieving infected, sore, or tired eyes as well as removing irritating objects. (Of course, caution should be used when removing a foreign object from the eye. Sometimes even small objects can tear the surface of the eyeball or cornea, and infection can result. So use common sense, and if the irritation is severe, soreness persists after removal of the object, or infection or inflammation follow the incident, seek prompt medical advice.) The folk treatments for treating conjunctivitis commonly employ drying substances, which give tone to swollen membranes around the eyes. Some of the herbs recommended also have antibacterial, antiviral, and anti-inflammatory properties.

Any persistent eye irritation or infection requires a medical checkup.

Remedies

TEA: Tea is used to treat eye conditions in the folk medicine of southern Appalachia; it is used in the folk medicine of India and Asia as well. Tea and tea leaves are used to treat all types of eyes irritations and infections, including runny eyes, conjunctivitis, particles in the eye, swollen eyelids, sticky eyelids, and eyes red from a hangover.

Tea is a virtual pharmacy of chemical constituents: The leaves contain 34 antibacterial substances, 16 antiviral substances, and 24 anti-inflammatory constituents. Tea leaves also have a strong astringent action, which soothes infected membranes.

☞ Directions: Make a tea using black or green tea bags or by adding 1 teaspoon of tea leaves to 1 cup of boiling water. Apply a tea-soaked cloth, a used tea bag, or wet tea leaves to the eyes. Keep in place ten to fifteen minutes. Repeat as desired.

WITCH HAZEL: Although eastern American Indians have used witch hazel *(Hamamelis virginiana)* to treat a variety of conditions, the Chippewa Indians used it specifically to treat sore, inflamed, or infected eyes. Contemporary New England folk medicine continues to use witch hazel in this manner.

Witch hazel is a tree native to North America. After colonists learned its importance from the Indians, its use for healing spread to Europe, where it is still prescribed today in professional British herbalism and in conventional German medicine. The German government, after reviewing scientific evidence, has approved its use for minor inflammations of the skin and mucous membranes. Witch hazel products are available in most drug stores and health food stores.

☞ Directions: Purchase witch hazel leaves at a health food store or herb shop. Do not use commercial alcohol-based preparations—the alcohol will irritate your eyes. Place 1 teaspoon of the leaves in a cup and fill with boiling water. Cover and let stand until the water reaches room temperature. Moisten a cloth in the tea and apply to shut eyes.

ROSE: Today, rose *(Rosa spp.)* is among the most often prescribed herbs in Unani Tibb, which is contemporary Arabic medicine. The use of rose as an eyewash may well have come to the American Southwest by way of the Arabs. The Arabs, who controlled Spain for the 800 years preceding the Spanish colonization of North America, had a profound effect on Hispanic culture and medicine.

Rose petals have a strong astringent action, toning up swollen and inflamed mucous membranes. This is their chief medicinal use in Arabic medicine.

Hispanics in northern New Mexico use rose petal tea as an eyewash. The rose oil in the leaves contains 15 bactericidal, 9 antiviral, and 7 anti-inflammatory constituents.

☞ Directions: Obtain rose petals from wild or garden-cultivated roses that are free of pesticides and chemicals. (Most commercial roses are sprayed with a variety of chemicals.) Place a handful of petals in a jar and add 1 pint of boiling water. Cover well to retain the aromatic oils, and let stand until the water reaches room temperature. Apply to the eyes with a clean cloth.

Pass the Cream

A New England remedy for treating a wide variety of eye problems—including tired, sore, itchy, ulcerated, or infected eyes—is to put a few drops of milk or cream in the eye. In the past, American Indians of the Rappahannock tribe used human breast milk in the same way. Today, contemporary residents of the southern Appalachians use the breast milk method. Human breast milk contains antibodies against many organisms and may help fight a local infection of the eye.

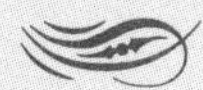

POTATO POULTICE: A remedy recorded in folklorist Clarence Meyer's collection of remedies, called *American Folk Medicine,* is the potato poultice. Presumably, the starch in the potato acts to soothe the inflammation in the eye. Small amounts of a number of other anti-inflammatory constituents are also present in the potato.

The potato is native to the Andes mountains in South America. Its use as a food spread throughout Europe in the 1700s. It is used today in European folk medicine to soothe painful joints, headaches, and other inflammatory conditions.

☞ Directions: Remove the skin from a whole, raw potato. Wash the potato and dry well. Grate as fine as possible. Place inside a clean cloth and fold to make a poultice. Place the poultice over the inflamed eye for fifteen minutes.

EYEBRIGHT: Eyebright *(Euphrasia officinalis)* is a plant native to Europe that traditionally has been used to treat conjunctivitis and other eye infections. It was first listed in British herbals in the 1500s, with the annotation that its flowers look like small yellow eyes. It is used as an eye remedy today in the folk medicine of Appalachia.

Like many of the other plants in this section, eyebright has both astringent and anti-inflammatory properties that may reduce inflammation in mucous membranes. Eyebright is very drying, so it should be used only on eye conditions that involve mucus or discharge. (It could increase the discomfort of dry, irritated eyes.) For this reason, the use of eyebright for eye problems has been discouraged by some authorities.

Here are directions for using eyebright from a German medical text called *Lehrbuch der Phytotherapie (Herbal Medicine)* by R.F. Weiss, M.D. The text is used in German medical and pharmacy schools.

☞ Directions: Place 1 tablespoon of eyebright leaves in 1 pint of water. Cover and simmer for ten minutes. Strain and apply to the eyes with a clean cloth. At the same time, pour the tea into a cup and drink. Do this twice a day.

GOLDENSEAL: During the second decade of the 19th century, American botanist Constantine Rafinesque traveled among the

continued on page 203

The Evil Eye

One of the most widespread folk beliefs in the world is the belief in the power of the "evil eye." Although explanations vary slightly, most people who hold this belief say that certain individuals have the power to cause evil to others just by way of looking at them. The person who casts the evil eye may not even know they are doing it. The most common cause for "overlooking," or putting a spell on someone, is envy. For example, if someone with "the power" envies another's good fortune, she may put the gaze on the person she envies. Her power results in bad luck or ill health for the person she "overlooked."

Children and pregnant women are considered to be likely targets for this kind of cursing. Not only are they naturally vulnerable, but someone with the power may well envy them. Praising a child without also touching or pinching him can be seen as a dangerous action. Sometimes a person who has complimented a child will spit or add a phrase like, "I mean no harm," to stop any unintentional envy she may be feeling.

The evil eye is a supernatural method of causing illness. As a result, virtually all preventions and treatments for evil eye also involve supernatural beliefs and practices. Cures are usually performed by women who have had the healing secrets told to them by older healers. Many people fear, however, that those women who can remove the curse can also cast the evil eye.

A wide variety of charms can be used to deflect the power of the evil eye. An amulet in the shape of an eye, a heart, a hand in a protective gesture, or a red horn can be worn as a defense. Garlic, salt, or written copies of religious texts can also be worn.

Hand gestures are among the most common ways of warding off "wasting sickness" and bad luck associated with the evil eye. Here's one gesture you can use when you believe the evil eye has been cast upon you: Point down with your index finger and pinkie finger extended straight and your thumb holding the middle two fingers down.

Colors That Protect

Red and blue are favorite colors for warding off the sicknesses and bad fortune caused by the evil eye. Among Christians and Jews in North and South America, red ribbons are attached to children's clothing or hair for this purpose. Some Christians will even embroider red crosses into children's underclothing as a hidden protection. In Europe and the Mediterranean, blue stones are often used as charms to deflect the negative power of the evil eye. One account even suggests tying a red ribbon to a new car to prevent it from being damaged by others' envy.

Treating Trachoma

Both goldenseal (*Hydrastis canadensis*) and Oregon grape root (*Mahonia aquifolium, Berberis aquifolium*) contain the constituent berberine. Berberine is used in Asia to treat eye infections caused by the organism *Chlamydia trachomatis*. This infection, called trachoma, is the most common cause of blindness in southern and southeastern Asia. Berberine sulfate was found in one clinical trial to be more effective than the most commonly used pharmaceutical antibiotic for the condition, especially when it is used to prevent recurrences. Berberine sulfate is also used to treat diarrheal infections in Asia.

Neither of the above plants have been tested in clinical trials in this country for their ability to treat trachoma, but both have been used to treat this condition in American folk medicine—goldenseal in the eastern United States where it grows, and Oregon grape root in the western states.

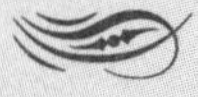

American Indians of the Ohio River and Mississippi River valleys, recording their uses of plants. His work resulted in *Medical Flora,* the first scientific book of medical botany in the United States. In his research, Rafinesque discovered that the Indians in the Midwest used goldenseal as a specific treatment for sore, inflamed, or infected eyes. They made an eyewash by boiling the root in water. This and other uses for goldenseal were quickly adopted by the European settlers in the eastern United States. A goldenseal eyewash is still used today in the folk traditions of Appalachia.

Part of goldenseal's medicinal action on the eyes is due to its constituents hydrastine and berberine (see sidebar). Like several other remedies in this section, it also has an astringent effect on swollen mucous membranes. Goldenseal is an endangered species in this country due to loss of habitat, overharvesting, and widespread use by the American public, who mistakenly take it as a treatment for cold and flu. In fact, treating eye infections is one of the few legitimate medical uses for goldenseal. Because goldenseal is no longer readily available, other berberine-containing herbs, including Oregon grape root, are less expensive, yet still effective, substitutes.

☞ Directions: Boil a handful of goldenseal root in 1 quart of water for twenty minutes. Let cool to room temperature. Apply to the eyes with a clean cloth.

OREGON GRAPE ROOT: A tea of the roots or leaves of Oregon grape root *(Mahonia spp., Berberis aquifolium)* was used as an eyewash by American Indians of both the mountainous American Southwest and the Pacific Northwest. The use of Oregon grape root for this purpose eventually spread to the settlers in those areas. Oregon grape root contains the alkaloid berberine, which acts as an antibiotic when used topically.

☞ Directions: Place ½ ounce of Oregon grape root in a pot and add 1 pint of boiling water. Let cool to room temperature. Apply to the eyes with a clean cloth.

CHRYSANTHEMUM BLOSSOMS: A Chinese treatment for tired, bloodshot, or sore eyes is a tea of dried chrysanthemum flowers.

Chrysanthemum *(Chrysanthemum indicum flos.)* is a popular beverage among Asians in the United States and can be found in almost any Asia market. The Chinese name for chrysanthemum is yeh-chu-hua, or simply chu-hua.

Chinese and Japanese researchers have found constituents in chrysanthemum tea that inhibit staphylococcus bacteria, a common cause of eye infection in some parts of the world. Chrysanthemum is also effective against a wide variety of other bacteria and viruses.

☞ Directions: Obtain chrysanthemum flowers from a health food store, herb shop, or Asian market. Purchase the whole dried flowers instead of a prepared tea. (The prepared products usually contain sugar or other additives that are not appropriate to put into the eyes.) Place a large handful of the flowers in a pot and add 1 quart of boiling water. Cover and steep for ten minutes. Strain, setting aside the still-warm flowers. Drink a cup of the tea. Wrap the still-warm flowers in a clean cloth, and, while lying down, apply to the eyes until the flowers cool.

URINE THERAPY: A North Carolina remedy for infected eyes—that is also used by Hispanic cowboys of the American Southwest—is to bathe the eyes in urine. Urine therapy for cleansing wounds and treating infection has appeared in the ancient medical systems of Mexico, Egypt, Persia, India, and China and in 17th and 18th century Europe.

Modern science suggests reasons why urine may be an effective disinfectant. Urine from a healthy person is as sterile as boiled water and thus is safe to apply to infected areas. Urine contains the substance urea, a disinfectant used today in pharmaceutical preparations to clean and disinfect burns

Whether Rain or Snow

Folk wisdom from throughout Appalachia calls for washing infected eyes with fresh rainwater or melted snow. The water, if collected carefully in a clean container, will not infect the eyes because it is sterile—not like the water collected from creeks or wells. The tradition tends to vary throughout the region. For example, some practitioners believe the remedy only works its magic if the rainwater is collected in the month of June. Others say the water must be collected during the first rain in May. Some Appalachians suggest that the remedy only works if water from the first frost or first snow of the year is used. Still others recommend using the last snow of the year or snow occurring in May.

Flaxseed

A common recommendation for removing tiny irritating objects from the eye is flaxseed. This method is found in the folk literature of North Carolina, Indiana, New England, and among the Michigan Amish. When flaxseed becomes moist, it also becomes very sticky. Small objects in the eye will adhere to the moistened flaxseed, making the object easier to remove. But the method should be used with caution, if at all, however. Sometimes even seemingly tiny objects in the eye can cause abrasions to the cornea. The tiny scratches can become infected and cause more serious eye problems. It's best to consult a doctor.

and wounds. Urea has strong drying properties and kills fungi, bacteria, and viruses by literally dehydrating them.

This may not be your remedy of choice for an eye infection, but it may come in handy if you have a serious eye infection while traveling in a third world country or are otherwise isolated from medical care.

☞ Directions: Allow about one third of the urine stream to pass. Catch the middle third in a cup or other container, and then let the last third pass as usual. The "middle catch" of urine is the most likely to be completely sterile. Apply warm to the eyes with a cloth.

EYE BATH: At the turn of the century, German immigrants recommended using an eye bath to remove objects from the eyes.

☞ Directions: Use a bowl large enough to completely immerse the face. Fill the bowl with cold water. Open the eyes underwater several times, until the object is washed out. Eye cups are still available in some pharmacies and are very convenient to use.

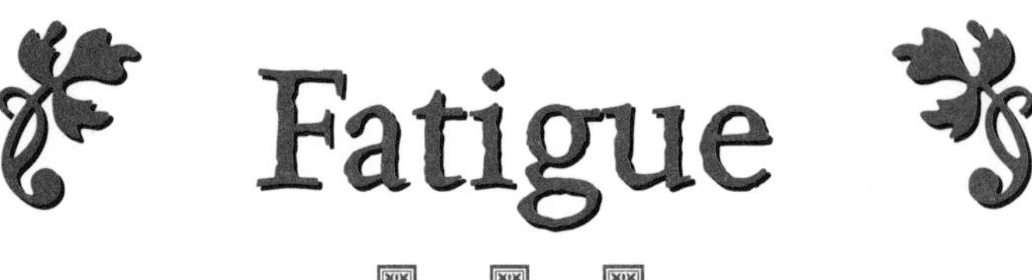

Fatigue

If you suffer from fatigue, try some of the folk remedies below—they're sure to get you moving again in no time

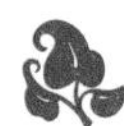

Fatigue may be physical or mental exhaustion, an overwhelming feeling of weariness, or a lack of energy and enthusiasm for even pleasant activities. Fatigue is a symptom of a vast number of diseases and disorders. More than 10 million people visit their doctors each year complaining of fatigue, making fatigue the seventh most common reason we make a doctor's appointment for a medical checkup. Between one-fourth and one-fifth of all Americans will seek medical advice for severe or chronic fatigue at some point in their lives.

The remedies in this section are appropriate for treating normal, brief periods of fatigue that are the result of some unusual stress or unexpected disruption of sleep. Any severe or long-lasting fatigue requires a medical checkup to determine the cause.

Fatigue and tiring rapidly with minimal activity are often among the early signs of an approaching illness. Fatigue is a warning sign of a variety of diseases and disorders, including the common cold, influenza, hepatitis, infectious mononucleosis, and other infectious diseases; heart disease; lung disorders, such as emphysema; some glandular diseases, such as diabetes; and anemia and nutritional deficiencies. Deficiencies of the minerals magnesium and zinc, the most common mineral deficiencies in the American population (affecting more than half of us), may cause fatigue in some people as well. Deficiencies of chromium, copper, folic acid, manganese, niacin, pantothenic acid, pyridoxine, thiamine, vitamin A, vitamin B_{12}, vitamin C, iron, and potassium may also be responsible. Overwork, either mental or physical, may also cause fatigue, as can psychological disorders or emotional stress. Sugar and caffeine consumption can also result in severe or chronic fatigue in some individuals.

Fatigue is best remedied by treating the physical disorder or psychological problem that is causing it. Some types of fatigue, particularly those due to physical overexertion, can probably be prevented by getting adequate exercise and rest. The average hours of sleep an American gets each night have been on the decline for the last 25 years. We now sleep an average of 7.5 hours a night. That's about an hour less than the average optimal amount of sleep. A third of Americans sleep less than six hours a night; many of them try to catch up by sleeping more on the weekends. A good alternative to sleeping more at night (or on the weekends) is to squeeze in naps during the day. Several folk traditions advocate napping on a regular basis to prevent or treat fatigue.

Remedies

BETONY: A folk source from 1824, listed in folklorist Clarence Meyer's *American Folk Medicine,* states that betony *(Stachys officinalis, Betonica officinalis)* is a good remedy for general debility that arises from disturbed digestion. The original source of this remedy was probably an immigrant from Europe, where betony had been used as a tonic since at least the time of the ancient Romans. In fact, the physician to the Emperor Augustus, who lived at the time of Jesus Christ's birth, listed 47 different diseases he thought betony would cure. The herb has remained so valued in Italy that a popular expression there advises you to "Sell your coat and buy betony."

Although betony is widely used in folk medicine in Europe even today, it has never been used to any extent by North American schools of medicine or by professional herbalists in North America. Betony is the first of the herbs in this section to be classified as a bitter tonic. Betony is also reputed to be a sedative, and its most common use in European herbalism today is for treating nervous tension, nervous headache, and accompanying exhaustion. Don't confuse this plant with North American betony *(Pedicularis spp.),* which grows in the mountainous

continued on page 210

Better Bitter Tonics

In North American herbal traditions, and in the medicine of the 19th century, bitter tonics have been one of the most often prescribed categories of herbs for fatigue and general debility. Bitter tonics are also commonly prescribed for these conditions by conventional physicians in Germany today.

Although these plants possess a mild to strong bitter flavor, they do not have strong medicinal properties. Many act as mild sedatives. The bitter principles in the plants stimulate the secretion of stomach acid and liver bile. Their reputed tonic effects may thus come from improved digestion and nourishment. (Because these herbs stimulate secretions, they are contraindicated if you have heartburn or other kinds of digestive pain.) The most famous of the bitter tonics in North American herbal history are goldthread *(Coptis trifola),* goldenseal *(Hydrastis canadensis),* Oregon grape root *(Mahonia aquifolium, Berberis aquifolium),* yellow dock *(Rumex crispus),* and dandelion root *(Taraxacum officinale).* Goldthread and goldenseal are practically extinct in North America, however. Betony, included in this section, is a common bitter tonic in British herbalism.

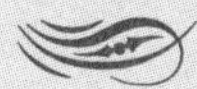

Sleep Paralysis

"What woke me up was the door slamming.... I was laying on my back just kinda looking up. And the door slammed, and I kinda opened my eyes. I was awake. Everything was light in the room.... But the next thing I knew, I realized that I couldn't move.... I kind of like gazed over to the door and there was no one there. But then from one of the areas of the room this grayish, brownish murky presence was there. And it kind of swept down over the bed and I was terrified!...It was like nothing I had ever seen before. And I felt—I felt this pressing down all over me. I couldn't breathe. I couldn't move. And the whole thing was that—there was like—I could hear the stereo in the room next to me. I was wide awake, you know.... And I couldn't move and I was helpless and I was really—I was really scared.... And this murky presence—just kind of—this was evil! This was evil!"

—Anonymous

Traditional beliefs that sickness and even death can be caused by a supernatural attack are universal. The account (at left) is typical: A person lying on their back is awakened by the sound of someone approaching, he finds he cannot move, and then he is aware of an evil presence that approaches and presses on him. It becomes difficult to breathe. The victim often fears that he will die, and he is overwhelmed by a sense of supernatural evil. What is surprising is that the young man in the previous quote had no idea that what had happened to him was actually a rather common occurrence.

The attack itself is an event medically called sleep paralysis. The paralysis is caused by a part of the brain that prevents movement during dream sleep so that the dreamer is not constantly awakened by movement. In sleep paralysis this same thing happens when a person is awake—just before falling asleep or just after waking up. Although the experience is terrifying, it is not dangerous. In fact, it is actually very common—at least one of six people have had sleep paralysis at least once—and it is not a symptom of disease.

Traditions vary on the causes and effects of these attacks. In the English-American tradition these attacks are believed to be the result of witchcraft. For example, during the Salem witchcraft trials, it was a common complaint that the alleged witch would enter the victim's sleeping chamber, paralyze him, and sit on his chest. This was called "witch riding," or "being ridden by a witch." Witches were once called "hags," so this attack was also called "hag riding." From this expression the phrase "hag rid" (that is, ridden by a hag) gradually evolved into the word haggard, meaning one who looks exhausted and disheveled—an understandable result of such attacks!

Many believe that this tiredness results from the stealing of their vital essence. Sometimes this is interpreted as theft of blood or of the soul. When the loss of blood or vital essence is believed to be involved, the attacker is often called a vampire. In the traditions of people from southeastern Europe, the vampire is generally believed to be a dead person who maintains an earthly existence by leaving his corpse in the grave and coming to his victims at night in a ghostly form. He magically removes either blood or vital energy from his helpless and frightened victims.

It is believed that the loss of blood or vital energy may result in sickness or in a weakened resistance to natural illnesses. In some traditions, including Mexican American and Arctic peoples, it is sometimes believed that one's soul can be taken. The loss of one's soul creates a very dangerous circumstance leading to chronic debilitation and eventual death. In Latino traditions such a victim is said to be *sustado*—without soul. The healer who helps such a person must either find the soul and lead it back or effectively call it back to its former owner.

Traditions found among some Filipino-American communities see the thief as more like a kind of witch; a living person who steals life substance. There are similar ideas among rural, southern African Americans (who use the English term "hag") and

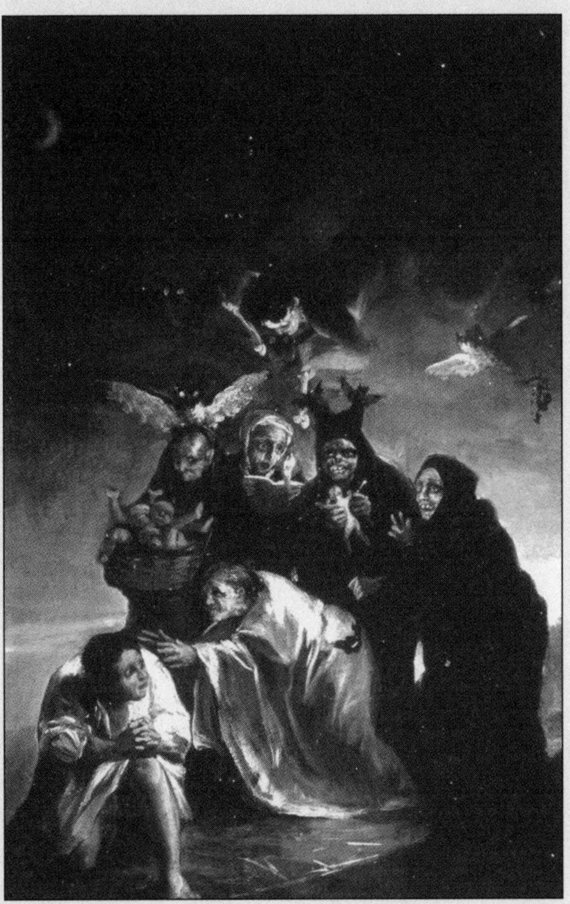

Sleep paralysis is believed to be caused by witchcraft.

some American Indian groups who describe their attacker using a term that can be translated as "skinwalker." The term skinwalker—or "slip skin"—is also sometimes found in various English-speaking traditions. A skinwalker is a person who can magically leave his skin behind either to become invisible or to put on an animal skin and travel as if he were a wolf or cat or other animal. Such "shape-shifting" is a common belief about witches, and it is frequently observed by victims of paralysis attacks. The earlier account (previous page), for example, describes a ghostly shape, but other victims describe very material-looking animals or people that sometimes change forms during the attack.

Sleep paralysis is indeed quite puzzling, even with all the current scientific knowledge about it. Why are the experiences so similar regardless of a person's beliefs and cultural background? Why do a majority of those who have had an attack insist that there was an evil presence with them during the paralysis? At present, no one knows. But knowing that the experience is found throughout humanity helps us to understand why some beliefs about sickness are universal and ancient.

areas of the West. *Pedicularis,* like *Stachys,* is a sedative, but does not have the bitter tonic properties.

☞ Directions: Place 1 tablespoon of betony leaves in a 1-pint jar and fill with boiling water. Cover and let cool until the water reaches room temperature. Drink the pint in 3 doses during the day, twenty minutes before meals, for seven to ten days.

NAPPING: The Amish have a saying that a half-hour nap in the afternoon is worth two hours of sleep at night. German immigrants at the turn of the century also advocated the afternoon nap, even if for only fifteen minutes, as an important way to restore energy and prevent exhaustion from overwork.

☞ Directions: Take a mid-to-late afternoon nap of fifteen minutes or more, lying down if possible.

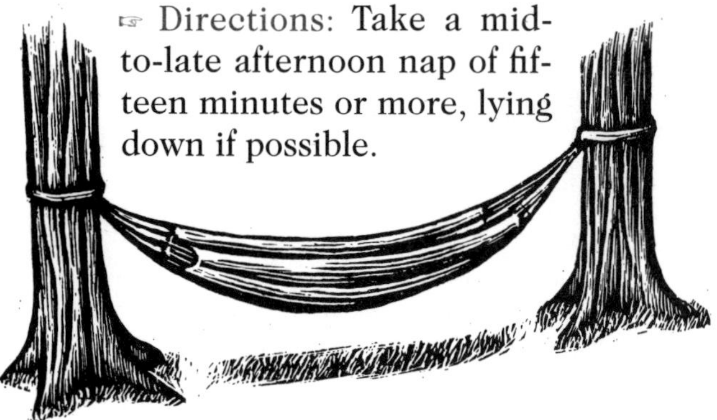

OREGON GRAPE ROOT: The American Indians of California and the Pacific Northwest used Oregon grape root *(Mahonia aquifolium, Berberis aquifolium)* to treat general debility. The herb acts as a bitter tonic. Although goldthread *(Coptis trifola)* and goldenseal *(Hydrastis canadensis)* are the most famous of the North American bitter tonics, these herbs have become practically extinct on the continent. Oregon grape root has become the most common substitute for these herbs among North American professional herbalists. Its action on the digestive system is due to its bitter alkaloid berberine, which is also present in goldthread and goldenseal.

☞ Directions: Place 1 tablespoon of Oregon grape root in 1 pint of water. Cover the pot and simmer for twenty minutes. Let cool to room temperature. Drink 1 ounce of the tea twenty minutes before meals for one to three weeks.

ASIAN GINSENG: Asian ginseng *(Panax ginseng)* has probably been used in Chinese folk medicine since about 3000 B.C. and remains the most famous and sought after herbal remedy in Chinese culture. In contemporary Chinese medicine, ginseng is used to restore strength when there is physical weakness or exhaustion resulting from a long-term illness. It is also used in folk medicine throughout the modern cities of China, Korea, Japan, and Southeast Asia to increase the individual's ability to resist the stresses of modern life.

Asian ginseng has been used in the folk medicine of Asian communities in North America for at least the last century. In the United States, it entered into mainstream society first through the counterculture movement of the 1960s and 1970s and then through the health food trade and the current natural healing movement.

Don't take Asian ginseng unless you are run down, because it can be overstimulating for a person with a normal energy level. Don't take it for chronic fatigue without first getting a thorough medical checkup, because the energy boost from the ginseng may simply temporarily mask the symptoms of a nutritional deficiency or a more serious underlying disease. And don't take ginseng if you also habitually use caffeine. If you begin to experience neck tension, insomnia, increased menstrual flow, or headaches, stop taking ginseng. Prolonged use after experiencing such symptoms can cause high blood pressure.

☞ Directions: Purchase a commercial ginseng product in a reputable herb shop. You'll generally find better quality ginseng there than in a health food store, supermarket, or pharmacy. Don't skimp on price—the more expensive products are usually the better quality products. Take 1 to 2 grams of ginseng powder a day, in 2 or 3 doses, for six weeks at a time. Take a two week break every six weeks.

Also, you can buy some whole ginseng roots—roots of average quality cost about $180 a pound in herb shops. An individual root costs between $6 and $12. Chop 4 ounces of the ginseng root and place in a quart of liquor such as vodka. Cover and let stand for five or six weeks in a cool dark place, turning the jar frequently. Don't strain. Take 1 ounce of the liquid each day, midmorning or just before lunch.

Adaptogens

An entire class of Chinese herbs—ginseng being the most famous of them—are used to restore the weary. These herbs and their beneficial actions were made more accessible to Westerners when Russian researchers investigated them in the decades after World War II. In fact, it was the Russians who coined the term "adaptogen." An adaptogen helps you "adapt" to different kinds of stress, whether from cold weather, overwork, or staying up at night with a crying baby. The Russians verified this adaptogen property in Asian ginseng, Siberian ginseng, schizandra berries, and several other herbs. Although they have been used in Asian communities in North America for more than a hundred years, these plants are now popular in various other communities throughout the United States as well. In fact, you can purchase various kinds of ginseng today in most pharmacies and supermarkets.

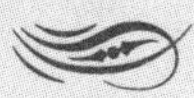

SIBERIAN GINSENG: Siberian ginseng *(Eleutherococcus senticosus, Acanthopanax senticosus)* has been used in Chinese medicine since the birth of Jesus Christ, but its properties as an adaptogen (see sidebar) were not clearly identified until after World War II. Russian ginseng researchers investigated the Siberian ginseng plant, looking for a less expensive alternative to Asian ginseng. Both animal and human trials showed that the plant increased response and adaptation to stress. The Siberian ginseng preparation remains a popular medicine in Russia today and is available over-the-counter. It is also sometimes prescribed by doctors in Europe.

The term Siberian ginseng was invented by marketers trying to sell the product in the United States in the 1970s, hoping to capitalize on the popularity of Asian ginseng. Siberian ginseng thus entered the folklore of North America through health food stores, and is now widely used in every region of the country. It is important to note that the *Eleutherococcus* plant is not actually a "ginseng," however, and it is nowhere near as powerful as Asian ginseng. But it is also less likely to cause overstimulation, insomnia, high blood pressure, or other side effects common to Asian ginseng. Because of its mildness, it is better suited for the average American than is Asian ginseng.

Unfortunately, much of the Siberian ginseng on the market is adulterated. The Canadian government recently examined three shipments arriving from Asia and found that two of them contained no *Eleutherococcus* at all; the other did, but also had 5 percent caffeine added. Most American products are also not made according to the specifications of the Russians and are weak by comparison to the Russian products, sometimes with only one-fifth the strength. For the best products, made according to the specifications of the Russian pharmacopoeia, look for a description such as "1:1 extract in 30% alcohol" on the label of the tincture bottle.

☞ Directions: Find a product matching the description above, and take a dropperful of the tincture three times a day for up to six weeks. Take a two-week break before starting another course of treatment.

AN EGG A DAY: Folklorist Clarence Meyer's collection of traditional American remedies called *American Folk Medicine* advises taking an egg a day to restore strength in cases of debility. Deficiencies of several nutrients—including iron, vitamin A, folic acid, riboflavin, and pantothenic acid—may cause fatigue. A single egg contains significant amounts of these nutrients.

☞ Directions: Beat a raw egg, flavor with a little sugar or honey, and drink it. If the texture is not appetizing, blend the egg in a glass of milk and drink it that way. Note: Some people caution that a raw egg may be contaminated with salmonella and should be cooked before eating.

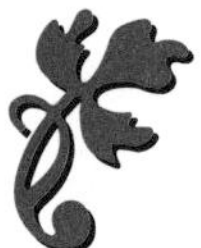

Fever

With the following remedies, you'll shed that fever faster

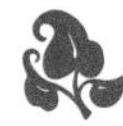

To understand what having a fever means, its helps to know something about how your body controls temperature. There is quite a range in what is considered "normal" in body temperature. (As you know, everyone has a temperature; when it rises above what is considered normal and stays there, it is then termed a fever.) The average human body temperature falls between 98°F and 98.6°F during daily activities, but normal temperatures can range anywhere between 97°F and 99°F. (And many healthy active children have normal temperatures as high as 99°F to 101°F.)

Your normal body temperature fluctuates about half a degree during the day, with the lowest reading usually occurring in the early morning and the highest in the late afternoon. The body temperature can be elevated to a range of 101°F to 105°F during fever (or during heavy exercise) and may also fall by about a degree below normal with exposure to cold.

Fever is regulated by a control center in the brain called the hypothalamus. The fever is activated when the hypothalamus senses tiny amounts of bacteria or bacterial toxins in the blood. The hypothalamus may also recognize chemical triggers in the blood that are sent out by white blood cells engaged in fighting off infection.

The hypothalamus is like the thermostat in your house—it is set for a certain temperature range. When it recognizes an infection or immune response, it turns the temperature up. Blood is shunted from the exterior of the body to the interior. As a result, the muscles may involuntarily shiver in order to replace the lost heat. Like a factory suddenly turned up to maximum production, the body's metabolism speeds up by as much as 30 percent in order to produce more white blood cells, antibodies, and other elements of the immune system. Once the infection is successfully fought off, the hypothalamus turns the thermostat back down and the body sweats to cool itself off.

Early in the 20th century, conventional doctors routinely suppressed all fevers with aspirin or related drugs. Modern medicine now recognizes that a fever is a beneficial healing response and mild fevers are no longer routinely suppressed. (Any fever that reaches 104°F or lasts more than three days requires prompt medical attention, however.) The best natural treatment for a simple fever is to support the body's response. Resting in bed, keeping warm, drinking plenty of liquids, and avoiding solid food helps the body to do its job to fight off the infection. Many of the folk remedies below help to induce a sweat to cool a fever.

Remedies

GINGER: A fever remedy popular in New England, Appalachia, North Carolina, Indiana, and China is ginger tea. Ginger tea is used to lower fever in the traditional medical systems of India and Arabia as well. Ginger *(Zingiber officinale)* induces sweating, which helps to cool the body during fever. It also contains many anti-inflammatory compounds, including some with mild aspirin-like effects. Thus, ginger may lower fever in more ways than one—it has both diaphoretic and anti-inflammatory effects. Several of these constituents in ginger have also shown to lower fever in animals.

☞ Directions: Thinly slice a fresh ginger root (the root should be about the size of your thumb). Place the ginger in 1 quart of water. Bring to a boil, then simmer on the lowest possible heat for thirty minutes in a covered pot. Let cool for thirty more minutes. Strain and drink ½ to 1 cup, sweetened with honey. Repeat three times a day as desired. As a precaution, don't take ginger in this dosage during pregnancy. (See "Pregnancy," page 324, for more details.)

PEPPERMINT: Peppermint *(Mentha piperita)* is a folk remedy used for fever in Indiana and by some Hispanics in the Southwest. In China, cornmint *(Mentha arvensis)*, a close relative of peppermint, is used in the same manner. Both plants, when taken as a hot tea, induce sweating, and help to cool a fever. Cornmint and peppermint also con-

Herbs That'll Make You Sweat

Many traditional folk remedies for fever are called *diaphoretics*—plants or foods that make you sweat. Constituents in the plants increase the blood circulation to the skin, which causes you to sweat (sweating helps cool the body during a fever). It is essential to drink plenty of fluids when taking these herbs, however, or dehydration may result. Anise, boneset, catnip, cinnamon, elder, ginger, mint, thyme, and yarrow are all reported diaphoretics. Take them as hot teas, go to bed, and wrap yourself in warm blankets. Continue to drink plenty of fluids.

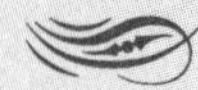

tain large amounts of antiseptic and cooling menthol. In addition, as the steamy hot tea is drunk and the fragrance is inhaled, the menthol may act as a decongestant. Thus, this treatment might be best for treating fever accompanied by congestion.

☞ Directions: Place ½ ounce of peppermint leaves in a 1-quart jar. Fill with boiling water and cover tightly. Let steep twenty minutes. While fever persists, strain and drink two or three cups a day. Wrap yourself in blankets and rest in bed after each cup.

ELDER FLOWERS AND BERRIES: Black elder *(Sambucus nigra)* is a famous flu and fever remedy from European traditional medicine. The plant's medicinal uses date back to the ancient Romans. Related elder species are native to North America. The Paiute and Shoshone Indians in the Rocky Mountains used the leaves and flowers of their local species for fevers, just as the Europeans used black elder. Elderberry was an official medicine in the *United States Pharmacopoeia* from the year of the book's founding in 1820 until 1909. The use of elder flower tea for fevers is still recorded in the folk medicine of the Amish, as well as in Indiana and by Hispanics in the Southwest.

The standard German medical textbook *Lehrbuch der Phytotherapie* describes elder as an immune stimulant. Elder flower tea is approved by the German government as a medicine for colds accompanied by cough. Recent research in Israel and Panama show that elderberry juice stimulates the immune system and can also significantly reduce the duration of an influenza attack.

The flowers contain anti-inflammatory constituents. (These constituents may also be present in other parts of the plant but have not yet been measured there. The bark and root of elder are very strong laxatives and should be avoided.) The flowers are traditionally taken as a tea, while the berries are made into syrups. Taking too much elder tea, however, whether in the form of flowers or berries, can bring about a feeling of nausea.

☞ Directions: Place ½ ounce of elder flowers in a 1-quart canning jar. Fill with boiling water. Cover and let steep for twenty minutes. Strain and pour a cup. Sweeten with honey. Take a cup every four hours for a fever, especially one accompanying the flu. Wrap yourself in warm blankets after drinking the tea. If the tea gives you a queasy feeling after a few doses, take less or stop taking it completely.

CATNIP: A fever remedy from the Seventh Day Adventists calls for drinking catnip tea while soaking the feet in hot water. Catnip *(Nepeta cataria)* is also a fever remedy in the folk traditions of New England and Appalachia. Catnip's warming aromatic substances are diaphoretic and help to induce a sweat. (Sticking the feet in hot water can induce sweating as well.) Catnip also purportedly acts as a sedative and may help you to rest and relax.

☞ Directions: Fill the bathtub or a smaller tub with hot water. Put the feet in the water while drinking the hot tea. (This remedy is contraindicated in diabetics because of the possibility of burning the feet.)

To make the tea, pour boiling water over 1 ounce of catnip leaves in a 1-quart jar. Cover tightly and let steep for ten to fifteen minutes. As the fever persists, soak your feet every three to four hours while drinking half a cup of the tea.

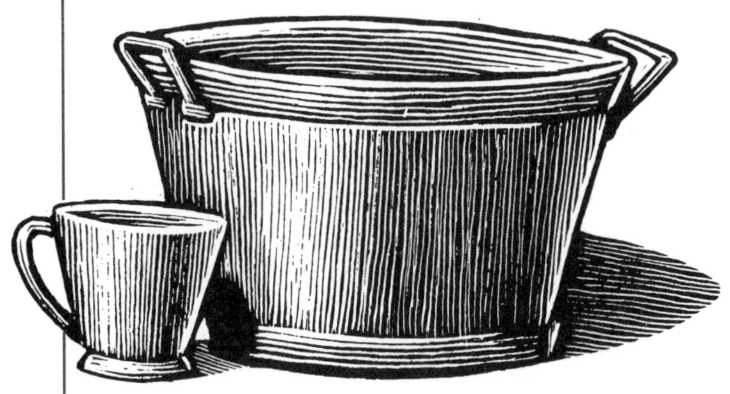

FEVERFEW: European scientific research investigated the folk use of feverfew *(Tanacetum parthenium, Chrysanthemum parthenium)* in the 1980s and early 1990s. As a result, the herb became popular in North American health food stores as a remedy for migraine headache. Feverfew is also famous in European and North American folk medicine—particularly in Indiana and Appalachia—as a treatment to lower fever (thus its name), reduce arthritis pain, or stimulate menstruation.

Research shows that its aromatic constituents contain anti-inflammatory properties that act similarly to corticosteroid drugs, although the constituents are not nearly as strong. The plant should be used as fresh as possible. If dried leaves are used, they should have a strong aroma and be prepared in a way that does not evaporate the leaves' aromatic constituents.

☞ Directions: Place ½ ounce of feverfew leaves in a 1-pint jar, fill with boiling water, and cover with a lid, tightly. Allow to steep for thirty to forty minutes. Drink half a cup every three to four hours.

BONESET: Traditional herbalist Tommie Bass of northern Georgia, who was the subject of a major study of Appalachian folk medicine during the 1980s, named the herb boneset *(Eupatorium perfoliatum)* as his favorite fever remedy. Boneset got its English name in the 1700s in Pennsylvania during an influenza epidemic. The flu was called "breakbone fever" in that area; the word breakbone referred to the fever's accompanying muscle aches and pains. Boneset proved to "set the bones" and relieve the muscle discomfort. The colonists learned the use of the plant from the Cherokee and Iroquois Indians and other eastern tribes.

continued on page 218

Jewish Folk Medicine in America

Prior to 1800, there were only about two or three thousand Jews in the United States. At the turn of the century, immigration began to increase slowly (especially from Germany), until the great wave of immigration began in the late 1800s. Between 1880 and 1930, over two million Jews (approximately one third of Eastern Europe's Jewish population), left Eastern Europe for America. Much smaller numbers came from the Mediterranean area. It is difficult to discuss Jewish culture. The groups within the culture are diverse, with different languages, customs, and experience. Yet the Jews remain a united people through a shared heritage of history and religion.

Throughout the centuries of diaspora the Jews adopted elements of the larger societies in which they settled, so that many folk beliefs they brought to the New World were the same as those of their non-Jewish neighbors. It is nevertheless possible to see distinctive themes in American-Jewish health lore, such as the emphasis on diet as a source of health. Many healing practices died out with the first generation of immigrants, however, because their better education and ability to read allowed them easier access to physicians and hospitals.

The folk cures that were specifically Jewish were, naturally enough, those associated with the Jewish religion. Names, for instance, have great significance in Judaism, which considers the ineffable name of God too sacred for human utterance. Thus, the name of a dangerously sick person, especially a child, might be changed. Some explain that this was done in order to deceive the Angel of Death, who would then be unable to find the person he had come for. Good choices for the child's new name were Chaim or Chiah, meaning "life"; Alter, meaning "long life" or "aged"; Baruch, meaning "blessed"; or Sarah, because the biblical Sarah lived to a ripe old age. The new name might be added as an extra or middle name. At one time the name change was made in a ritual religious event, but American sources describe more informal venues. It might be done by a rabbi on a hospital visit, a friend's errand to the temple, or at the grave of a relative.

A related custom was the "selling" of a sick child. Since children were identified by the parents' names as well as their own (Isaac, son of Abraham and Sarah), the Angel might only be diverted if it came looking for the couple and found they had no children! Thus, a symbolic "sale" of the child was made, usually to a couple who had healthy children. This might also be done with a new baby, if the couple had other unhealthy children or children who had died. The figure of the Angel of Death is not universally affixed to these cures; some people said it was evil spirits who had to be fooled.

Parents of a sick child could also visit the grave of a loved relative or grandparents to ask for their assistance. Less seriously ill children might be given an amulet to wear, which could consist of coral beads, coins or medals, or garlic or salt tied in cloth. The most common amulets were in the form of Hebrew writings—a kind of portable version of the mezuzah, or Hebrew prayer, that is traditionally affixed to doorposts of a home. (During World War I, many Jewish soldiers carried a mezuzah in their pockets.) Rabbis often opposed the use of amulets, which may be why amulets are said to be especially powerful if given by a pious person. Adults who were ill could make a present to the temple—a bible, perhaps, or their own weight in coal. Or they could promise to do something charitable.

The religious rites of Judaism have until very recently been in the hands of men. It is fascinating to read in anthropologist Melvin Firestone's book, called *Sephardic Folk-Curing in Seattle,* the description of healing practices, known as "endurcos," which were conducted almost solely among the Sephardim women of Seattle. The immigrants came from Rhodes early in the century. Although the rituals were no longer performed, some people still knew the words of the long incantations in Ladino (a kind of medieval Spanish) and the ceremonies, which could extend over several days. In this country, these rituals were used mostly to treat emotional problems, such as those conditions caused by the evil eye. These rituals had psychotherapeutic value, for in addition to the lengthiness of treatment, they often involved special foods, fasting, or isolation—all things that would make a dramatic break with the patient's previous state of mind. The practitioners, however, were not eager to pass their knowledge on. "The people have doctors in this country; they don't need it," one said.

Jewish tradition has always placed high value on learning and the written word. In medieval Europe, Jewish physicians were considered so superior that they were sought out even when their services were outlawed. Their very skillfullness, however, also made them feared as sorcerers. Jewish scholars translated important medical works, and compiled manuscripts of customs and remedies, which, in the age of print, became handbooks for the conduct of everyday life. In North America, the prestige of physicians and the absorption of Jewish immigrants into American culture, however, worked against the persistence of a distinctively Jewish folk medicine.

Jewish Women in Healing

Jewish women have traditionally dispensed the most famous Jewish folk medicine—chicken soup, which is sometimes referred to as "Jewish penicillin." But first-generation immigrant women sometimes had more specialized healing roles: A Cleveland woman of Russian-Jewish descent recalled that her grandmother was known as a "Sprecherke," or "one who can speak things," and that people came from all over town to have her pray over them, especially for toothache. And, in St. Louis early this century, a child who cried too much might be taken to an old woman who would "absprechen ein hora"—that is, act against the evil eye.

Constituents have been identified in boneset that are both immune-stimulating and anti-inflammatory. Today, boneset is used in the folk medicine of Indiana and southern Illinois as well as Appalachia. In Europe, boneset is used to treat colds and flu. Physicians in Germany use boneset to treat acute viral infections. Do not overdo it with boneset, however, because it can induce vomiting if taken in large quantities. Boneset was actually used for that purpose during the 18th and 19th centuries.

☞ Directions: Place 1 teaspoon of dried boneset leaves in a cup and fill with boiling water. Let steep for fifteen minutes. Strain and drink the cup while still warm. Go to bed immediately and wrap yourself in warm blankets. Don't take more than one cup every four hours and no more than three cups a day. Stop taking boneset tea if you begin to feel nauseous.

Starve a Fever

In the medicine of many North American Indian tribes, the standard treatment for fever was rest with either a liquid diet or no food at all. The admonition to "starve a fever" remains in many folk traditions today, including those of New England, the southern Appalachian mountains, and Indiana.

Starving a fever was also a firm tenet of early 20th century naturopathic medicine. Henry Lindlahr, M.D., N.D., the founder of a naturopathic medical school and a 200-patient nature cure hospital in Chicago, wrote in 1914 that a patient with a fever shouldn't eat "so much as a drop of milk" until the fever subsides. This approach, recorded in Lindlahr's book *Natural Therapeutics* (Volume II), has a sound physiological basis. Fasting reduces energy expenditures by the body that are normally required to produce digestive enzymes and absorb and eliminate the food. That energy can instead be used to fight the infection. Drinking plenty of liquids is important to prevent dehydration, however.

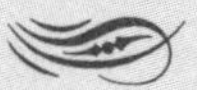

LEMON BALM: In Indiana, lemon balm *(Melissa officinalis)* is a folk remedy for fever. The plant, which was native to southern Europe and northern Africa, arrived with the colonists and spread throughout North America. It has been used as a relaxing and sweat-inducing herb at least since the 12th century in Germany, where it is approved today as a medicine for digestive complaints or sleeping disorders, though not specifically for fevers. Of the sweat-inducing herbs included in this section, lemon balm is probably the mildest herb and is the most suitable for use in children. Lemon balm is also a mild sedative and can help relax the restless patient with cold or flu.

☞ Directions: Pour boiling water over 1 teaspoon of the dried herb in a cup. Fill and let steep for ten minutes. While the tea is steeping, inhale the steam from the cup.

Mal Ojo

In the Hispanic traditions of the American Southwest, the "mal ojo" or "evil eye" is believed to be one possible cause of high fever. "Ojo" can occur when a person with a powerful gaze looks admiringly at someone without touching them. Children are most susceptible.

The symptoms of ojo can include sudden onset of high fever, vomiting, headache, fainting, or convulsions. The diagnosis of ojo can be made by examining the contents of a fresh egg that's broken after it's passed over the patient's body. If the contents of the egg appear to be cooked, or the yolk appears to have the image of an eye, the person is a victim of the strong person's gaze. The perpetrator must touch the patient as soon as possible to cure the condition. Various methods are used if that individual is not available. The condition caused by mal ojo can be prevented by making sure that, if a child is complimented, the caregiver is sure to touch him or her.

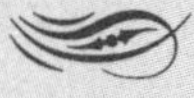

Strain and drink the tea, sweetened with honey as desired, up to four cups a day.

WILLOW BARK: The Greeks used willow bark *(Salix spp.)* to treat pain more than 2,400 years ago. American Indians of the Alabama, Chickasaw, Houma, Montagnais, Shoshone, and Thompson tribes and the Ninivak Eskimos were using willow bark for the same purpose before the arrival of the European colonists. Scientific investigations of willow bark during the 19th century led to the isolation of its pain-relieving and fever-lowering constituents, and, ultimately, to the synthesis of aspirin in 1898. (Willow bark itself does not contain aspirin, but similar milder compounds.)

Willow bark is used to lower fever or reduce pain in the folk medicine of Indiana, New England, and the Southwest, as well as by professional medical herbalists of North America and Great Britain. The German government has approved the use of willow bark by its conventional physicians for treating pain and fever. Besides its aspirin-like constituent salicin, willow bark contains other anti-inflammatory constituents as well.

☞ Directions: Purchase some willow bark capsules in a health food store or herb shop. Take as directed on the label. Alternately, place 2 teaspoons of powdered willow bark in a cup, fill with boiling water, and let steep for fifteen to twenty minutes. Sweeten with honey as desired, and drink up to four cups a day for as long as the fever persists.

HORSEMINT AND THYME: Both horsemint and thyme are stimulating diaphoretics; they induce sweating, which helps to reduce a fever. The herb horsemint *(Monarda punctata)* is used as a folk remedy for fever in Appalachia. Related *Monarda* species, such as bee balm *(Monarda menthafolium),* which grows in the Rocky Mountains, is used for the same purpose in the folk medicine of that region. Plants of the *Monarda* species contain large amounts of the aromatic constituent thymol, which has anti-inflammatory properties. Thymol is also a major constituent of garden thyme *(Thymus vulgaris)*.

Thyme tea is recommended as a treatment for fevers in the folk medicine of Indiana and China. Thymol is also a powerful antiseptic, and the vapors of thyme tea are inhaled in some folk traditions to kill the organisms that cause colds and flu. Thus, you may want to try thyme to help reduce fever that accompanies a cold.

☞ Directions: Put 1 teaspoon of dried thyme leaves in a cup and fill with boiling water. Let steep for five minutes while inhaling the fumes through both the nose and mouth. Then strain, sweeten with honey, and sip the tea slowly. Go to bed and bundle yourself in blankets.

HERBAL FORMULAS: According to *Herbal Medicine Past and Present* (Volume I), by John K. Crellin and Jane Philpott, a fever-reducing herbal formula from traditional Appalachian herbalist Tommie Bass of northern Georgia is a combination of equal parts of boneset *(Eupatorium perfoliatum)*, horsemint *(Monarda punctata)*, and catnip *(Nepeta cataria)*. Thyme leaves *(Thymus vulgaris)* can be substituted for horsemint.

☞ Directions: Place one handful each of the three herbs in a 1-quart jar and fill with boiling water. Cover tightly and let stand for twenty to thirty minutes. Take 1-cup doses of the tea every three to four hours. Be sure to drink plenty of liquids and wrap yourself in blankets.

YARROW: The ancient Greeks used yarrow *(Achillea millefolium)* to reduce fevers. The plant's use has persisted in Europe ever since. At least 18 American Indian tribes from all corners of the continent also used yarrow (and its close botanical relatives) for the purpose of reducing fever. The early colonists throughout North America used yarrow to treat a wide variety of ailments—most of them infectious or inflammatory in nature. Using yarrow tea to fight colds and flu survives today in the folk medicine of New York, Appalachia, North Carolina, Indiana, and the American Southwest.

☞ Directions: Place 1 ounce of dried or fresh yarrow in a 1-quart canning jar. Fill the jar with boiling water and cover tightly. Let steep for twenty minutes. Strain and pour a cup. Sweeten with honey. Take two or three cups a day while fever persists. Wrap yourself in blankets and rest in bed after each cup.

DANDELION: A common herb used to reduce fever in Chinese folk medicine is dandelion. (In traditional Chinese medicine, dandelion is classified as a "heat clearing" herb.) The Chinese dandelion *(Taraxacum mongolici)* and this country's common backyard dandelion *(Taraxacum officinale)* have similar appearances and constituents. Like many of the herbs in this category, dandelion contains several anti-inflammatory constituents. But, unlike the other herbs listed above, dandelion does not induce sweating. Its fever-reducing activity, if any, comes from some other mechanism. Dandelion has not been tested for fever-lowering properties by conventional scientists.

☞ Directions: Pick some dandelions, taking the whole root and leaf. (Be sure to harvest them away from lawns or fields that may have been sprayed with chemical pesticides.) Wash the roots well with running water. Place 1 to 2 ounces of the plant in 1 quart of water. Bring to a boil and cover. Simmer on the lowest heat for thirty to forty minutes. When suffering from fever, drink the quart in 3 to 4 doses during the course of a day. If your fever is not better within three days, be sure to see a doctor. Don't take dandelion if you suffer from indigestion or heartburn.

AMERICAN GINSENG: Another herb used to treat feverish illnesses in Chinese folk medicine is American ginseng *(Panax quinquefolium)*. It is also used by residents of Appalachia.

Although American ginseng has never been used much in American medicine, it is a very popular remedy in China. Hundreds of tons of American ginseng are shipped from farms in Michigan and Wisconsin to China every year. (American ginseng, also reputed for its sedating effects, is often more popular than Asian ginseng in Chinatowns throughout North America.) The Chinese use the American ginseng species for different purposes than their own native Asian ginseng *(Panax ginseng)*. They view American ginseng as a "cooling" plant; they take it during hot summer weather and to cool feverish illnesses. Other than the basic identification of its constituents, very little scientific research has investigated American ginseng. Its "cooling" properties have not been examined or demonstrated.

☞ Directions: Chop 3½ ounces of ginseng and place in 1 quart of liquor such as vodka. Cover and let stand for five or six weeks in a cool dark place, turning the jar frequently. When fighting a fever, take 1 ounce after dinner or before bed.

LEMON: Lemons in the form of hot lemonade is a folk remedy for fever and influenza in New England and Indiana. The ancient Romans used lemons in the same way. No one has performed clinical trials to see if this method really works, but the constituents of lemon and its fragrant oils may indeed be helpful for treating fever and infection.

Lemon juice is an expectorant, increasing the flow of healthy mucus to infected mucous membranes. Other constituents of lemon are antimicrobial and anti-inflammatory. It is not known whether clinically significant levels of these constituents are present in hot lemonade, however.

☞ Directions: Pour 1 cup of boiling water over a blended whole lemon—skin, pulp, and all. Let the mixture steep for five minutes. While the tea is steeping, inhale the fumes. Drink one cup. Do this at first onset of a fever, and repeat three to four times a day for the duration of the infection.

ONIONS: Although onions *(Allium cepa)* appear to be a near-universal remedy for treating fever, recommendations for their use vary. In folk medicine, it has been recommended that onion slices be placed on the bottoms of the feet; put under the bed; eaten raw, roasted, or boiled; taken in teas, milk, or wine; worn in the sock or in a bag around the neck; or applied to the chest as a poultice. In every region of the country, American Indians used wild onions to lower fever. The use of onions continues today in the folk traditions of New England, New York, North Carolina, Appalachia, Indiana, and China.

The onion's constituents may explain its widespread use for treating fever, colds, and flu. Onions are also expectorant—they induce the flow of healthy and cleansing mucus. It is possible that, in the traditional "chicken soup" cure for the common cold, it is the onion that actually does the trick, not the chicken!

☞ Directions: Cut up 1 whole large onion, and simmer in a covered pot for twenty minutes. Drink a cup of the tea three to four times a day while your fever lasts. After each cup, go to bed, wrap yourself in blankets, and keep warm.

REACTIVE HYDROTHERAPY: Here is a fever-reducing method from Gypsy traditions that is taught in North American naturopathic medical colleges. This type of treatment—which includes warm coverings over mild cold applications—is called *reactive hydrotherapy*. In reactive hydrotherapy, the body reacts to a mild cold application by sending blood to the area of the cold stimulus.

☞ Directions: Take cotton socks, soak them in cold water, wring them out, and put them on the patient's feet. Cover the cold socks with one or two pair of warm wool socks. Leave in place for at least forty minutes, or overnight.

BLANKETS: A tradition from North Carolina calls for simply wrapping the patient in warm blankets and putting him to bed. When you wrap the patient warmly, his body does not have to work as hard to produce a fever. (Normally the body has to produce shivers and chills to raise the temperature. The blankets reduce the need for this.) Plus, rest in bed conserves energy and frees the body to fight infection.

☞ Directions: Wrap the patient in 1 to 3 layers of blankets, and let him rest in bed.

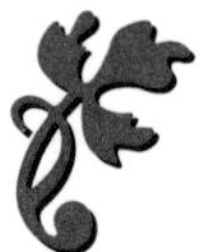

Foot Problems

One of the most common foot conditions is athlete's foot. But, in this section, you'll find remedies for cold feet and ingrown toenails, too

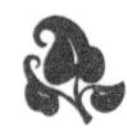

The most common foot problem mentioned in the literature of folk medicine is athlete's foot, a fungal infection of the feet. The organisms that cause athlete's foot normally reside on the skin but thrive in a hot, moist setting. An actual outbreak of athlete's foot may be due to either poor hygiene—failing to keep the feet clean and dry—or to a systemic weakness of the immune system.

Antifungal creams and ointments as well as improved foot hygiene make up the conventional treatment for athlete's foot. Many of the folk remedies for athlete's foot increase local circulation to the feet, thus increasing the presence of the body's own blood-borne immune agents that help fight infection. Other folk treatments include antifungal and anti-infective herbs and foods. These folk remedies are effective against the most common infecting organisms—members of the *Trichophyton* and *Microsporum* genera of fungi—but are ineffective against many other infectious agents. Some of the folk remedies to follow may be more effective than others. For example, the garlic foot bath may be more effective than some of the recommended creams and ointments, because garlic kills a wider range of organisms. Garlic and other antiseptic herbs may also kill the bacteria that can infect and complicate a case of athlete's foot.

Other foot problems covered in this section include cold feet and ingrown toenails. Proper methods to rewarm cold feet were of great interest to our ancestors because many of them worked as farmers, often in cold temperatures. You'll also discover a few treatments for curing ingrown toenails. (If a stubborn ingrown toenail causes persistent discomfort, however, a visit to a podiatrist—a foot doctor—may be in order.)

Remedies

ATHLETE'S FOOT

PLANTAIN: A favorite remedy for foot infections among American Indians of the Southwest is plantain *(Plantago major).* (Plantain is used in many cultures to treat wounds, bites, and stings.) Plantain leaf contains several identified anti-inflammatory and bacterial properties as well as analgesic and antiseptic properties. It also contains the constituent allantoin, which promotes cell proliferation and tissue healing. This four-leaved plant is a common weed found in lawns and along sidewalks throughout North America.

☞ Directions: Crush fresh plantain leaves and rub the juice directly onto the infected area.

ALOE VERA: Although aloe vera juice is best known for its ability to treat burns, it is also recognized as a folk cure for athlete's foot. In experiments testing aloe vera's ability to heal burns, scientists found that the plant juice not only promoted the growth of healthy tissue, but also acted as a disinfectant, reducing bacterial counts in the burns. Both of these properties are also beneficial for treating athlete's foot.

☞ Directions: Break off a part of the leaf. Apply the juicy sap to the infected area. If you don't grow your own aloe vera plant, you can purchase aloe vera gel at a health food store or drugstore.

GARLIC: Calvin Thrash, M.D., and Agatha Thrash, M.D., teachers of the folk remedies of the Seventh Day Adventist religion, suggest that garlic water can cure a fungal infection. Scientific experiments have shown that garlic's main antimicrobial constituent, allicin, kills more than 40 different types of bacteria, viruses, molds, fungi, and parasites. In fact, allicin is the plant's natural defense against the microorganisms that attack it! Allicin seems to work against most of the organisms that attack humans as well.

The allicin is only released when a clove is cut, crushed, or otherwise broken apart. Thus, the best method for releasing the maximum amount of allicin is to pulverize the garlic cloves in a blender. A hot garlic-water footbath helps soften the superficial layers of the skin so the garlic can penetrate to the full depth of the infection. The hot water and the mild irritation of the garlic also draw circulation to the feet, enhancing local immune resistance in the area.

☞ Directions: Blend 2 whole garlic bulbs in a blender and add to 1 quart of hot water. (The bulbs do not have to be peeled.) Fill a small tub with enough hot water so that the feet will be covered. Add the quart of hot garlic water to the bath. Soak the feet for twenty minutes, once a day, in the evening. Towel the feet briskly after the treatment to brush away any dead skin and dry the feet.

LICKING YOUR WOUNDS: A folk remedy from contemporary Indiana suggests the cure for athlete's foot is letting a dog lick your feet. As outrageous as this may seem, allowing dogs to disinfect your wounds with their saliva is a widespread practice throughout the world and has been practiced among North American Indian tribes and by Europeans at least since the 1500s. Modern science also supports the use of dog saliva.

Saliva is part of the immune system, and it contains a number of antimicrobial substances, including those with such names as mucin, fibronectin, beta-2 microglobulin, lactoferrin, salivary peroxidase, histatin, and cystatin. (These antimicrobial substances are part of the reason why dogs can eat substances right off the street or out of a neighbor's garbage can and not get sick.) Another antibacterial substance found in saliva, lysozyme, has been developed into a drug for commercial use in Europe for treating wounds and infections. Saliva also contains antibodies. Finally, saliva contains healing agents that promote the growth of new cells. These saliva-based growth factors are being tested by pharmaceutical companies for possible use as wound-healing drugs.

☞ Directions: Take off your shoes and socks, wash your feet, and let your dog start licking.

BLEACH: A remedy for athlete's foot from New England is to soak the feet in bleach water once a day. The same remedy was recommended by the naturopathic physician John Bastyr in the 1980s. Bastyr Health Sciences University in Seattle was named after this doctor, whose medical career—which included the use of natural remedies—spanned more than sixty years.

☞ Directions: Using ¼ cup of bleach for each quart of water, prepare enough bleach water to cover the feet in a small tub. Soak for fifteen to twenty minutes.

URINE: Fungal infections of various sorts are sometimes treated in the folk medicine of New England, the Southwest, and the Midwest with urine. Urine therapy for cleansing wounds and treating a variety of infections has appeared in the ancient medical systems of Mexico, Egypt, Persia, India, and China. The remedy was even used in Europe in the 17th and 18th centuries. During World War II in North Africa, British soldiers were shocked to see their Arab allies urinating on the wounds of injured soldiers.

Modern science suggests reasons why urine may be an effective disinfectant. Urine

continued on page 226

Rheumatism and Arthritis

In everyday conversation, the words "arthritis" and "rheumatism" tend to be used interchangeably to refer to joint pain and stiffness. In fact, though, rheumatism comprises a wide variety of disorders in which connective tissue is inflamed, including arthritis (where it is the joints that are affected). Arthritis can be chronic (a result of rheumatic disease) or it may be the cumulative result of wear and tear on the joints that commonly occurs in many older people. Medically, these distinct disorders may receive quite different treatment, but they tend to be lumped together in folk medicine.

In folk medicine, counterirritants are often used to soothe painful arthritis. A counterirritant is anything that produces one irritation with the intention of relieving another. Counterirritants, when they are applied to the surface of the body, work by bringing more blood to the surface of the skin. In many parts of North America, this affect was achieved by cooking mullein leaves in vinegar and then applying them as a poultice.

A different "warming" treatment recommended taking alcohol "for medicinal purposes." Alcohol has long been a standby in folk medicine, and it is included in many rheumatism recipes. In Indiana, for example, pokeberries and anise were added to gin for rheumatic patients, while in Illinois, it was a snake placed in whisky!

Wearing copper, usually as a bracelet, is widely known as a rheumatism preventive and treatment. There are also beliefs about electricity and healing, especially regarding the use of copper, a metal widely associated with electricity because of its use as a conductor in wires. Folk uses include wrapping copper wire around sore joints.

Folk tradition also provides a long list of magical treatments for arthritis and rheumatism, most of them involving some kind of transference of the disease from the patient to something else. One of the most common treatments is based on the belief that if the rheumatic patient sleeps with a dog, the sickness will pass into the dog and leave the patient well. In the American West, a local twist is added by specifying that the dog must be a Chihuahua. In Europe, one rheumatism remedy involved tearing a mole in half and applying the still warm innards to the stiff joints. In a similarly grotesque ritual, an Illinois remedy instructs the sufferer to split a chicken in half, leaving the entrails in, and then stand with your right foot inside the chicken carcass. The blood of the chicken will draw out the "poison" causing the rheumatism.

Though the symbolic logic of transfer to an animal is clear enough to some, the reasoning behind many other treatments is not. For example, all over North America, it is believed that carrying a buckeye or horse chestnut in a pocket prevents or cures rheumatism. A bit messier is the same practice using an Irish potato. An equally obscure but far more romantic preventive comes from Georgia. It is said that on his wedding day, the groom should place a pierced dime on each side of his bride to protect her from arthritis.

from a healthy person is as sterile as boiled water; therefore, it is safe to put on an infected area of the skin. Urine also contains the substance urea, a disinfectant used today in pharmaceutical preparations to clean and disinfect burns and wounds. Urea has strong drying properties and kills fungi, bacteria, and viruses by literally sucking the water right out of them. (If you are revolted by the idea of putting urine on the skin, consider this: Many modern cosmetic skincare products contain urea derived from the urine of cows.)

☞ Directions: Cover the infected areas of your feet with your own urine each time you urinate. A recommendation from New England says not to wash off the urine for several days in a row.

COLD FEET

HOT FOOT BATH: Perhaps the most obvious treatment for cold feet, once back indoors, is to soak them in warm water. A hydrotherapy treatment from German immigrants at the turn of the century called for a 15 minute bath in 102°F water. It's best to measure the temperature of the water with a thermometer, however. Don't just stick your feet right in because the temperature-sensing nerves of cold feet may not be able to detect if the water is too hot.

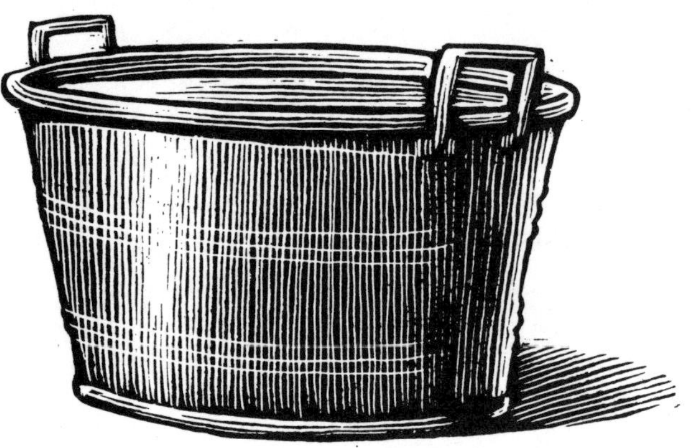

☞ Directions: Run hot bath water in a small tub or bathtub. Measure the temperature of the water with a thermometer, and then add cold water until the temperature is about 102°F degrees. Soak the feet for fifteen minutes.

RED PEPPERS: A suggestion from North Carolina folklore for warming cold feet for those who must remain outdoors for work or play is to put red pepper pods in the shoes. The mild irritation of the capsaicin in peppers draws warming blood to the area. Capsaicin also alleviates local pain. Recent studies show that capsaicin can deplete substance P, which is involved in pain transmission. Hispanic cowboys from the Southwest often use powdered cayenne pepper *(Capsicum annuum)* instead of the unbroken pods.

☞ Directions: Sprinkle a small amount of cayenne pepper in your socks before going out into the cold. Bring a clean pair of socks along just in case the red pepper becomes irritating or painful. Commercial capsaicin ointment is also available for topical application to control pain from shingles and arthritis.

CINNAMON: Much of China endures cold winters, so Chinese folk traditions have a lot to say about cold feet. Most Chinese preventives and remedies for cold feet are herbs that stimulate circulation. The Chinese recommend cinnamon *(Cinnamomum cassia),* taken internally, to prevent cold hands and feet in those who work outdoors or who have cold dispositions.

☞ Directions: Stir 1 gram of powdered cinnamon (the amount in two average-size gelatin capsules) into a glass of hot water and let steep for a few minutes. Drink three times a day.

GINSENG: A famous remedy from China for rewarming cold limbs is Asian ginseng *(Panax ginseng)*. In traditional Chinese medicine, ginseng is indicated for those men or women who are run down and fatigued and who also feel cold and have cold hands and feet. Animal experiments have demonstrated that Asian ginseng helps the body to resist chilling and hypothermia.

☞ Directions: During the winter months, purchase an Asian ginseng product at a health food store, herb shop, or Chinese or Korean market. The potency of commercial ginseng products varies widely, but the rule of thumb is that you will have to buy a more expensive product if you want to get good results. (Cheap ginseng products tend to contain almost no ginseng.) On the other hand, beware of paying for expensive "rare" ginseng roots, a scam common in some herb shops. And make sure that you are buying Asian ginseng, and not American ginseng *(Panax quinquefolius)* or Siberian ginseng *(Eleutherococcus senticosus* or *Acanthopanax senticosus)*, which have different medicinal properties. A top-of-the-line encapsulated product is probably your best buy. Take 1 to 3 grams a day during the winter months.

Keep Your Feet Dry

Both conventional and folk medicine alike recommend keeping the feet dry to prevent the development of athlete's foot. Here's a prevention program from New England folk medicine for doing just that: Wash the feet thoroughly, dry them, and change socks twice a day. Each time you wash your feet, dust them with cornstarch, which will absorb moisture. If the feet still get wet or sweaty, dry them more often. Also, rotate wearing two pairs of shoes, allowing each pair to dry for a full twenty-four hours before wearing them again. You can also keep shoes dry by dusting the insides with cornstarch.

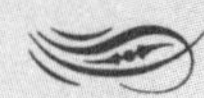

ASTRAGALUS: Another popular remedy for cold hands and feet in Chinatowns throughout North America is astragalus *(Astragalus membranaceus)*. The herb's long, yellowish root slices look like tongue depressors or large popsickle sticks. Wild North American astragalus species are sometimes called "loco weed," because of its overstimulating effect on cattle that eat too much of it. The Chinese hold that astragalus is a better "tonic" than Asian ginseng for those who are exposed to the wind and weather. NOTE: Don't purchase alcohol-based astragalus tinctures available in many health food stores. The traditional Chinese take astragalus as a tea, and the medicinal properties of astragalus extracted in alcohol are unknown.

☞ Directions: Purchase whole astragalus root slices at a health food store, herb shop, or Asian market. Place 3 or 4 slices in 1 pint of water, bring to a boil, and simmer until one third of the water is gone. Drink two cups a day during cold weather.

INGROWN TOENAILS

HOT SOAK AND A TRIM: Here's a treatment for ingrown toenails from folklorist Clarence Meyer's *American Folk Medicine*.

☞ Directions: Soak the foot in hot soapy water for fifteen minutes, until the nail becomes soft. With a knife, scrape the nail until it is very thin on the upper surface. This will supposedly cause the nail to assume its proper shape and flatten out.

YARN: An ingrown toenail treatment from New England calls for raising the toenail up from the nail bed with a piece of yarn.

☞ Directions: Using a piece of wool yarn like dental floss, work it as deeply as possible under the corner of the toenail that's growing inward. Cut the yarn and leave it in place. This will make that corner of the nail grow straight. If in doubt, or to avoid infection, however, you may want to consult a podiatrist.

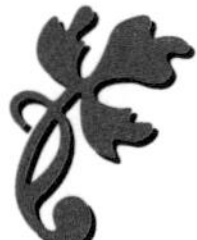

Headaches

If you are prone to headache pain, read on. The remedies that follow can help you feel better—fast

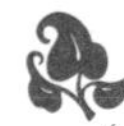

A headache is a symptom of disease, and not a disease in itself. Rarely is a headache the symptom of a serious illness—most headaches are caused by minor conditions, such as muscle tension in the neck and around the skull or inflammation of blood vessels in the brain.

There are three basic types of headaches. The vascular headache occurs when blood vessels in the head enlarge and press on nerves, causing pain. The most common vascular headache is the migraine. The second type of headache is the muscle contraction headache, which results when the muscles of the face, neck, or scalp contract and tighten. A tension headache is an example of a muscle contraction headache. The third kind of headache is the inflammatory headache. Such a headache is the result of pressure within the head. The causes range from relatively minor conditions, such as sinusitis, to more serious problems, such as brain tumors.

Headaches are most often treated with aspirin and nonsteroidal anti-inflammatory drugs (NSAIDs) such as ibuprofen or acetaminophen. Treatment of a migraine already in progress usually consists of a drug therapy program chosen from a variety of painkillers, sedatives, and special drugs and remedies, including vasoconstricting drugs and caffeine. Tension headaches can be treated by eliminating the tension or correcting the physical problem that is causing the headaches. This can sometimes be done through physical manipulation of the spine or skull by a chiropractic or osteopathic physician.

The herbal folk remedies for headaches, which are still used today by alternative physicians in the United States and by some conventional doctors in Europe, fall into four categories: pain-relievers, anti-inflammatories, sedatives, and digestive herbs. The pain-relieving and anti-inflammatory herbs may relieve most types of headaches. The sedatives work well for relieving tension headaches. The digestive herbs and laxatives are most useful for treating headaches that accompany digestive sluggishness or constipation.

Feverfew?

Scientific studies in the 1980s popularized the use of the herb feverfew (*Tanacetum parthenium*) for treating migraines. But think twice before investing large amounts of money in this herb, however. Although it proved more effective than the placebo in the clinical trials, feverfew actually helped fewer than half of the people who took it—and it didn't even help them very much. In fact, for most people, it didn't prevent migraines at all. It only reduced their occurrence—from four migraines a month to three. Besides, further studies have demonstrated that the active constituent in feverfew (the one that helps lessen migraine occurrences) is not even present in most commercial products.

If you want to try feverfew for your migraines, try this original British folk usage: Eat 2 to 3 leaves a day, rolled up in bread. For some people, this dosage prevents migraine headaches and reduces the severity of the headaches when they do occur. Feverfew is not recommended during pregnancy or for people with known pollen hypersensitivity.

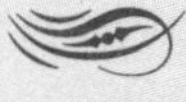

Remedies

WILLOW BARK: More than 2,400 years ago, the Greeks used willow bark *(Salix spp.)* to treat headache pain. American Indians of the Alabama, Chickasaw, Houma, Montagnais, Shoshone, and Thompson tribes and the Ninivak Eskimos used it for the same purpose, even before the arrival of the European colonists. Willow bark is still used to treat headache pain in the folk medicine of Indiana, New England, and the Southwest. It is recommended by professional medical herbalists of North America and Great Britain. The German government has approved its use by conventional physicians for treating pain and fever.

The most important active constituent in willow bark is salicin, but the bark also contains at least three other anti-inflammatory constituents. In Germany, the suggested dose is about one gram of the powdered bark—the amount in about two average-sized gelatin capsules. Willow bark is not as

Where Aspirin Came From

Aspirin is perhaps the best-known drug for treating headaches in North America today. In fact, per-capita consumption of aspirin in the United States is one tablet per person per week. Aspirin was "discovered" after chemists studied plants such as willow bark, sage, and pennyroyal. These plants, and others, have traditionally been used to treat pain.

The first of the plants to be studied was willow bark, which had been used by both the ancient Greeks and by the American Indians to treat pain. The pain-relieving constituent of willow bark, salicin, was isolated in the 19th century. Similar aspirin-like compounds were later found in other plants as well. In fact, chemists created acetylsalicylic acid—aspirin—from salicylic acid obtained from meadowsweet.

Further study in the 20th century has led to a whole new class of drugs, called *nonsteroidal anti-inflammatory drugs* (NSAIDs), which have anti-inflammatory properties similar to those of aspirin. NSAIDs are useful in the treatment of athletic injuries, postoperative pain, rheumatoid and osteoarthritis, and skin, bone, and teeth disorders. We owe our knowledge of this new class of medicines to the original folk use of plants for pain.

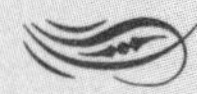

potent as aspirin, but it is less likely to cause stomach upset.

☞ Directions: To make a tea, place 2 teaspoons of powdered willow bark in a cup and fill with boiling water. Let steep for fifteen to twenty minutes. Sweeten with honey as desired. Drink up to 4 cups a day. Note that salicin can cause skin rashes in some people.

Alternately, you can purchase willow bark capsules in a health food store or an herb shop. Take as directed on the product label.

ROSEMARY AND SAGE: A folk remedy for treating headache pain is to drink a tea of rosemary *(Rosmarinus officinalis)* and sage *(Salvia officinalis)*. Rosemary has been a popular medicine in Europe for treating pain at least since the time of the ancient Greeks. Among the Greeks, rosemary had a reputation for improving the memory.

Today, rosemary is used to soothe headaches in the folk medicine of China, and, in the United States, it is used for the same purpose in Indiana and among the Amish. The German government has approved the use of rosemary for pain. There, rosemary is often used externally, in preparations such as salves and baths. It is a common folk use to apply rosemary to the temples in the form of a poultice to relieve headache pain.

Sage is not often used in folk medicine as a pain reliever, but it has an important chemical constituent in common with rosemary—rosmarinic acid (see sidebar, "Rosmarinic Acid"). In addition, the combination of rosemary and sage contains more than 20 anti-inflammatory constituents, although some of these exist only in minute amounts. Seek medical attention for any headache that lasts longer than three days. Do not ingest rosemary in any amount exceeding those usually found in foods because of the herb's reputed abortifacient and emmenagogue effects (see page 232).

☞ Directions: Place 1 teaspoon of crushed rosemary leaves and 1 teaspoon of crushed sage leaves in a cup. Fill with boiling water. Cover well to prevent the escape of volatile substances. Let steep until the tea reaches room temperature. Take ½-cup doses two or three times a day for two or three days. You don't have to mix rosemary and sage to find pain relief. You can also try drinking either rosemary or sage teas separately.

AMERICAN PENNYROYAL: Pennyroyal tea *(Hedeoma pulegioides)* is a headache remedy of the Onondaga Indians. In European folk medicine, a European species of pennyroyal *(Mentha pulegioides* L.) is used for pain relief. In fact, the 17th century British herbalist John Gerard wrote of pennyroyal: "A Garland of Pennie Royall made and worne about the head is of great force against swimming in the head, and the paines and giddiness thereof." The use of pennyroyal for treating headaches persists today in the folk medicine of Appalachia and Indiana.

Pennyroyal contains significant amounts of the anti-inflammatory substance diosmin.

☞ Directions: Place 1 teaspoon of dried pennyroyal leaves in a cup and fill with boiling water. Cover well to avoid the loss of volatile constituents. Let steep. Take ½-cup doses as desired, up to four times a day. Seek medical attention for any headache that lasts longer than three days.

MINTS: The mints—peppermint *(Mentha piperita)* and spearmint *(mentha spicata)*—are used as headache remedies in the

continued on page 234

Rosmarinic Acid

Rosmarinic acid is a nonsteroidal anti-inflammatory agent similar to aspirin, ibuprofen, and acetaminophen. High amounts of rosmarinic acid are contained in many plants used in folk medicine to treat pain, including rosemary, sage, mint, basil, and thyme. Some folk traditions advise crushing these plants (to release the rosmarinic acid) and applying the plant material to the temples or forehead. This type of application may sound somewhat odd, but animal studies have shown that rosmarinic acid is readily absorbed through the skin. You can add rosemary to your bathwater as well. The German government has approved the use of rosemary as a topical agent for pain relief.

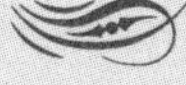

Menstruation and Folk Medicine

Most menstrual folk medicine is concerned with maintaining a comfortable, moderate, and above all, punctual period. Published collections of remedies are often vague as to the exact nature of the "menstrual difficulties" in question, however. "Motherwort is good for women's troubles" is a typical entry, for example. Most lists of home remedies do not identify premenstrual syndrome (by any name) as a problem, but it was probably one reason to hurry menstruation along. Information available that is more specific often discusses "delayed" menstruation.

The most common solutions to menstrual problems were herbal. There were herbal teas made from pennyroyal, tansy, ginger, nutmeg, mallow, feverfew, horseradish, bloodroot, bark of cotton root, carrot and carrot blossom, oregano, coriander, and rue. The length of the remedy list reflects the prevalence of the complaint! Other substances taken for menstrual problems were honey, garlic, crushed avocado stone, quinine, and Epsom salts. Remedies for cramps were much the same as those listed above, and also included chamomile, sage, horsemint, avocado leaf, and blackhawk bark teas; olive oil; onion; wintergreen oil; sugar; water boiled with black and red peppers; and hot wine.

Of course, "bringing on a late period" can also be a euphemism for deliberately inducing a miscarriage. More extreme methods for causing an abortion (like jumping off a roof or drinking turpentine) had no choice but to be frank, but herbal abortifacients could go in the name of treating "irregularities." In contrast to the long list of emmenagogues (menstrual-inducers), prescriptions to prevent miscarriage are rare.

Warming properties were the essence of most flow-enhancing plants because warming enhances circulation. If heat could encourage menstruation, a chill could stop it cold—and for good. A common belief was that a menstruating woman should avoid cold in any form. She should not drink iced beverages, for instance, lest they "freeze the flow." A combination of cold and wet was especially risky: If swimming was bad, swimming in cold water was even worse! These and other prohibitions—she should not ride a bike or drink tomato, lemon, or orange juice or anything acidic—stemmed from the belief that she was more vulnerable to illness or upset during this time.

Another common view saw the menstrual discharge as a general "cleansing," removing excess blood and other undesirable elements from her body. Its stoppage, according to this view, led to backed-up blood that could cause a headache or stroke or, worst of all, tuberculosis.

Thus, many of the restrictions urged on a menstruating woman in the past were sincerely believed to be in the best interest of her health. Some beliefs surrounding menstruation, however, were more concerned with the health of those things around her. These beliefs were based on the idea that a menstruating woman was "unclean," spreading pollution wherever she went. Outdoors, it was believed, young plants withered in her presence and seeds wouldn't sprout. In the kitchen, milk curdled and bread wouldn't rise. She shouldn't pick up a newborn baby. And she certainly shouldn't have sex, because her partner might get sick, possibly with a venereal disease! The underlying belief was that menstruation was something dirty or noxious.

According to one old saying, when a girl had her first period it was good luck for her mother to slap her in the face. One person explained that the reason for the slap was to "initiate her into life and its shocks."

Were there any positive beliefs about menstruation? An old English source stated that it was good for the fields to have a menstruous woman walk through them—because the crop-eating insects would die! Another antique belief, still practiced among California teenagers, is that menstrual blood is a powerful love charm when mixed into a man's food.

But the power of menstrual fluid was double-edged: It could also be used by a woman's enemy against her in a curse or spell, so, in some places, she was careful to burn used cloth or padding. Most of this magical thinking, however, has little to do with the physiological process of menstruation. Although there are many physical remedies to coax a missing period along, there are no magical remedies. No magical charm known to womankind can bring on a missing period!

And what about when periods go missing in the natural course of time? Remedies for menopausal symptoms are not widely noted as such, but the topic may be included in those vague categories called "women's troubles." One pleasant-sounding Mexican remedy for hot flushes is orange blossom tea laced with alcohol.

Menstrual Dangers

Ideas about the dangers of animals smelling a woman's menstruation are very widespread. Today, according to contemporary camper lore, the most unhealthful thing that can happen to a menstruating woman is an encounter with a grizzly bear. A menstruous woman should not ride a horse either, according to one American source, because the woman's scent will make the horse hard to handle. Some women avoided farm animals like pigs or sheep for this reason.

In a recent study of Amazonian dolphin lore in Brazil, the anthropologist Candace Slater noted that dolphins are believed to be angered by the menstrual scent and will pursue a boat with a menstruating woman aboard. Slater found this belief unlikely, though, because the dolphin has a weak olfactory system. Slater's informants were more convinced of their experiences, however. In legendary stories, the dolphin can take on human form and have human lovers. Thus, in this enchanted state, if the woman is menstruating and has ignored the taboo of going near the water, it is believed the male dolphin may force himself on her.

folk medicine of the particular regions where they grow. American Indians of both eastern and western North America, including the Cherokee, Iroquois, Gosuite, and Paiute tribes, used these mints as headache remedies. Some tribes crushed the plant and inhaled the fumes; others placed the plant on the forehead or temples in the same way rosemary is used (see "Rosemary," page 230).

Today, mints are used in the folk medicine of China, Mexico, Appalachia, and the American Southwest to treat headaches. The mints contain about the same levels of the anti-inflammatory rosmarinic acid as do rosemary and sage (see sidebar, "Rosmarinic Acid," page 231).

☞ Directions: Place 1 ounce of dried mint leaves in a 1-quart jar and fill with boiling water. Cover tightly to prevent the escape of the aromatic constituents. The dose is ½ cup of tea, two to four times a day. If a headache persists for more than three days, a visit to the doctor is in order.

YARROW: Yarrow *(Achillea millefolium)* has been used as a universal pain and headache remedy among various American Indian tribes, including the Cheyenne, Chippewa, Gosuite, Iroquois, Lummi, Mendocino, Navaho, Paiute, Seneca, and Shoshone. Yarrow contains at least 18 anti-inflammatory constituents, including salicylic acid, an aspirin-like substance.

☞ Directions: Place 1 ounce of dried or fresh yarrow leaves in a 1-quart jar and fill with boiling water. Cover tightly to prevent the escape of the aromatic constituents. The dose is one-half cup of the tea, two to four times a day. If any headache persists for more than three days, see your doctor.

COFFEE AND TEA: Coffee and tea are recommended as headache cures in several traditions. Caffeine is the medicinal constituent responsible for the benefits. Caffeine is also used in conventional medicine to treat migraine headaches. It works by con-

Using Your Head

A German herbal that was used by turn-of-the-century immigrants suggested binding mint across the forehead, a practice that American Indians also used for treating headache pain. Folk traditions from every region of North America and Europe recommend applying substances to the head to treat headaches. For example, from New England to the Southwest, folk remedies suggest applying camphor spirits and vinegar to the head to treat headache pain. In New England, practitioners of folk medicine apply witch hazel to the forehead or spread sauerkraut on the temples. Other North American traditions call for applying raw onions or boneset leaves to the forehead. We don't know if any these methods really works, but some medicinal substances, such as the anti-inflammatory rosmarinic acid found in mint, are easily absorbed through the skin.

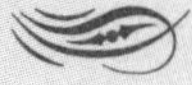

Ergot Alkaloids

During the Middle Ages in Europe, a disease called "St. Anthony's Fire" swept whole villages. The cause of the disease was rye bread that had been contaminated with a fungus called ergot *(Claviceps purpurea)*. In A.D. 994, a St. Anthony's Fire epidemic in France killed more than 40,000 people.

St. Anthony's Fire was characterized by hallucinations similar to those produced by the hallucinogenic drug lysergic acid diethylamide, or LSD. (In fact, derivatives from ergot fungus led to the discovery and manufacture of LSD.) Another symptom of St. Anthony's Fire is gangrene of the fingers and toes. A constituent of ergot constricts the blood vessels and cuts off blood circulation, causing intense pain and death of the tissues in the extremities.

Ergot alkaloids are used today in small doses to treat migraine headaches. These alkaloids, given in the form of drugs called vasoconstrictors, act by constricting the dilated vessels of the brain that accompany migraines. Mexican folklore advocates using the ergot fungus itself to cure migraine, which is a risky practice.

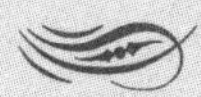

stricting the vessels of the brain, which are sometimes dilated during a headache attack. Tea is recommended in New England, and strong black coffee in Appalachia. Black coffee is a famous cure throughout Europe and North America for the type of headache that accompanies hangover. Note that habitual use of caffeine can cause headache on withdrawal, however.

☞ Directions: Make a pot of strong black coffee or tea and drink 1 to 2 cups to relieve an acute headache.

LAXATIVES: A collection of remedies by folklorist Clarence Meyer called *American Folk Medicine* suggests taking low doses of laxatives to cure a headache. This remedy is best used on headaches that accompany constipation. The habitual use of laxatives is not recommended, however.

☞ Directions: Place ¼ teaspoon of senna leaves in a cup. Add ¼ teaspoon of sage leaves and ¼ teaspoon of powdered ginger. Fill the cup with boiling water. Let steep until cool. Drink a cup every four hours. Do not exceed 3

continued on page 237

Beating Headache

Today, headache is the leading cause of time lost from work. The prevalence of headache is often blamed on the hectic pace of modern life, but it was just as common in the past, to judge from the myriad beliefs and practices that grew up around it. Wear gold earrings, swallow a spider web—anything seemed worth a try in pre-analgesic days.

Suspected causes were even more diverse: If you threw your hair outdoors and birds put it in their nest, it was believed a headache would result. And, if you cut your hair in March, it was likely you would have a headache all month.

Some magical causes and cures may fall into the category of simple "old sayings," but others were taken seriously. Being stared at was sometimes thought to cause headache, especially among people of Italian or Mediterranean backgrounds who believed in the evil eye. The person with the "bad eye" did not necessarily do damage on purpose—their unconscious envy of the "victim" was a kind of independent force of its own. Cures for headache caused by the evil eye were often small rituals using water, salt, and oil (three drops of oil in a pan of water swirled three times, for example).

Folk tradition often mixes magic and material methods, even for ordinary pains. Most cures for headache, naturally, focused on the head, which could be anointed (with oil or water); bound (with a stocking that has been worn but not washed or a hat with a snakeskin band); or poulticed (with tea leaves or vinegar and brown paper). The aromatic properties of vinegar are found in compounds like ammonia, camphor, or turpentine. All of these compounds were used to help sinus conditions and were all used in folk headache cures.

Interestingly, the feet might be used to treat head pain as well. An English cure suggests tying freshly killed pigeons to the soles! Some people still swear by soaking the feet in hot or cold (or alternating) water.

Many procedures probably work just by making the sufferer slow down long enough to do them. Since most headaches are caused by tension, anything that reduces stress can help.

Head Herbs

In the past decade, the herb feverfew has been the subject of clinical trials for treating and preventing migraine headaches, though its effectiveness is still in question. (In the folk traditions of the United States, feverfew has not often been used to treat headache, but instead to promote menstrual flow. Current pharmaceutical guidelines, noting that it causes abortion in cattle, have therefore recommended against its use by pregnant women.) For treating headache, there are other traditional American herbs you can try, including boneset, basil, borage, and hop.

Water Treatments

A variety of "water cures" for headaches are mentioned in North American folk literature. Little consistency exists between the treatments, however. For instance, Indiana folklore suggests applying a hot cloth to the forehead. New England tradition suggests applying cold water or ice to the area. Perhaps the method that makes the most sense for migraines—a method that is recommended by the Amish and is also taught in today's North American naturopathic medical colleges—is the hot foot bath. When heat is applied to the feet, it increases blood circulation there, moving blood away from the dilated vessels in the brain and easing the head pain. Sometimes a cold cloth is applied to the head, or a few teaspoons of mustard powder are added to the foot bath, to reinforce the action.

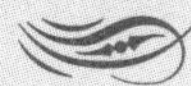

doses in a day. Do not repeat the treatment for a second day. If the constipation and headache persist, see a physician. Do not use laxatives during pregnancy.

BONESET: During the 1700s, the herb boneset *(Eupatorium perfoliatum)* was one of the most common household remedies in the eastern colonies. The colonists learned the plant's uses from the American Indians, who used it to treat a wide variety of conditions, including colds, flu, and arthritis pain. The use of boneset for headaches, especially migraine headaches, persists today in southern Appalachia and in Indiana.

Several constituents of boneset have been shown to be anti-inflammatory, but their clinical significance is not clear. Boneset contains bitter substances that promote the secretion of digestive enzymes, so boneset can be used as a mild laxative. Thus, boneset may be most appropriate for headaches that accompany or follow digestive disturbances.

☞ Directions: Place 1 tablespoon of dried boneset leaves in a cup and fill with boiling water. Let stand until cool (room temperature). Strain and drink the liquid in 3 divided doses during the day, away from meals. Note: Boneset taken in larger doses has been shown to cause nausea.

WORMWOOD: Plants of the *Artemisia* genus *(Artemisia spp.)* have been used as pain remedies by at least 22 American Indian tribes throughout North America. Some tribes received the pain-relieving properties of the plants by burning them and inhaling their smoke and aromatic oils. To treat a headache, others made a tea of the leaves and used them as a wash on the forehead and temples. The use of the *Artemisia* species is recorded today in the folk medicine of northern New Mexico. The European species *Artemisia absinthum* (or wormwood) is approved as a digestive stimulant by the German government. Excessive use in large amounts can lead to brain damage, however.

The active constituents of plants in the *Artemisia* species include bitter digestive stimulants and anti-inflammatory volatile oils such as azulenes. These constituents are also present in yarrow and chamomile.

Vinegar and Brown Paper

Using vinegar to treat headaches is a common remedy in traditional folk culture throughout the eastern United States. North Carolina folklore suggests wetting a brown paper bag with vinegar and placing it on the head. Some North Carolina variations of the remedy call for using a vinegar-soaked towel instead of a paper bag, but the paper bag method also appears in Amish folklore and in the remedies of contemporary Indiana folk medicine. A Vermont method is to drink the vinegar—a tablespoon in a glass of water along with a tablespoon of honey. Another Indiana method is to mix equal parts of water and vinegar, bring to a boil, and inhale the vapor, taking 75 breaths. There is no apparent scientific rationale for any of these practices.

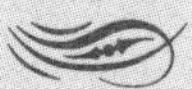

Bitter Herbs for Healing

Many traditional folk remedies for headaches require the use of bitter herbs. Such traditional medical systems as Ayurveda (from India), Unani Tibb (from Arabia), and traditional Chinese medicine consider the bitter flavor of the herbs to be "cooling." In these systems of medicine, inflammatory headaches such as migraines are universally treated with bitter digestive herbs. The concept is that the herbs cool the "fire" in the digestive system and prevent it from "rising" to the head and causing a headache. Bitter herbs in this section include yarrow, senna, boneset, hop, and chamomile.

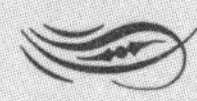

☞ Directions: Place 1 teaspoon of wormwood leaves in a cup of water and fill with boiling water. Cover well. Let cool to room temperature. Take ½-cup doses every three hours for up to three days. If the headache persists, see a doctor.

HOP: The herb hop *(Humulus lupulus)*, which is responsible for the bitter flavor of beer, has been used as a pain reliever by the Cherokee, Dakota, and Mohegan Indian tribes. It is approved by the German government for use as a sedative and may be best suited to relieving stress-related headaches or headaches that interfere with sleep.

☞ Directions: Place 1 teaspoon of hop flowers in a cup and add boiling water. Cover and let stand for ten minutes. Drink two or three cups a day for up to three days.

Also, you can crush 1 ounce of dried hop flowers, sprinkle with alcohol, and place inside a pillow. Sleep with the pillow close to the face.

CHAMOMILE: Chamomile tea *(Matricaria recutita)* is recommended for headaches today in the Hispanic folk medicine of the Southwest. Chamomile contains bitter digestive stimulants, anti-inflammatory compounds, and sedative constituents. It may be especially appropriate for soothing stress-related headaches. Other activities of this tea have shown to be antibacterial, anti-inflammatory, antispasmodic, and antiviral.

☞ Directions: Place ½ ounce of chamomile flowers in a 1-quart jar. Fill the jar with boiling water and cover. Let steep until the tea reaches room temperature. To soothe a headache, strain and drink ½-cup doses every three hours.

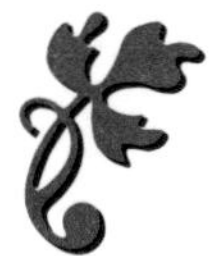

Hemorrhoids

Hemorrhoids (often called piles) are enlarged veins inside or just outside the anal canal. As the veins swell, they can cause discomfort. The remedies below will help you find relief

In some cases, hemorrhoids are the result of poor toilet habits. Habitual postponement of bowel movements can lead to loss of rectal function and undesirable straining during elimination. Straining puts increased pressure on the veins and slows the flow of blood, thereby contributing to swelling and inflammation of the veins. If bowel movements are postponed, the stools retained in the bowels may lose moisture. When feces becomes dry and hard, the added strain of constipation favors the development of hemorrhoids.

Another source of hemorrhoidal irritation comes from pressure on the veins due to disease of the liver or heart or due to a tumor. Pregnancy may also contribute to the development of hemorrhoids, because the en-

Salves

Salves, often called ointments, are fat-based preparations used to soothe abrasions, heal wounds and lacerations, protect babies' skin from diaper rash, and soften dry, rough skin and chapped lips. Homemade salves are also widespread among the folk treatments for hemorrhoids. Salves are made by heating an herb with fat or vegetable oil until the fat absorbs the plant's healing properties. These salves can be quite easily made from lard or butter, which are the most common ingredients. You simply begin by chopping, powdering, crushing, or grinding the herbal material as small as possible and place it in a skillet or a crock pot. Place enough lard or butter in the pan or pot to cover the herb. Leave the mixture over the very lowest heat for a while—at least ten to twenty minutes for a leafy substance, forty to sixty minutes for roots. Let the ointment cool, and store in the refrigerator. These traditional ointments, because they are made from perishable foods, don't keep very well. For a more permanent salve, use beeswax instead of lard or butter. Also, beeswax will stay solid at room temperature, so you don't need to refrigerate it.

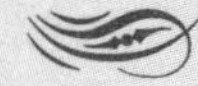

larged uterus increases pressure on the veins. Diet also plays a major role in the development of hemorrhoids. A diet containing a high proportion of refined foods, rather than foods with natural roughage, increases the likelihood of constipation, and therefore, the likelihood of hemorrhoids. And lack of exercise is one of the strongest contributing factors to the formation of hemorrhoids because exercise ensures robust circulation in the abdominal venous system.

Hemorrhoids occur "universally," according to *The Merck Manual,* a standard medical text. If they do not cause pain or other symptoms, no treatment or surgical removal is necessary. Conventional treatments include giving bulk laxatives to soften the stool (see "Constipation," page 141), warm sitz baths, topical anesthetics for itching or pain, and witch hazel compresses (a remedy we adopted from the American Indians). Other treatments include tying off the hemorrhoids and removing the hemorrhoids by surgical means. Folk remedies include all of these treatments—except the tying off procedure and the surgery. In folk medicine, the laxative effect is often achieved by taking certain herbs or foods.

Remedies

WITCH HAZEL EXTRACT: A commercial witch hazel extract *(Hamamelis virginiana)* has been a popular over-the-counter remedy for hemorrhoids in North America since the mid-1800s. The story of this commercial product is one of the best documented cases of an American Indian medicine that was adopted by both the medical profession and the general public. In the early 1840s, Theron Pond of Utica, New York, saw the local Indians of the Oneida tribe using an herbal preparation to treat burns, boils, wounds, and other afflictions of the skin. After making the acquaintance of their medicine man, Pond learned that the preparation was made by steeping witch hazel bark in an ordinary tea kettle over an open fire and collecting the steam. The result was a clear liquid with a golden color and strong aroma. Pond went into partnership with the medicine man to produce the product for local sales. They added alcohol to stabilize the product. Called Golden Treasure, the product was put on the market in 1848. Pond died a few years later and, ultimately, the product was renamed Pond's Extract.

Pond's family physician, a homeopathic doctor named Frederick Humphrey, M.D., obtained some of the medicine and tried it out. With his recommendation, its use soon spread rapidly among the other homeopaths of New York. Eventually the product's use spread even further amongst the medical profession. It became a popular over-the-counter remedy throughout the United States and in Europe. By the late 1880s it was a standard toiletry item in hotels in Paris and London. Pond's Extract Company survived into the 20th century. It is the source of the famous Pond's cold cream, which, in its original formula, also contained witch hazel extract.

Witch hazel bark contains astringent compounds that help shrink swollen tissues, although these are not the medicinal ingredients in the witch hazel extract sold in stores today. The bark also contains small amounts of the substance phenol, which escapes with the steam and is captured in the extraction process. Large amounts of phenol are poisonous, but tiny amounts can be used medicinally as a topical anesthetic, antiseptic, and anti-itching agent.

☞ Directions: Purchase some witch hazel extract at a pharmacy. Moisten toilet paper and apply to painful or itching hemorrhoids every time you go to the bathroom.

RASPBERRY LEAF TEA: In folklorist Clarence Meyer's *American Folk Medicine,* a source suggests applying a tea of raspberry leaves *(Rubus idaeus)* to hemorrhoids. Raspberry leaf is astringent and promotes the shrinking of swollen and inflamed tissues.

☞ Directions: Simmer 1 ounce of raspberry leaf in 1 pint of water for twenty minutes. Let cool to room temperature. With a bulb enema, inject half a cup of the tea into the anus and retain for ten to fifteen minutes. Do this four times a day for as long as hemorrhoids are painful or bleeding.

MULLEIN LEAF: Mullein leaf *(Verbascum thapsus)* is used as a remedy for hemorrhoids in the folk medicine of New England and by Hispanics in the Southwest. The leaf consists mostly of soothing demulcent starches as well as several anti-inflammatory substances. Various folk methods include wiping the affected area with the leaves, applying a leaf poultice and leaving it in place, and applying mullein tea directly to hemorrhoids with a cotton cloth.

☞ Directions: Place 1 ounce of mullein leaves in a 1-quart jar and fill with boiling water. Cover and let stand until it

continued on page 244

Fighting Cancer

Cancer describes a broad group of diseases in which certain body cells grow out of control. Because the symptoms of cancer vary a great deal, and because cancers can occur anywhere in the body, the term *cancer* has been used to describe a number of conditions. Before modern times, it was difficult to distinguish tumors from other swellings, such as goiter and various ulcers and sores. As a result, many folk "cancer cures" have actually been used to treat conditions that were not really cancer.

Cancer gets its name from the Latin word for crab, perhaps because of the crablike appearance of the swollen veins around a visible tumor. Also, astrological use of Cancer the Crab in the zodiac has long kept the disease associated with crabs (and crablike animals) in folk tradition. For example, in Europe and North America, folklorists have recorded the belief that when dead crabs decayed they created a poison gas that caused cancer. Pennsylvania folk medicine tradition attributed cancer to worms or evil, gnawing crabs. Powdered crab claws, on the other hand, have been used to treat cancer in folk medicine, both as a salve and as an internal remedy.

Cancer and its causes are mysterious. Even now this dreaded disease is only partially understood by medical science. It is not surprising then that folk tradition associates cancer with the supernatural. In folk tradition, there are many stories of people developing cancer as a result of being touched, or even slapped, by a ghost. But folk tradition contains beliefs about the physical causes of cancer. Medical research into folk use of plants for cancer has shown that a number of these remedies do have anti-tumor activity. For example, the Indians in Maine used Mayapple resin (podophyllum) to treat skin cancer. Today a descendant of that remedy is used for the same purpose.

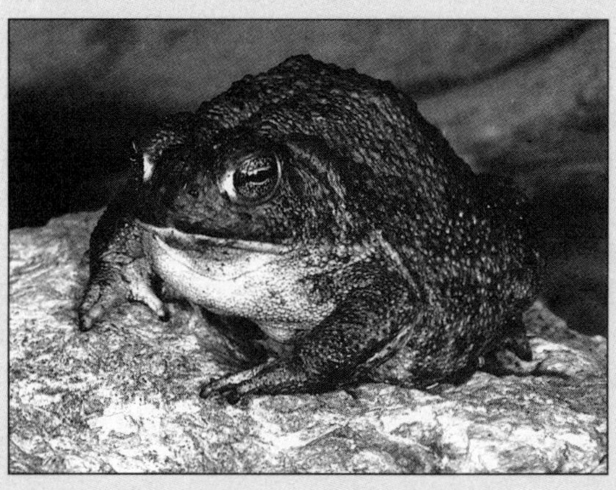

Toads have been used to treat skin cancer.

Modern medicine has identified more and more risk factors of cancer. (It sometimes seems that absolutely everything can cause the disease.) Folk tradition also believes that many things can cause cancer. The water in which eggs have been boiled was believed to cause cancer and other diseases. The persimmon tree has also been blamed. And, in 1988, a Florida newspaper reported the belief that just walking past a nutmeg tree could cause cancer! Interestingly, many folk beliefs about cancer have turned out to be true and are now widely accepted by modern medicine. For instance, as early as the 19th century, folklorists reported the

Conventional Combos

The search for effective folk medicine cancer treatments is nothing new among physicians. In the mid-19th century, physicians developed a procedure that used both surgery and a paste made from bloodroot (*Sanguinaria canadensis*). The use of bloodroot in cancer treatment was based on reports of the American Indians' use of the herb. (The practice was also documented in Russian folk medicine). In 1857, the bloodroot method was reported as substantially superior to surgery alone in the treatment of breast cancer. But the technique was debunked as "practically useless" in 1880. By 1962, however, a similar chemosurgical technique using a salve of bloodroot was being employed in conventional treatment of superficial cancers.

Many other kinds of salves for the treatment of cancer, most of them caustic, have been reported in folk tradition. Frequently these remedies included arsenic or even lye. It is no wonder that many folk cures for cancer were said to "hurt like Hell!"

belief that tobacco, once a common ingredient in folk medicine, could cause cancer of the lips and tongue. On the other hand, folk belief has also credited chewing tobacco with the prevention of cancer!

In folk tradition, the search for cancer remedies (and other herbal treatments) included the observation of animals that were believed to have cancer. For example, the "Hoxsey Treatment" was the result of just this kind of research. Harry Hoxsey marketed this unproven cancer remedy, which became very popular in the 1920s and remained widely used until it was outlawed in the 1960s. Hoxsey said his grandfather had developed the product after observing plants eaten by a horse that had a tumor on its leg. The elder Hoxsey maintained the horse was cured by the plants. He bottled and sold the remedy as the Hoxsey Treatment.

There are many cancer remedies in folk medicine. Many folk cures for external cancers involved ointments or powders. From the Midwest came a recipe for an oil made by placing a live toad in unsalted butter in a sealed can and leaving it in the sun for several days. Other cures were more magical. An Ozark remedy called for placing powdered human bones on a skin cancer.

Many folk cures and preventives are indistinguishable from those used in other diseases. For instance, the skin or dried foot of a mole worn between the breasts was a preventive for breast cancer in the American South, where mole amulets were used to ward off all sorts of diseases. And, echoing many other folk ideas of disease, cancer has been said to be caused by "bad blood." In part this idea resulted from the observation that some cancers run in families. Before the role of genes in inheritance was understood, folk tradition attributed familial inheritance to substances in the blood.

reaches room temperature, shaking the bottle from time to time to mix the contents. Apply the tea directly to the hemorrhoids with a cotton cloth each time you use the bathroom.

CHAMOMILE OR YARROW TEA: Chamomile tea *(Matricaria recutita, Anthemis nobilis),* applied directly to the hemorrhoids, is a treatment from German folk medicine. Chamomile contains strong anti-inflammatory substances that may reduce the pain or itching of hemorrhoids. Yarrow tea *(Achillea millefolium)* may also do the trick: Yarrow contains some of the same anti-inflammatory constituents as chamomile.

☞ Directions: Make enough strong chamomile or yarrow tea to use in a sitz bath. (Use 1 ounce of either herb for every 2 quarts of water.) Put the hot tea in a bucket or tub just big enough to sit in. There should be enough tea in the bucket to cover the hemorrhoids. Soak in the tea for fifteen minutes, two to three times a day, for an acute hemorrhoid attack. Alternately, you can make a quart of the tea and apply it hot to the hemorrhoids with a cotton cloth each time you use the bathroom.

HORSE CHESTNUTS: Indiana folklore suggests soothing hemorrhoid pain with an ointment made from horse chestnuts *(Aesculus hippocastanum),* also called buckeyes. Horse chestnut extracts are used in European conventional medicine for hemorrhoids and varicose veins. These extracts, which contain standardized amounts of aescin, are available in some United States health food stores. The constituent aescin tightens swollen veins.

☞ Directions: Split six buckeyes, remove the shells, and chop up the contents as small as possible. Place in a skillet, cover with lard, and simmer for an hour. Allow to cool until the ointment is solid. Apply to the hemorrhoids several times a day. Alternately, you can look for ready-made horse chestnut ointments at your health food store or herb shop.

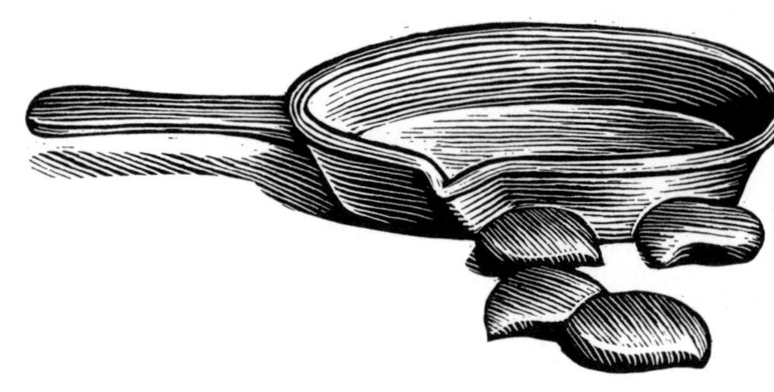

CALENDULA: The Amish suggest using an ointment of calendula flowers *(Calendula officinalis)* to treat hemorrhoids. Calendula, which is also called pot marigold, is a different plant from garden marigolds *(Tagetes erecta)* and it contains different constituents. Calendula contains anesthetic and anti-inflammatory constituents as well as other constituents that promote the healing of wounds. Calendula-based ointments made with beeswax are readily available in health food stores and herb shops and are often combined with other herbs.

☞ Directions: Purchase a commercial calendula ointment at a health food store or herb shop and apply to the hemorrhoids each time you use the bathroom.

ALOE VERA: Aloe vera is best known as a pain-relieving remedy for mild burns. But it may also be effective for the pain and itching of hemorrhoids. The same anti-inflammatory constituents that reduce blistering and inflammation in burns may also reduce the irritation of hemorrhoids.

☞ Directions: Break off a piece of an aloe vera leaf. Apply the clear mucilage (and not the yellow sap under the leaf) to the hemorrhoids each time you use the bathroom. Alternately, you can purchase aloe vera gel at a health food store or drugstore.

RED CLOVER: A salve made from red clover blossoms is a hemorrhoid remedy from the Amish and also from the folk medicine of New England. The blossoms of red clover, like mullein leaf above, contain the topical anti-inflammatory constituent coumarin. The clover blossoms also contain a variety of other aromatic anti-inflammatory constituents.

☞ Directions: Chop ½ ounce of red clover blossoms and spread on the bottom of a skillet. Add enough lard to cover. Apply just enough heat to melt the lard, and stir the clover blossoms into the lard. Remove from the heat and allow to stand until the salve becomes solid. Apply to the hemorrhoids each time you use the bathroom.

OINTMENT FORMULA—GREASE ONESELF: An ointment for hemorrhoids that combines several other herbs in this section was suggested by a Mr. P. Smith in 1812, according to Clarence Meyer's *American Folk Medicine.* The remedy is slightly modified here to include only the plants that are likely to be available for purchase in stores today.

☞ Directions: Take one handful each of plantain leaf, burdock root, and mullein leaf. Powder the roots in a coffee grinder, and crumble the leaves. Place all the items in a skillet, and add a pound of butter. Melt the butter, and simmer on the lowest heat for thirty to forty minutes. Remove from the heat and let cool to room temperature. Place in another container and put in the refrigerator until the butter is solid. "Grease onesself," said Smith.

DANDELION ROOT TEA: Dandelion root tea *(Taraxacum officinale)* is sometimes used in the folk medicine of Hispanics in the Southwest as a laxative for constipation accompanying hemorrhoids. The root stimulates the flow of bile, which in turn promotes normal elimination. As a laxative, dandelion root is very mild, making it appropriate for use with hemorrhoids. Dandelion is approved in Germany as a digestive aid and liver stimulant. Don't take dandelion root if you have gallstones or pain and inflammation in the digestive tract, however.

Mild Laxatives

Conventional doctors recommend the use of mild laxatives to treat constipation that often accompanies hemorrhoids. Mild laxatives also appear widely in folk medicine as internal treatments to accompany the various external remedies for hemorrhoids. It is important not to use strong stimulating laxatives when suffering from hemorrhoids because these laxatives can irritate the inflamed tissues. The mild laxatives burdock root (*Arctium lappa*), dandelion root (*Taraxacum officinale*), psyllium seed (*Plantago spp.*), and yellow dock (*Rumex crispus*) are recommended and appear in this section.

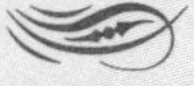

☞ Directions: Place 1 ounce of dandelion root in 1 quart of water. Cover the pot, bring the water to a boil, and then simmer on the lowest heat for forty minutes. Remove from heat and let cool to room temperature. Drink the quart of tea in 3 or 4 doses during the day. Continue for up to three weeks.

Garlic Clove

Several folk sources mention the practice of inserting a peeled garlic clove into the anus to treat hemorrhoids. This method is also mentioned in some contemporary herbal texts. But it's best to avoid this method, because raw garlic can cause skin burns, including serious second- and third-degree burns. The area just inside the anus has no nerve endings, so you could burn your rectum with the garlic and not even realize it. Garlic should never be left on the skin for more than 20 to 30 minutes at a time.

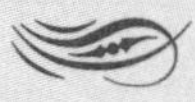

BURDOCK ROOT: Burdock root *(Arctium lappa)*, along with dandelion root, is one of the top ten herbs prescribed by North American professional medical herbalists today. Burdock is mild in its actions, and herbalists consider it to be the best choice when mild actions are preferred, as in the case of constipation accompanying hemorrhoids. Burdock increases the flow of bile from the liver and has mild laxative and diuretic effects. It also gently increases the blood circulation to the skin and, presumably, to the swollen hemorrhoids. When taken as a tea, burdock's complex carbohydrate constituents may also feed the "friendly" bacteria in the bowels, helping to restore balance and correct constipation due to any bacteria imbalances.

☞ Directions: Place 1 ounce of burdock root in 1 quart of water. Cover the pot, bring the water to a boil, and then simmer on the lowest heat for forty minutes. Remove from heat and let cool to room temperature. Drink the quart of tea in 3 or 4 doses during the day for three weeks.

PSYLLIUM SEED: According to Hispanic folklore of the American Southwest, psyllium seed *(Plantago spp.)* is recommended as a bulk laxative for bleeding hemorrhoids. Psyllium seed is beneficial for bleeding hemorrhoids because it softens the stool, reducing the irritation and pressure on the swollen veins. Today, conventional doctors throughout the United States recommend psyllium-based laxatives for constipation accompanying hemorrhoids.

☞ Directions: Purchase a psyllium-based laxative at a pharmacy, supermarket, or health food store. Follow the instructions on the label.

YELLOW DOCK: Yellow dock *(Rumex crispus)* has been used both internally and externally for treating hemorrhoids in North American folk traditions. Taken internally, yellow dock is a mild laxative. Its laxative effect comes partly from small amounts of constituents that stimulate the smooth muscles of the colon, and partly from the effect of its bitter constituents, which promote the flow of bile from the liver. Bile, in turn, promotes elimination. Although yellow dock is considered a stimulating laxative, and stimulating laxatives are generally avoided with hemorrhoids because they can irritate the inflamed tissues, the doses here are quite small and are not likely to have that effect. Yellow dock can be used externally to treat hemorrhoids, too. The Amish suggest using it in a salve, mixed with other herbs.

☞ Directions: For internal use, boil 1 ounce of yellow dock root in 1½ quarts of water. Allow to cool to room temperature, then strain. Take a 2-ounce dose, morning and evening, on an empty stomach before meals.

To make a salve, combine some powdered yellow dock with an equal amount of butter, lard, or melted beeswax. Mix well. Apply to hemorrhoids.

CARROT BOLUS: A hemorrhoid remedy from New England calls for a grated carrot bolus. This bolus is a herbal preparation that is inserted into the anus to treat protruding hemorrhoids. The pressure of the grated carrot bolus works by pressing the hemorrhoids back into the tissue surrounding the rectum. The carrot is grated and used for its firm texture.

☞ Directions: Grate a small carrot. Mix it with enough lard to hold the soft mass together. Insert the bolus into the anus and hold it in place as long as possible.

ONIONS: Several North American folk sources suggest eating onions for hemorrhoids. In their book *Home Remedies: Hydrotherapy, Massage, Charcoal, and Other Simple Treatments,* Agatha Thrash, M.D., and Calvin Thrash, M.D., physicians who are affiliated with the Seventh Day Adventist religion, recommend eating cooked onions to stop the bleeding of hemorrhoids. Russian folklore calls for steaming the hemorrhoids with the fumes of cooked onions. It is conceivable that anti-inflammatory compounds in cooked onions could reduce the inflammation and itching of hemorrhoids.

☞ Directions: Place 4 large onions, peeled and chopped, into a half gallon of milk in a large pot. Cover and heat the mixture in an oven on low heat. Remove the pot from the oven, remove the lid, and cover with a toilet seat. Take a seat and let the onion fumes steam the hemorrhoids. (Be careful not to burn yourself on the hot pot.) Complete the treatment by applying Vaseline to the hemorrhoids.

HEAT AND STEAM: New England residents report that the application of heat, in the form of steam, hot baths, or other hot applications, can relieve the discomfort of hemorrhoids. The Seventh Day Adventists recommend taking a hot sitz bath for hemorrhoid pain. Conventional physicians say the same. The physiological action of the hot water increases circulation in the veins around the anus, removing the stagnancy of blood that contributes to the swelling and discomfort of hemorrhoids.

☞ Directions: Run enough hot water in a tub to cover the hips when seated. For acute hemorrhoids, sit in the tub with your feet out of the water for ten to fifteen minutes twice a day.

COLD BATH: At the turn of the century, German immigrants, who arrived here with their own system of folk water cures, recommended treating hemorrhoids with cold sitz baths instead of hot ones. The cold baths are indicated, according to the Germans, *between* acute attacks—not when there is active pain, inflammation, or swelling in the hemorrhoids. The baths work by constricting the blood vessels of the hemorrhoids.

☞ Directions: Run enough cold water in the bathtub to cover the hips when sitting. Between acute hemorrhoid attacks, sit in the tub with your feet out of the water, for forty seconds to two minutes, depending on your tolerance to the cold water. Do this in the evening before bed three times a week.

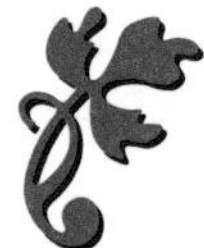

Hiccups

Experts say hiccups are most often a reaction to common digestive disturbances. And luckily, they're usually more of a nuisance then anything else

A hiccup is an involuntary spasm of the diaphragm followed by a sharp intake of air, which is abruptly stopped by a sudden, involuntary closing of the glottis (an opening between the vocal cords). The consequent blocking of air produces the repeated sharp sound, which sounds like *hic*.

The cause of short episodes of hiccups is unknown. Episodes of prolonged or recurrent hiccups may be the result of swallowing hot or irritating substances, pneumonia, alcoholism, certain prescription drugs, disorders of the stomach, pregnancy, or even some emotional disorders.

According to conventional medicine, a high blood level of carbon dioxide inhibits hiccups. You can bring on a high blood level of carbon dioxide by holding your breath, a solution to hiccups that is used in many folk traditions. Modern medicine and folk medicine also suggest stimulating the *vagus nerve,* one of the nerves that activates the diaphragm, which can be done simply by swallowing.

Some serious illnesses can cause persistent hiccups, but the occasional passing episodes are no cause for concern. However, if your hiccups persist for longer than eight hours, or you suspect that a prescription drug may be causing your hiccups, give your doctor a call.

Remedies

GYPSY HICCUP CURE: A Gypsy folk tradition suggests drinking the following tea to cure hiccups. The herbs used in the tea have sedative, anti-inflammatory, and antispasmodic properties. Whether these properties have an actual effect on the nerves or muscles responsible for producing hiccups is not clear. In any case, it is a nutritious and relaxing tea.

☞ Directions: Take a handful each of valerian root, blackberry leaf, fennel seeds, chamomile flowers, peppermint leaf, and sage leaf. Crush and mix well in a bowl. Place 2 tablespoons of the dried herbs in a 1-pint jar. Fill with boiling water and cover. Steep for ten to fifteen minutes. Strain and drink 1 cup of warm (not hot) tea three times a day for up to ten days.

DILL SEED: Several entries in folklorist Clarence Meyer's *American Folk Medicine* suggest taking dill seeds *(Anethum graveolens)* to cure hiccups. The same treatment is mentioned in contemporary Indiana folklore. How the remedy works is not clear. It may be that some properties of the seeds are at work, or that the difficulty in swallowing them stimulates the vagus nerve to terminate the hiccups.

☞ Directions: Chew and swallow a teaspoon of dill seeds.

LEMONADE: A North Carolina remedy for hiccups calls for taking nine swallows of lemonade. Another suggestion from the same state calls for nine sips of water. (Thus, it seems to be the repetition of swallowing, not the substance sipped, that's important.) Taking so many sips involves not only repeated gulping, but it requires holding the breath for a while—both of which are conventional mechanisms for stopping hiccups.

continued on page 251

Things to Swallow

According to conventional medicine, the simple action of swallowing can end a case of the hiccups. Swallowing stimulates the vagus nerve, one of the nerves that controls the diaphragm and other muscles involved in breathing. Folk traditions recommend a wide variety of things to swallow to cure hiccups, including: dill seeds, peanut butter, sugar, lemonade, strong coffee, water, crushed ice, and cold soda water. It is not clear whether it's the substance that is swallowed or the action of swallowing that is responsible for the remedy's benefits.

Morning Sickness

Morning sickness, which ranges from nausea to actual vomiting, is a common complaint among pregnant women. (The term morning sickness is actually a misnomer because the symptoms can happen at any time of day.) According to present day medical opinion, the cause is still unclear. Some findings, however, do suggest that increased production of the HCG (human chorionic gonadotropin) hormone is a contributing factor and slowed digestion, anxiety, and emotional stress can make the problem worse. Today's physicians and midwives recommend eating a carbohydrate, such as crackers or a banana, before rising to prevent nausea and eating small amounts of non-greasy foods throughout the day. Other specialists also recommend taking a B_6 vitamin supplement daily or eating natural sources of B_6, such as Brewer's yeast and yogurt. Eating ginger, an ancient herbal treatment for nausea, is now also recognized by modern medicine as being helpful.

Although nausea is a problem for most women only during the first trimester, it is so common that folk remedies and explanations abound. Herbal and food remedies to prevent morning sickness are very common. One folk remedy recommends eating two soda crackers before getting up in the morning—exactly the remedy prescribed by today's health specialists! The Cherokee Indians used goldenseal (*Hydrastis canadensis*), which grows wild in the woods of eastern North America, for morning sickness. A preventive from Indiana is to drink one teaspoonful of apple cider vinegar mixed in a glass of water. One from Utah recommends eating a chocolate candy bar before getting out of bed. Another Utah remedy is to eat raw eggs, a recommendation that many queasy pregnant women might find hard to follow! More advice from Utah is that the pregnant woman should just accept morning sickness because it is actually an indication that the infant will be healthier and the delivery easier. Some medical evidence does in fact indicate that those women who experience nausea in early pregnancy are less likely to have miscarriages.

Folk belief also suggests that morning sickness can indicate the sex of the baby. In Utah, if morning sickness is pronounced, then you are sure to have a girl. In other parts of the country, it is believed the opposite will result. Another belief in Utah ascribes the color of the pills taken for nausea during pregnancy to be the determining factor in the sex of the child. It is believed that blue pills will bring a boy and pink pills, a girl. In Utah, it is also believed that the baby's sex can be predicted by the physical symptoms that the father feels (called the couvade syndrome). If, instead of the mother, the expectant father feels nauseous, it is believed the baby will be a boy.

☞ Directions: To cure hiccups, make some lemonade and take 9 consecutive sips.

SUGAR OR HONEY: Eating sugar or honey is one of the most widespread folk cures for hiccups. The ancient Aztecs recommended swallowing honey; this same practice persists today in the folk traditions of Mexico and the American Southwest. A spoonful of sugar is preferred in North Carolina and Indiana folklore. Both substances are difficult to swallow, which may stimulate the vagus nerve and help stop the hiccups.

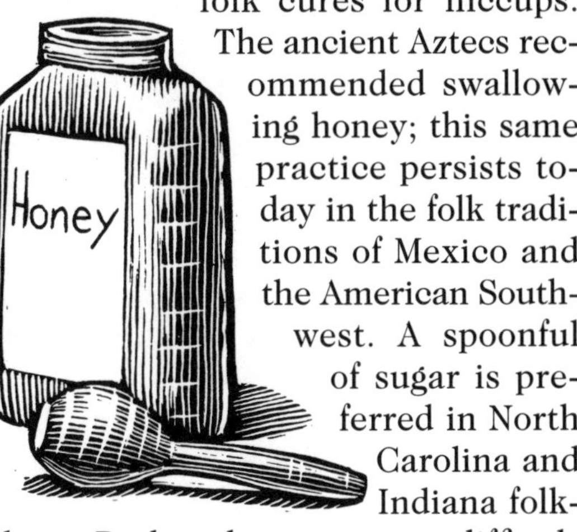

☞ Directions: Take 1 teaspoonful of dry sugar into the mouth and swallow it. Or, swallow 1 tablespoon of honey.

HOLD UP: A North Carolina hiccup remedy recommends holding your arm above your head. This action may change the tension in the muscles used in breathing, thus breaking the rhythm of the hiccups. The posture may also stimulate the vagus nerve, which descends through the muscles that connect the neck to the shoulder. An Indiana variation of this remedy calls for holding up both arms and shaking them overhead.

☞ Directions: Hold your arms over your head and shake them. It may help to hold your breath as long as possible while doing so.

Water Cures

Drinking water is a universal remedy for hiccups, mentioned not only in conventional medicine, but also in folk traditions throughout North America. The variations of this remedy are plentiful: Sip water without taking a breath. Drink a glass of water while holding the nose. Drink as many swallows of water as you can without taking a breath. Block the ears with one finger from each hand while taking five sips of water from a glass on a table. (The number of sips varies from tradition to tradition—five, seven, eight, or nine sips are all cited.) Drink a cupful of cold water in nine gulps. Drink cold soda water instead of tap water.

Interestingly, you don't always have to *drink* the water to cure yourself of hiccups. According to one North Carolina remedy, simply staring into a glass of water is enough to cure you of the affliction!

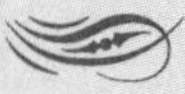

HOLD YOUR BREATH: In his collection of folk cures called *American Folk Medicine*, folklorist Clarence Meyer calls for simply holding your breath. This remedy is also recommended in conventional medicine, because holding the breath increases the carbon dioxide level in the blood, which helps to end the hiccups. This method is also mentioned in the folklore of New England, Indiana, Kentucky, and Louisiana.

☞ Directions: Hold the breath as long as possible. Repeat until the hiccups are cured.

BOO!: Scaring someone with the hiccups is a well-known cure. This remedy's benefit may be due to the person's suddenly inhaling and holding his breath. A remedy used in Kentucky folk medicine suggests surprising the sufferer by suddenly popping a paper bag behind him.

☞ Directions: Find some suitable—but safe—way to frighten or surprise the sufferer.

THUMBS BEHIND THE EARS: A remedy from North Carolina suggests placing the tips of the thumbs behind your ears and pushing inward on the scull bones. This region behind the ears is where the vagus nerve exits the skull and descends toward the respiratory muscles. So pressure in that area may actually have a physiological effect on the respiratory system. The area is, in fact, the region of the liver meridian, which is the meridian that is sometimes stimulated in Chinese acupuncture to treat hiccups.

☞ Directions: Place the thumbs behind the ears and press inward until hiccups subside.

THINK OF THE ONE YOU LOVE: Possibly the most pleasant of the folk hiccup cures, practiced by individuals in both Indiana and North Carolina, is to think about the person you love the most. The North Carolina version of the remedy claims that if the person you love loves you back, the hiccups will stop.

☞ Directions: Focus on the one you love.

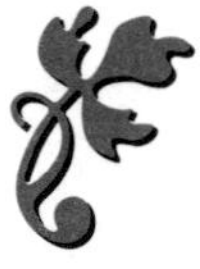

Indigestion and Heartburn

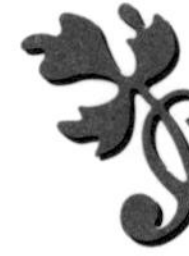

Indigestion and heartburn may occur simultaneously, but different folk remedies are usually prescribed for each

Painful indigestion and heartburn are so common in the United States today that antacids are among the top-selling categories of over-the-counter drugs. This section deals specifically with digestive pain rather than sluggish, inefficient digestion. Although the two conditions may occur simultaneously, different folk remedies are usually prescribed for each. For instance, bitter herbs are commonly prescribed for sluggish digestion, but they are contraindicated if pain is present. Bitter herbs increase the secretion of digestive juices, which can increase pain (see "Digestion," page 175).

Simple digestive pain can come from two main causes: inflammation of the wall of the stomach or intestine, or spasms of the intestinal muscles, often in response to a buildup of gas. The most common causes of digestive inflammation are irritation of the digestive lining by the body's own digestive secretions, infection by a bacterium known as *Helicobacter pylori,* or irritation by offending foods. Persistent indigestion pain should be a cue to visit the doctor, who will help you experiment with your diet to determine and remove the cause.

Heartburn—a gassy, burning sensation in your upper abdomen, sometimes accompanied by the regurgitation of sour, bitter material into your throat or mouth—actually has nothing to do with your heart. Heartburn indicates that the lower part of your esophagus, the upper part of your stomach, or the first section of your bowel has become irritated, and the contents of your stomach have started to back up into the esophagus. Most cases of heartburn aren't serious. The easiest way to avoid a simple case of heartburn? Moderation. Heartburn is generally the result of eating too much too fast.

Eating while under stress is also a major cause of indigestion and heartburn. When relaxed, the body secretes its own antacids from the pancreas and bile ducts in response to food entering the intestine. In a state of stress, these secretions shut off. Thus "acid" indigestion may not be due to excess acid, but to a deficiency of the neutralizing secretions. The best way to turn these secretions back on is to relax for at least ten minutes before eating. Persistent inflammation of the digestive tract can cause ulceration. Ulcers can have serious and even fatal complications if they bleed or if the ulcer eats entirely through the intestine.

The most common categories of folk remedies for digestive pain and heartburn are demulcent herbs (slimy mucilaginous plants that coat and soothe inflamed tissue), herbs containing anti-inflammatory substances, and carminative herbs, which reduce the spasms of intestinal cramps that often accompany gas.

Remedies

SLIPPERY ELM: Slippery elm bark *(Ulmus fulva)* is used in modern European and North American professional medical herbalism as a soothing treatment for gastritis and ulcers of the digestive tract. The bark, when mixed with water, makes a slimy mucilaginous mass that is soothing to inflamed tissues. Please note that ulcers can cause internal bleeding and have serious health consequences. If you suffer from ulcers, be sure to see a doctor.

☞ Directions: Place 1 tablespoon of powdered slippery elm bark in a cup. Fill with boiling water. Let steep for ten minutes. Stir, without straining, and drink the whole cup. Do this as needed for pain.

GINGER: Ginger *(Zingiber officinalis)* is a near-universal remedy for pain in the digestive tract, appearing in the folklore of New England, North Carolina, the southern Appalachians, Indiana, the Southwest, and

continued on page 256

African-American Folk Medicine

The great majority of African Americans are descendants of people taken from Africa by force and brought to America for the purpose of enslavement. For generations, African Americans lived in this country in conditions that suppressed their culture. Because the plants in America were very different from those at home, and the first generation of enslaved Africans spoke a variety of languages, it was hard to retain the African heritage. But, despite tremendous obstacles, much was preserved and passed down orally from generation to generation. One part of that important African heritage is folk medicine.

African-American folk medicine was appreciated by some white colonists. For example, the famous Puritan minister in Massachusetts, Cotton Mather, wrote that he learned how to inoculate for small pox from an enslaved African. Rarely were whites so impressed that they gave an enslaved person freedom in gratitude for a remedy, however. But, in one such case in South Carolina, a man named Cesar was freed and given a pension because of his remedy for rattlesnake bite. In other cases, slave owners forbade and opposed the traditional herbal practice of enslaved Africans. (Some enslaved Africans, for example, used certain herbs to produce abortion because of the economic value of enslaved children.)

In 1865, ratification of the Thirteenth Amendment to the U.S. Constitution finally ended slavery. By then, African Americans had added to their knowledge of folk medicine by learning about North American medicinal plants and by adopting some of the folk medicines of the whites.

Emancipation did not bring an end to the persecution of blacks by whites, however, and even now, disparities in the medical care of African Americans continue to be documented. From the end of the Civil War to present time there have been understandable fears by blacks of medical mistreatment. Up until World War I, African Americans feared "night doctors" (also known as "Ku Klux Klan doctors" and "student doctors"), who were believed to prowl at night looking for bodies to be used in medical education and research. These beliefs and concerns, reflecting a public uneasiness about the new development of anatomic dissection in medical schools, were shared by some in the white community as well. Bodies for research were in fact hard to come by during that period, and grave robbing did supply some of the corpses used in medical schools—a practice which resulted in riots in some American cities.

Such distrust of the medical community continues to the present, fueled more recently by the infamous Tuskegee Syphilis Study, a federal project carried out in Alabama over a period of more than thirty years. Poor black men diagnosed with syphilis were simply told that they had "bad blood," a general folk term covering a variety of conditions, and were studied rather than treated. The study continued and was not stopped until the 1970s, when it was exposed in newspapers. This study, carried out under federal supervision, has led many African Americans to reject vaccination programs and even AIDS prevention and treatment efforts for fear of once again being treated as "guinea pigs."

The mistrust of medicine, in addition to poverty and segregation, has made access to medical care and physicians difficult and uncommon for some blacks. This, in turn, has made folk medicine all the more important in the African-American community. Like other cultures, African-American tradition combines natural and supernatural theories and practices. African-American culture has always had a very strong spiritual dimension, which is reflected in its approach to healing.

Some of the oldest influences in African-American folk medicine come from the combination of West African religions and the Roman Catholicism of white slave masters (both French and Spanish), especially in the Caribbean and Latin America. These influences led to the development of distinctive religions with strong African roots, such as *voodoo,* also called "Voudun" after the West African deity of that name. Voodoo is a very widespread religion among the people of Haiti, and it has influenced American folk belief as well, especially within Louisiana where French influence remains strong. Unfortunately, voodoo has been both popularized and misrepresented in American cinema, where its reputation is often evil rather than religious. The word *voodoo,* and the related word *hoodoo,* tend to be used in American folk tradition to refer primarily to methods of harming others by sorcery, although the words are sometimes attached to healers who combat such curses. A related term is "rootwork." Placing a spell is called, by some, "working a root" (the "root" may be an item such as a feather or an actual root). There are also rootwork healers, called "rootworkers." In the same principle, there are "evil-eye healers" in traditions where the evil eye is believed to be a cause of disease. The confusion between cursing and healing, and the evil reputation produced by Hollywood—partly because of racist stereotypes—has led to the rejection of these older traditional terms by many people who use folk medicine. Today, there are other names for healers that are more acceptable, such as "treater" or, in Louisiana, "Secret Doctor."

African-American folk medicine has a rich and varied herbal tradition in the rural South. Herbs are used for both natural illnesses, such as those caused by exposure to the cold, and also for some treatments of "unnatural" illness—that is, curses and spells. But African-American migration to the cities has made it difficult for many people to learn about and obtain healing plants, although some cities have herbal shops that help to fill this void. Shops called "botanicas" combine herbal and spiritual traditions, and these are patronized by African Americans as well as Latinos. But perhaps the most dominant form of healing among African Americans is prayer—prayer by the patient, by the family, by the pastor, and by the congregation. A deep and abiding faith in the power of God underlies most of African-American folk medicine, and prayer is always available.

China. The plant contains both antispasmodic and anti-inflammatory constituents. It also contains topical anesthetic compounds that may directly reduce pain in the digestive tract. In clinical trials ginger has shown to be effective in treating some kinds of nausea.

☞ Directions: Thinly slice a fresh ginger root. (The root should be about the size of your thumb.) Place the slices in 1 quart of water. Bring to a boil, and then simmer on the lowest possible heat for thirty minutes in a covered pot. Let cool for thirty minutes more. Strain and drink ½ to 1 cup, sweetened with honey as desired.

If you don't have fresh ginger, stir ½ teaspoon of ground ginger into 1 cup of hot water. Let stand for two to three minutes. Strain and drink, as desired.

Baking Soda

A do-it-yourself antacid remedy of questionable safety from various streams of North American folklore is to ingest baking soda. Habitual consumption of large amounts of baking soda can cause salt imbalances in the body, however. A safer method is to use commercial antacids, which contain measured amounts of bicarbonate and provide instructions for safe use on the label.

FENNEL: Today, in the professional medical herbalism of Great Britain, North America, and New Zealand, fennel *(Foeniculum vulgare)* is a commonly prescribed herb for abdominal cramping and gas in adults. It appears in the folk medicine of both New England and China. Fennel is an approved medicine in Germany for mild gastrointestinal complaints. It contains at least 16 chemical constituents with antispasmodic properties.

☞ Directions: Crush 1 teaspoon of fennel seeds with a mortar and pestle or grind them in a coffee grinder. Place the cracked seeds in a cup and fill with boiling water. Cover and let sit for ten minutes. Strain and drink 3 cups of the warm tea each day on an empty stomach. Do this as often as desired.

CARAWAY SEEDS: North Americans know caraway seeds (*Carum carvi*) as the tiny seeds coating the crust of rye bread. Caraway seeds are known throughout the Arabic world and in European folk medicine as a treatment for painful intestinal gas. The German government has approved caraway as an official medicine for that condition. The seeds are used for the same purpose in the folk medicine of North Carolina, Appalachia, and Indiana.

☞ Directions: Place 1 teaspoon of crushed caraway seeds in a cup and add boiling water. Cover the cup and let stand for ten minutes. Strain and drink 3 cups of warm tea a day on an empty stomach. Alternately, you can simply chew on the seeds. Do this as often as desired.

CHAMOMILE: Chamomile *(Matricaria recutita, Anthemis nobilis)* is a popular folk remedy for treating stomachaches in New England, Indiana, and the Southwest. It is an approved medicine for this purpose in Germany. Chamomile contains at least 19 antispasmodic constituents as well as five sedative ones. A 1993 clinical trial showed that the plant was effective in relieving infant colic as well.

☞ Directions: Place 1 tablespoon of chamomile flowers in a cup and add boiling water. Cover the cup and let stand for ten minutes. Strain and drink warm three times a day on an empty stomach. Do this for two to three weeks, and then take a break for a week or two. Note: In general, chamomile poses no health threat. If you have suffered previous anaphylactic shock reactions from ragweed, however, talk to your doctor before using this herb.

MINTS: Different types of mints, including peppermint and spearmint, are recommended for indigestion in the folk literature of New England, New York, North Carolina, Appalachia, Indiana, New Mexico, and California. Mints have also been used as carminatives by members of at least seven major North American Indian tribes. Mint is an official digestive aid in German medicine. Peppermint contains antispasmodic compounds. (It is better suited to treating abdominal cramping than heartburn. It can sometimes make heartburn worse.)

☞ Directions: Place 1 teaspoon of the dried herb in a cup and add boiling water. Cover the cup and let steep for ten minutes. Strain well and drink 1 cup three times a day on an empty stomach. Do this as often as desired.

FORMULA: The following formula, from contemporary North American professional medical herbalism, combines four of the remedies in this section.

☞ Directions: Place 1 tablespoon each of chamomile flowers, mint leaves, fennel seeds, and slippery elm bark in a 1-pint jar. Fill the jar with boiling water and cover. Let stand until the water reaches room temperature, shaking the bottle occasionally to mix its contents. Strain and drink the quart during the course of the day (on an empty stomach) between meals. Do this as often as desired.

CATNIP: Catnip is a widespread folk medicine for intestinal cramping and colic. It is included in the folk literature of New England, Appalachia, North Carolina, Indiana, and New Mexico. It is used by blacks throughout the deep South and by Hispanics in the Los Angeles area. Like chamomile, above, catnip contains both antispasmodic and sedative constituents. It was an official medicine in the *United States Pharmacopoeia* from 1840 until 1870.

☞ Directions: Place 1 teaspoon of the dried herb in a cup and add boiling water. Cover and let stand for ten minutes. Strain and drink 3 cups a day, on an empty stomach, before meals. Do this as often as desired.

 Insomnia 

If disturbed sleep leaves you feeling fatigued and not up to par the next day, you may be suffering from insomnia. Here's how to get some shut-eye

At some point in our lives, between one third and one half of all Americans have a serious bout of chronic insomnia, which is the inability to sleep the desired amount at least three nights a week for a month or more. Insomnia may mean difficulty falling asleep, waking up periodically during the night, or waking up too early. Length of sleep is not a measure of insomnia, because different people require different amounts. So, if disturbed sleep leaves you feeling fatigued and not up to par the next day, you may be suffering from insomnia, even if you slept for eight hours. Brief spells of insomnia may accompany worry, stress, changes in job shifts, or other temporary life situations. Habitual coffee drinking, even if only a few cups a day, may also cause or contribute to insomnia. Chronic insomnia may accompany such conditions as depression; chronic pain; or withdrawal from nicotine, alcohol, drugs, or sleep medications; or life passages such as menopause. Because some of these conditions become more prevalent as we age, insomnia is common among the elderly.

Insomnia can be the first sign of nutritional deficiencies, appearing before more serious diseases arise. It may indicate a deficiency of the minerals calcium, magnesium, or potassium, all of which are common deficiencies in the American diet. Deficiencies of the B-vitamins (niacin, pathothenic acid, folic acid, biotin, and pyridoxine) or of vitamin E may also cause insomnia.

Chronic stress can also lead to insomnia. Our body possesses hormonal mechanisms to respond to brief periods of stress throughout the day. At night, our body is given a break from these mechanisms to recuperate. When the body adapts to persistent stress, however, we end up physically prepared to run from a bear, even at bedtime, when we should be resting. Many of the folk remedies in this section help send cues to the brain, body, and glandular system that we are safe and that it is now time to relax and recuperate in order to meet the challenges of tomorrow.

Conventional medical treatment for chronic insomnia includes drugs in the benzodiazepine class, such as Valium and Xanax. These drugs may be appropriate to induce sleep during a brief crisis, but withdrawal from them may worsen the insomnia or induce anxiety, and use for as little as six weeks may cause addiction. These drugs, as well as over-the-counter sleep medications, can also disrupt patterns of sleep, interfering with the deepest stage of sleep known as deep delta wave sleep. During this part of sleep, the body normally recovers from stress, rebuilds its immune system, and repairs tissues. Chronic drug use can result in a constant feeling of fatigue, however. Before you turn to prescription or over-the-counter medications, you may want to try one of the folk remedies below for a healthier, more natural snooze.

Water Cures for Insomniacs

Water cures were widely used to treat insomnia and many other ailments in 19th century America. Such treatments eventually became institutionalized at health spas throughout the country. In Germany and France today, these treatments are considered part of conventional medicine—a patient may receive prescriptions, paid for by insurance, to spend up to three weeks resting and receiving daily hydrotherapy sessions at a spa. Treatments for insomnia include applications of hot, cold, or neutral-temperature water. You will need to experiment to find the water temperature that helps you get to sleep, however, because different people and different types of insomnia require different treatments. In general, very hot or very cold treatments tend to stimulate rather than sedate, so it's best to use moderate temperatures.

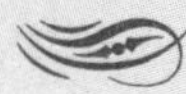

Remedies

REACTIVE HYDROTHERAPY: As the name implies, hydrotherapy is therapy with water in any of its forms—ice, cold water, hot water, steam, freshwater, or water imbued with special minerals. Reactive hydrotherapy uses cool water treatments to provoke an increase in circulation in a certain area. Cold initially drives blood out of an area, but eventually the body reacts by flooding the area with blood to warm it up. In Clarence Meyer's *American Folk Medicine* it is noted that reactive hydrotherapy will often "Soothe the wary brain, and quiet the nerves better than an opiate." Some forms of insomnia are accompanied by excess circulation to the brain, such as might accompany mental stress. A cool compress on the neck draws blood away from the brain, helping to soothe the mind.

☞ Directions: Put a cloth soaked in cold water on the back of the neck, and cover it with a warm towel. Keep the cloth in place for no more than fifteen minutes.

HOT FOMENTATION: An alternate treatment from the Seventh Day Adventists, a 150-year-old religious group that has long influenced folk medicine throughout North America, is to apply hot water to the back. In contrast to reactive hydrotherapy (see above), this method uses heat to directly draw blood to the area.

☞ Directions: Soak a cloth in moderately hot water and rest it on the spine for twenty to thirty minutes before bedtime.

HOT FOOT BATH: Another Seventh Day Adventist water treatment is the hot foot

continued on page 262

Curanderismo

Curanderismo is the Spanish name for a folk healing system found primarily among Mexican Americans and Mexican nationals. The healers are called *curanderos* (*curanderas* if the healers are female), which simply means "curer." Although other Spanish-speaking populations also have folk healers called curanderos, and many of the beliefs and practices are very similar, the name curanderismo is particularly applied to the folk-healing system of Mexico. This system bears the influences of the beliefs, healing practices, and medicinal plants of both the New World and its native peoples, and of the Spaniards who conquered and governed Mexico in the 16th and 17th centuries.

As is typical in folk medicine, curanderismo blends material and magical as well as natural and supernatural elements in its approaches to prevention and healing. A person's health is considered to include physical, mental, emotional, and spiritual aspects and all of these aspects are believed to interact. For example, a physical sickness or a set of symptoms can be brought on by emotional or spiritual causes; an emotional illness or spiritual crisis can be brought on by physical illness. And, as might be expected, the act of healing also focuses on these aspects. In fact, healing is usually approached through two or more of these avenues, despite what the diagnosis is.

While the system of curanderismo focuses on all of these aspects, most curanderos work primarily on what they call "the material level." The healers use herbs, massage, and other physical treatments. They also use some form of prayer as well as several other approaches that may not seem "material" to those outside curanderismo.

A smaller number, usually healers who are considered to have special gifts, may specialize in spiritual or "mental level" diagnosis and treatments, similar to psychic healing efforts. The skills of these spiritual specialists are often sought by family members of someone who has been ill for a very long time, who has a degenerative or terminal disease, or whose health problems seem to be mainly mental, spiritual, emotional, or behavioral in nature. Curanderos often refer patients to regular medical doctors, in addition to offering treatments themselves.

When people go to a curandero, they usually have already tried some form of first aid and self-care and have not been satisfied with the results. People go to these respected community healers to be treated for every kind of sickness, from common childhood complaints such as colic, thrush, and measles to cancer and tuberculosis, as well as specific folk illnesses (see "Latino Folk Illnesses," page 362). People may also seek the services of a curandero when they have reason to believe that the cause of their troubles is magical or supernatural in origin. In this tradition, as in many folk medical traditions, it is believed possible to be made sick by such influences as the evil eye or hexes.

The curandero will listen to the patient's description of the problem (and the descriptions given by their accompanying family members), ask probing questions, and try to understand the history of the presenting illness. The healer will then make his or her own diagnosis. In addition to looking, listening, and questioning, diagnosis can involve the healer's intuition, help from guiding spirits, and sometimes a form of divination, such as breaking an egg into a glass of tap water or holy water, passing the glass over the patient and interpreting the behavior of the egg in the water (sinking, rising, yolk separating from whites, etc.) to understand the nature of the problem. Spirits and divinations, if they are used, typically apply to cases in which there seems to be an important spiritual aspect to the sickness.

Once the diagnosis is made or confirmed, the curandero will usually give some treatment on the spot, as well as prescribe treatments and actions to be followed by the patient later. Treatments may include administration of herbal teas, wrapping the patient in blankets to "sweat out the illness," massages of specific parts of the body, prayers, counseling and encouragement, and "sweeping" of the body with specific herbs, raw eggs, or other objects. The principle at work in the sweepings is that of transference: It is the idea that disease, impurities, or evil elements may be transferred out of the body of the patient and into the sweeping substance, which can later be safely discarded. Particularly when the disease is strong or the causes are spiritual or supernatural, eggs may be used for sweepings. Because the eggs contain the cells of life, sickness and other bad elements may transfer into these potential living forms instead of remaining with the patient.

Scared to Death

Susto, which means "fright," is one of the best known of the Latino folk illnesses, and it is specifically treated by curanderos. It is caused by severe fright or emotional shock—such as the startle one gets when stepping absentmindedly into the street and nearly being hit by a car, witnessing an accident, or receiving unexpected bad news. It is believed that this shock may cause a person's soul to be separated from their body (see "Soul Loss," page 182). If the soul cannot return, the person will begin to feel depressed and disinterested in life, he will lose sleep and his appetite, and become nervous or anxious at small things.

The friends and family members of an individual who has susto should bring him to a curandero promptly, because susto is a serious condition, especially if proper treatment is delayed. Studies done in Mexico confirm that people with susto recover better when they are treated by a curandero than when they are treated by a psychologist or psychiatrist.

bath. The treatment draws blood away from the brain and upper body toward the feet. This is also a treatment for headaches due to congestion and menstrual cramps, so it may be especially helpful for insomnia that accompanies those conditions. You can add crushed mustard seeds to the water to increase the heating effect. Be sure to wrap the upper body in a blanket to avoid chills and promote sweating. You can also cover the head with a cloth soaked in cool water to decrease circulation to the brain. (Caution: People with insulin-dependent diabetes should not use this treatment due to the possibility of burning the feet.)

☞ Directions: Soak the feet in hot water. The water should be moderately hot, but not so hot that you pull back from it. Continue soaking for about fifteen minutes before bedtime.

THE NEUTRAL BATH: A standard Seventh Day Adventist water treatment for insomnia and nervous exhaustion is the neutral bath. Scientific studies have shown that taking a full immersion bath quiets the production of the "fight-or-flight" hormones from the adrenal glands. Thus, this treatment is proven to relax you when you're all wound up.

☞ Directions: Fill the tub with water at or just below body temperature, about 94–98°F. Soak for as long as one hour before bedtime.

COLD HIP BATH: A hydrotherapy treatment used to treat insomnia by German immigrants of the late 19th and early 20th centuries was the cold hip bath. The body reacts to a short, cold stimulus by pulling blood away from the brain toward the site of

Valerian

Valerian is one of the most famous herbs for treating insomnia; it is still used today in folk remedies in New England, Appalachia, and Indiana. Scientific studies show that, for some people, it is as effective as the drug Valium in inducing sleep. It doesn't work for everyone, however, and can actually produce insomnia in some people.

United States physicians of the last century listed valerian as a sedative, but also called it a cerebral stimulant, which means it increases the blood flow to the brain. Herbal texts of the time recommended it for restless individuals with cold constitutions (those with a pale face, cold hands and feet, and a desire for warm drinks and extra layers of clothes). It was not recommended for "hot-headed" individuals (those with a red, flushed face and a desire for cold drinks and fewer layers of clothes). Today, valerian is usually combined with another herb such as hop to avoid the occasional stimulating effects of valerian.

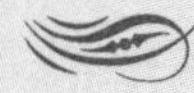

the stimulus. The treatment is still recommended today by some naturopathic physicians. It has not been tested in formal scientific trials.

☞ Directions: Sit in a tub filled with cool, but not extremely cold, water. The water level should reach just above your navel. Rest your feet on the edge of the tub so the water just covers your hips and abdomen. This position may be easier to negotiate in a large bucket or laundry tub. (If you do this, place the bucket or laundry tub in the bathtub to catch any water that spills when you get in.) Soak for forty seconds to two minutes before going to bed.

HERBAL BATHS: Herbal baths were popular among German immigrants, and they remain popular in Germany today. When you bathe with herbs, your skin absorbs their essential oils. An herb's aroma may also help to induce a peaceful state of mind. You can add relaxing herbs to any of the baths previously described. Avoid using oils such as peppermint, clove, and cinnamon, however. These hot oils can burn sensitive skin.

☞ Directions: Place 1 ounce of valerian, hop, chamomile, or lavender in a pot and cover with 1 quart of boiling water. Strain and add the water to the bath. Another approach is to add 1 or 2 drops of essential oil to the tub water. Remember that herbal oils are highly concentrated, so a little goes a long way. Enjoy an herbal bath right before bedtime.

THE HOP PILLOW: A widespread folk cure for insomnia is the hop pillow. Hop *(Humulus lupulus)* has been used for centuries as a mild sedative. German and British immigrants, Seventh Day Adventists, Indiana farmers, and residents of the American Southwest have all used hop to help induce sleep. Hop was listed as an official medicine in the *United States Pharmacopoeia* from 1820 to 1926.

☞ Directions: Cut two 8×11-inch squares of muslin fabric. Place 1 muslin square on top of the other and pin together around the edges. Sew ½-inch seams along the two long sides and 1 short side of the fabric, leaving the second short side open. Turn the seams to the inside. Take 4 ounces of hop, the fresher the better. Sprinkle it with a small amount of alcohol to bring out the active principle, but not enough to make it soggy. Add the herb to the muslin pillow case. Spread the herbs evenly within the pillow. (You will place it in your bed pillow, so you don't want it to make a lump.) Turn the raw edges under and pin the opening shut to enclose the content of the pillow securely.

Hop can also be used to make a soothing tea. Place 1 tablespoon of the herb in a cup and cover with boiling water. Cover the cup and let stand for ten minutes. Strain and drink before bedtime.

DILL SEEDS: A folk remedy from China is to wash the head in a tea of dill seeds *(Anethum graveolens)* so you'll inhale the fumes of the tea. Dill contains a number of sedative constituents in its volatile oil, which may explain the value of the plant for insomnia. Dill itself has not been tested by scientists for these purposes.

☞ Directions: If you don't want to smell like a pickle all night, here's a modified version of this remedy: Put 8 to 10 drops of essential oil of dill in 1 ounce of another oil, such as almond oil. Apply the mixture to a cloth, and keep it near your nose while you sleep. No direct application to the head is necessary. To avoid burns and blisters, never apply an essential oil in its concentrated form directly to the skin.

ROSE OIL: An aromatic remedy from the Amish is to apply diluted rose oil to the forehead. The pleasant fragrance somehow tricks the brain into relaxing the body. Apply and leave on throughout the night.

☞ Directions: Place 8 to 10 drops of concentrated rose oil in 1 ounce of almond oil. Apply a small amount to the forehead before going to bed.

PINE, JUNIPER, AND SAGE: A very common American Indian aromatherapy technique to induce sleep uses the scents of pine *(Pinus spp.)*, juniper *(Juniperus spp.)*, or sage *(Artemesia spp., Salvia spp.)*. The remedy requires burning and then inhaling the fresh or dried needles or leaves of the herbs. Also, you can inhale the scent by pouring a tea made from the dried plant over hot rocks.

☞ Directions: You can adapt this technique for household use by burning the dried needles or leaves like incense. Take some dried needles or leaves of pine, juniper, or sage, light them with a match, blow the flame out, and put the smoking embers in an ashtray. Inhale the fragrance as it fills the room.

EXERCISE: According to the Seventh Day Adventists, the best way to put yourself to sleep is to make yourself tired.

☞ Directions: Get twenty to forty minutes of proper moderate physical exercise each day. Try going for a brisk walk or participating in a sport or a hobby you enjoy.

MASSAGE: Another Seventh Day Adventist method to induce sleep is to give the person with insomnia a gentle stroking massage. Scientific research shows that massage can induce relaxation and ease stress.

Aromatherapy for Insomniacs

Aromatherapy is the use of inhaled fragrances to induce physiological actions or states in the body. The substance inhaled may be from a simple aromatic herb or an extracted plant oil.

Aromatherapy with essential oils is an accepted medical technique in France and is used there in hospitals as an adjunct to other treatments, especially to induce relaxation. The chemicals in the inhaled fragrances reach the bloodstream through the lungs, just as the nicotine in a cigarette does. The scent may affect the higher regulatory centers in the brain to trigger a relaxed state. The scents of hop, rose, dill, sage, and juniper have all been used to treat insomnia in American folk medicine.

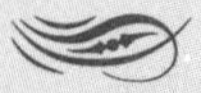

☞ Directions: Massage the patient gently, with the strokes always moving in the direction of the heart.

DEEP BREATHING: Another Seventh Day Adventist technique is to take slow, deep breaths. Breathing techniques are used throughout the world to relax the body and slow the mind. Research into the breathing techniques of yoga shows that deep breathing actually changes the brain waves, inducing a more relaxed state.

☞ Directions: Take 10 to 20 slow, deep breaths of fresh air at an open window or while lying in bed.

CATNIP: Catnip *(Napeta cataria)* tea has been a popular sleep aid in America since the arrival of the first European immigrants. The plant arrived with the colonists and became rapidly naturalized here. Indian tribes, including the Onondaga and Cayuga, used it to calm sleepless and peevish children.

The Seventh Day Adventists continue to use catnip today to induce sleep, and a 1995 poll of contemporary professional herbalists concluded that catnip remains one of the most prescribed herbs for insomnia.

☞ Directions: Place 1 to 3 teaspoons of the dried herb in a cup and cover with boiling water. Cover and let sit for ten minutes. Strain and drink before bedtime. When making the tea, contemporary Appalachian herbalist Tommie Bass suggests combining catnip with passion flower, sage, peppermint, or skullcap.

PASSION FLOWER: From the southern Appalachians to the American Southwest, people have long used passion flower *(Passiflora incarnata)* as a sedative to aid in sleep. The Amish combine it with chamomile. Passion flower contains sedative alkaloid constituents that help you relax.

☞ Directions: Place a heaping teaspoon of passion flower in 1 cup of water and steep ten minutes. Strain and drink before retiring for the night.

HOT MILK: Drink a cup of hot milk before bed. This New England remedy has doubtlessly appeared wherever milk is consumed and persists today in the folk medicine of the United States. How does it work? The warm milk may trigger instincts of safety associated with nursing at the breast. Variations of this remedy include adding ½ teaspoon of nutmeg or 2 teaspoons of honey. (Note: Nutmeg has psychoactive constituents that can induce unpleasant hallucinations in doses of only several teaspoons.)

☞ Directions: Warm the milk and drink before bedtime. It'll cultivate pleasant, relaxing thoughts.

CHAMOMILE: Chamomile tea *(Matricaria recutita, Anthemis nobilis)* is one of the most popular commercial beverages used today to induce relaxation and sleep. The plant came to North America with the colonists and is now native to many areas of the country. It has been used in folk medicine in New England, Appalachia, the Midwest and Southwest, and possibly everywhere in between. Chamomile's constituents, which have both anti-inflammatory and antispasmodic actions, also promote digestion. It may be especially suited for insomnia that accompa-

continued on page 267

Beliefs on Bedwetting

Childhood can be a difficult time in any culture, and many folk remedies are aimed at curing common problems for children. One concern is bedwetting. Sometimes bedwetting can be a symptom of infection or other physical difficulty. Other times, children just don't wake up when they need to urinate. Not only is bedwetting messy, but it can be embarrassing to both child and parent. Some of the folk remedies used to cure it, however, are even more embarrassing. For example, draping the wet sheet over the child's head and making him stand outside in the sun until it dries is one recommended remedy!

Some say a child playing with hot ashes before going to bed at night will suffer the affliction. But you can cure him of bedwetting by heating a brick and having the child urinate on it.

It is believed that what you do with the umbilical cord when a child is born can cause or prevent a child from becoming a bedwetter. Laying an umbilical cord down will cause the child to be a bedwetter. Some say that if you burn the "navel string" the child won't wet the bed.

Belief in the curative power of corpses is widespread. So is the idea that burying something in a grave will cure the person associated with the item. Some people have even tried to get a child to urinate in an open grave to cure bedwetting. Another related remedy involves putting a bottle of the child's urine in a grave before the grave is closed up. Put a small hole in the bottle's cork so the urine can drip out. When it does, the bedwetting will be cured.

Seeds and teas are commonly used in folk remedies. Feeding a child watermelon seeds or pumpkin seeds is said to cure bedwetting. Both corn silk and gum bark teas have also been tried. A rare parent or two has even squeezed the urine from the sheets, mixed it with milk and sugar, and made the child drink that! This remedy could actually poison a child and lead to much worse problems than bedwetting!

Mouse Tea?

Some of the most peculiar cures for bedwetting use rats or mice. Boiling a mouse for a tea is one method. Roasting or frying a mouse or rat and having the child eat part of it, sometimes in a sandwich or pie, is another treatment. The strangest use is to wrap a mouse in a cloth and bite off its head, then tie the cloth, with the head in it, around the child's neck—and leave it there for several days. With all the diseases we can catch from rodents and their fleas, these treatments could make a child, or you, very sick!

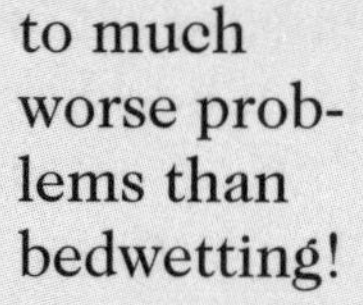

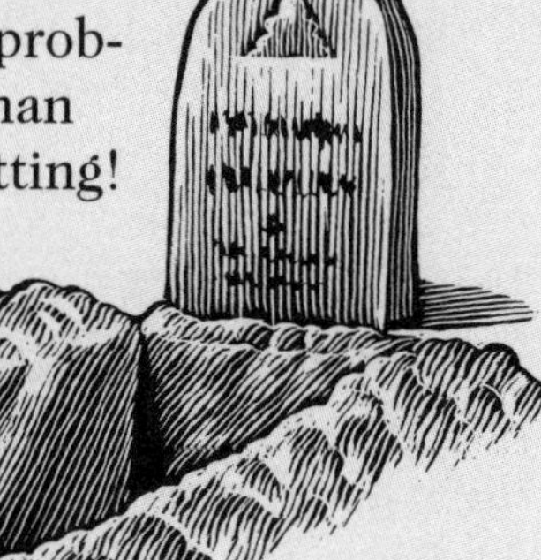

Herbs for Insomnia

Today, medical herbalists often use plant medicines as minor sedatives. In general, herbs will not force you to sleep like some of the stronger pharmaceutical medicines used for the same purpose. Instead, herbs may gently trigger your innate sleep response. It is best to take them as warm teas, because warm fluid in the stomach also has a relaxing effect. Take a ½-cup dose an hour before bedtime to help calm you, and then take a second dose just before going to bed. For severe insomnia, try adding a one-third dose just after dinner, and keep a fourth dose by the bed in case you awaken during the night. Sedative herbs may work better in combinations of three or more; different herbs help induce sleep through various mechanisms.

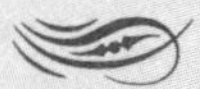

nies inflammation or digestive upset. (Note: Chamomile is not appropriate for habitual use because it may suppress normal and healthy inflammatory responses. Occasional use is safe, but don't use daily for more than two to three weeks. In addition, chamomile flowers may cause symptoms of allergies in some people allergic to ragweed and related plants, although the risk of this is quite low.)

☞ Directions: Put a heaping tablespoon of chamomile flowers in a cup and add boiling water. Cover and steep for ten minutes. Strain and drink before turning in for the night.

GINSENG WINE: For insomnia that results from chronic stress or an illness, especially a feverish illness, try making an herbal wine out of American ginseng *(Panax quinquefolium)*—not Asian ginseng. American ginseng in various forms is used in Chinese folk medicine and throughout Chinatowns in North America today.

☞ Directions: Chop 3½ ounces of American ginseng and place it in 1 quart of liquor such as vodka. Let the mixture stand for five to six weeks in a cool dark place, turning the container frequently. Then, take 1 ounce of the solution after dinner or before bed. (You don't need to strain the liquid in this remedy. The root is heavy and will settle at the bottom of the container.) Be sure to use American ginseng, not Asian ginseng, in this remedy.

HERBAL FORMULA: Folklorist Clarence Meyer's *American Folk Medicine* calls for equal parts of skullcap, blue vervain, hop, and chamomile with ½ part of valerian. This balanced formula is typical of what might be prescribed for chronic insomnia today by a North American or British medical herbalist. Valerian can be stimulating to some individuals, but the amount in this formula will be overridden by the other herbs (see sidebar, "Valerian," page 262). The multiple sedative actions of the various herbs in this remedy may be more effective than taking any of these single herbs alone.

☞ Directions: Mix the dried herbs in a bowl. Then place a heaping tablespoon of the mixture in a cup. Cover with ½ cup boiling water, and steep for ten minutes. Strain and drink before bedtime.

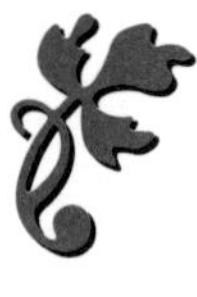

Itching and Rashes

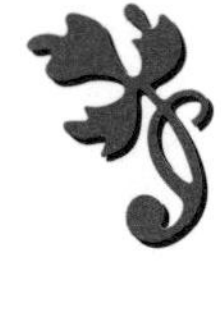

Once you've discovered the cause of your skin condition, it's likely there's a good folk remedy ready to treat it

An itch may be due to local irritation of the skin. Local irritation may be caused by insect bites, stings, or infestation; by an allergic reaction to a plant, animal, or synthetic substance; or by infection from molds, yeasts, or other microorganisms. Sometimes itching can be simply due to dry skin. Many prescription drugs can also cause itching.

An itch may also be due to a systemic disease—one that's irritating the skin from the inside out. For example, disorders of the blood, kidneys, or thyroid can cause itching. An itch from a systemic disease may affect only a small area of the skin, as in cases of eczema or psoriasis or allergies to substances that have been eaten. Sometimes a systemic disease will cause itching over large areas of the body or itching that moves from one place to another.

Conventional treatment of itching and rashes first requires an investigation of the cause of the skin condition. For example, if itching is the result of an allergic sensitivity to a certain fabric, avoiding that particular fabric is likely to be recommended. If prescription drugs are responsible for your discomfort, your physician may prescribe a different medication. Folk remedies traditionally rely on herbs to treat and soothe the skin. If your doctor has diagnosed your skin condition as one that can be self treated, you may want to try some of the remedies below.

Remedies

JUNIPER AND CLOVE: Folklorist Clarence Meyer's *American Folk Medicine* suggests using a salve of juniper *(Juniperus spp.)* and clove *(Eugenia carophyllata)* to soothe itchy skin. Juniper berries have been used to treat itching by American Indians of the Paiute, Shoshone, and Cherokee tribes. Clove has been used throughout Asia, the Middle East, Mexico, and the American Southwest to treat itchy skin conditions. Juniper contains anti-inflammatory volatile substances, and clove contains the substance eugenol, a topical anesthetic widely used by dentists. The eugenol presumably affects the itch by numbing the nerve endings in the skin. The following salve is modified slightly from the one in Meyer's collection.

☞ Directions: Melt 3 ounces of unsalted butter in a sauce pan. Then, in a separate pan, melt a lump of beeswax about the size of 2 tablespoons (it is difficult to get beeswax actually into the tablespoon). When the beeswax is melted, add it to the melted butter and stir well. Add 5 tablespoons of ground juniper berries and 3 tablespoons of ground clove to the butter/beeswax mixture and stir. (Instead of purchasing the herbs as powders, it is best to grind the herbs yourself because the volatile substances are preserved better in the whole berries and clove.) Allow the mixture to cool and become solid. Apply as a salve to itchy skin.

BASIL: A wash of basil tea *(Ocimum basilicum)* is used in Chinese folk medicine to treat itching from hives. Basil, like cloves, contains high amounts of eugenol, a topical anesthetic.

☞ Directions: Place ½ ounce of dried basil leaves in a 1-pint jar and fill with boiling water. Immediately cover to prevent the escape of the aromatic eugenol from the tea. Allow to cool to room temperature. Strain, dip a clean cloth in the tea, and apply to itchy areas as often as desired.

MINT: Another remedy from Chinese folk medicine for treating itchy skin rashes or hives is a wash of mint tea. In China, cornmint *(Mentha arvensis)* is the type of mint used. In North America, peppermint *(Mentha piperita),* which has constituents similar to cornmint, is preferred. Both peppermint and cornmint contain significant amounts of menthol, which has anesthetic and anti-inflammatory properties when applied topically. In general, mint also contains high amounts of the anti-inflammatory rosmarinic acid, which is readily absorbed into the skin.

☞ Directions: Place 1 ounce of dried peppermint leaves in a 1-pint jar and fill with boiling water. Immediately cover the jar to prevent the escape of the aromatic eugenol from the tea. Allow to cool to room temperature. Strain, dip a clean cloth in the tea, and apply to the itchy area as often as necessary.

THYME: A remedy from Chinese folk medicine, similar to the two above, uses garden thyme *(Thymus vulgaris)*. Thyme contains large amounts of the volatile constituent thymol, which gives thyme some of its fragrance. Thanks to thymol's anesthetic and anti-inflammatory properties, it numbs the nerves that cause the itch while reducing local inflammation. A Chinese tradition suggests mixing thyme with dandelion root.

☞ Directions: Place 1 ounce of dried dandelion root and ½ ounce of dried thyme leaves in a 1-quart jar. Fill with boiling water and cover with a tight lid. Allow to cool to room temperature. Strain, dip a cloth in the tea, and apply to the affected areas.

CLEAVERS: Cleavers *(Galium aparine)* has been used to treat skin ailments since the time of the ancient Greeks. American Indians of the Iroquois and Chippewa tribes later used cleavers for the same purpose. Today, teas made from the plant remain a common prescription by professional

continued on page 272

Unconventional Wart Cures

Warts are infectious growths in the outer layers of the skin. They are contagious and can spread from person to person. Most warts are not health-threatening, but they can be a nuisance, and most who have them are eager to get rid of them. Even Mark Twain wrote about a remedy for warts. When Huckleberry Finn buried a dead cat in a crossroads at midnight, he was taking part in just one of the many strange wart cures found throughout American folk medicine.

One of folk medicine's most bizarre wart cures involves graveyards, not crossroads, however. In the southern and western United States, according to folklorists, some residents attempt to cure warts by taking a dead cat to a graveyard at midnight. (Whether or not the cat is killed for this purpose is not always specified in the folk literature.) When a noise is heard, the cat is thrown in the direction of the sound. In Tennessee, people believe the sound heard is the devil—"coming to get his people." As the person throws the cat, he or she must say, "Cat follow the devil, warts follow the cat."

Wart cures are a popular part of folk medicine. That's probably because warts have plagued humanity for centuries. In ancient times, people weren't sure where warts came from, so they invented causes for the malady. For example, the belief that warts were caused by touching toads is probably due to the similarity between a wart's appearance and a toad's lumpy, wartlike skin.

Today, we know warts are caused by the human papilloma virus (HPV). Scientists once thought warts were caused by just one kind of virus; now we know there are at least 60 types of HPVs that cause a wide variety of warts, from plantar warts that grow on the feet to the warts that

Wart Cures

There are some wart cures that are gruesome as well as dangerous. Many of these cures require the use of blood, either drawn from the wart or applied to it. In one remedy, blood drawn from a wart by repeatedly pricking it with a pin is to be put on grains of corn that are then fed to chickens. (Presumably the chicken then gets the warts—but perhaps not before the sufferer gets an infection!) In another remedy, warm bloody meat from a freshly killed hog is applied directly to the wart. Another remedy suggests rubbing the wart with the head of a recently killed cock; the cock is then buried under the eaves of your home or barn. Finally, a recommendation from Pennsylvania that is both gruesome and dangerous: Wash the warts in water from cattle dung!

most often appear on the hands and fingers. Warts can emerge anywhere on the skin including the genital and anal areas, even internally.

Some wart cures seem medicinal, like those that require the use of dandelion or milkweed juice. Other treatments appear ritualistic: A treatment from North Carolina instructs patients to gather seven different kinds of leaves, rub each on the wart twice, and bury the leaves where no one will find them. But most folk cures have a magical element. Take, for instance, the blacksmith's water cure. Water into which a blacksmith has plunged his hot iron has an ancient reputation as a magical remedy for many things. Iron supposedly had supernatural properties, so a blacksmith's water was therefore thought to be magical. Iron has long been used in the folk traditions of many cultures.

Why are wart cures so popular? Probably because they seem to work. Even if left alone, most warts will disappear on their own in a few months. By the time a person is annoyed enough with a wart to seek a remedy, the wart is probably already in its final stages and it will soon disappear. Most folk cures capitalize on this fact. One cure from the southern United States says to rub warts with the sole of a shoe. As the leather wears away, so will the warts. A cure from Pennsylvania directs the patient to put a chalk mark for each wart on the back of an old iron wood-burning stove. When the chalk marks wear away, the warts will be gone. In both of these cases, the remedies are likely to work—simply because of patience and the passage of time.

Cures for warts often involve physical contact with certain items, as in the shoe example above. Similar cures call for rubbing the wart with a potato, onion, or dish rag. The item used to rub the wart is then hidden in a place where it will decay; for example, under the eaves of a house. If a dishrag is the chosen item, the remedy often specifies that the dish rag be stolen from the individual's mother. (Children tend to acquire warts more often than adults.)

There is little evidence that some of these cures actually have the medical ability to cure warts. More likely, it is the power of suggestion—and the passage of time—that is so successful in curing warts. For these reasons, many ancient wart cures continue to be practiced and passed from one generation to the next.

Unwelcome Warts

Many magical wart cures are uncharitable to say the least, especially when they involve the intent of giving the warts to someone else. This sort of behavior can be illustrated in a cure that requires an individual to rub his warts with a penny and leave the penny in the road–whoever picks up the penny is believed to take the warts along with him!

Another wart cure involves rubbing the warts with a penny until they bleed. The treatment is believed to be more powerful because of blood's magical reputation. But leaving the bloody penny in the road is uncharitable, and the action of rubbing the warts also carries with it the risk of infection.

herbalists in North America for treating skin ailments.

No constituents with specific anti-inflammatory or anti-itch properties have been identified in cleavers. Herbalists theorize that the constituents work by "purifying the blood"—that is, by treating the itch from the inside out. No scientific evidence for such an action is apparent, however. Its constituents include tannins, which may account for the mild astringent action it possesses. Dried cleavers is rich in mineral nutrition, with an ounce of the herb providing significant portions of the daily requirement of such minerals as calcium, magnesium, and iron.

☞ Directions: Place 1 ounce of dried cleavers in a quart of water, and simmer for twenty minutes. Strain and drink as a beverage throughout the day. Sweeten with honey if desired. Drink 3 to 4 cups a day for two to three weeks and see if your skin condition improves.

Poke Root

Poke root *(Phytolacca decandra)* appears to be a universal topical remedy for itching. References to teas made from poke root that were designed to treat itching appear in American Indian lore and in the folk traditions of Appalachia and the South, where the plant grows. Poke root is not appropriate for internal use, however, except under medical supervision—the berries are a relatively common cause of poisoning among children.

Poke root is not usually found for sale in herb shops or health food stores. If it grows in your area, you can dig up the plant, wash and dry the roots, and chop the roots into small pieces. To make a wash, use 1 ounce of the root to 1 quart of water. Be sure to keep the plant away from children, and do not take poke root internally.

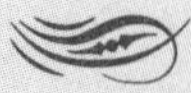

BAKING SODA BATH: A baking soda bath is recommended for itchy skin conditions in the Hispanic folklore of the Southwest. The same treatment is used in New England. Contemporary Seventh Day Adventists, a religious movement that advocates natural remedies and alternative medicine, also use baking soda baths for treating itchy skin conditions, eczema, and sunburn.

☞ Directions: Add 1 cup of commercial baking soda to a tub of 94–98°F water. Stay in the tub for thirty to sixty minutes. Let the skin dry naturally without toweling.

LEMON JUICE: Rubbing lemon juice on itchy, inflamed skin is recommended in American folklorist Clarence Meyer's *American Folk Medicine*. The same method is used in the Hispanic folklore of the American Southwest. The aromatic substances in lemon have anesthetic and anti-inflammatory properties, which may be responsible for its medicinal activity, if any in fact exists.

☞ Directions: Juice a lemon. Apply undiluted to itchy skin.

continued on page 274

Healing Burns

Burns are a very common injury. They are always painful, they can be disfiguring, and even relatively minor burns can be life-threatening if they become infected. It's no wonder, then, that folk medicine traditions always include burn remedies.

All sorts of herbal remedies have been suggested to treat burns. Some, like lavender, can provide at least symptomatic relief because they contain mild anti-inflammatory substances. Others, like tea, contain soothing tannins. But such remedies have never been tested for safety or efficacy, and some treatments, such as bittersweet bark, are known to be toxic if taken internally. These herbal treatments were usually combined with greases or oils, including lard, butter, or axle grease. The mixture was often slathered on a leaf to make a poultice. Another topical application that has been used in the treatment of burns is mud, and although it provides a cooling sensation, it is extremely unsanitary. Today, doctors strongly urge against using any such application. These applications increase the risk of infection and make cleaning the wound much more difficult. For the treatment of a major burn, see your doctor. For minor burns, try aloe vera gel.

Magical Means

Magical treatments for burns can be as dangerous as some herbal treatments. Some healers believed that burns should not be cooled too quickly. (That is an unfortunate belief, however, because cold water is the most effective first-aid treatment for burns. Its application can actually reduce the severity of a burn if applied immediately.) These healers instead recommend a sort of "like cures like" technique—they often call for the burn to be warmed near a fire. One healer in Utah actually held his victims' burns over a fire for this purpose. The belief was that the burn would be "drawn out" into the fire.

Folk treatments for burns are not limited to applying medicinal substances. Religious and magical treatments abound as well. In fact, one of the most interesting folk treatments of burns involves "fire doctors," as they have been called in the South. Fire doctors are individuals who use prayers and rituals to "talk fire out of burns."

In the traditions of some Christian groups, short prayers are used to treat burns. Sometimes called "charms," these prayers usually invoke "the three highest names"—that is, the Father, Son, and Holy Ghost. These prayers are sometimes in the form of rhyme.

The healers who use such charms usually refuse payment. Some say that the patient must not even say "thank you," or the treatment will not work. Many burn patients claim their recovery was rapid and painless after treatment by a fire doctor.

PLANTAIN: Plantain *(Plantago major)* was called "Englishman's footprint" by the American Indians and by residents of the Southwest because the herb came to North America with the immigrants from the British Isles and rapidly spread to wherever the immigrants went. Today it can be found in lawns and along sidewalks throughout North America. Foot baths of "English" plantain are used in the folk medicine of northern New Mexico to alleviate itchy feet. Plantain teas are also recommended in the southern Appalachian mountains to treat itchy skin conditions. Plantain contains small amounts of at least 14 different anti-inflammatory constituents, which, acting together, might be responsible for its itch-reducing effects.

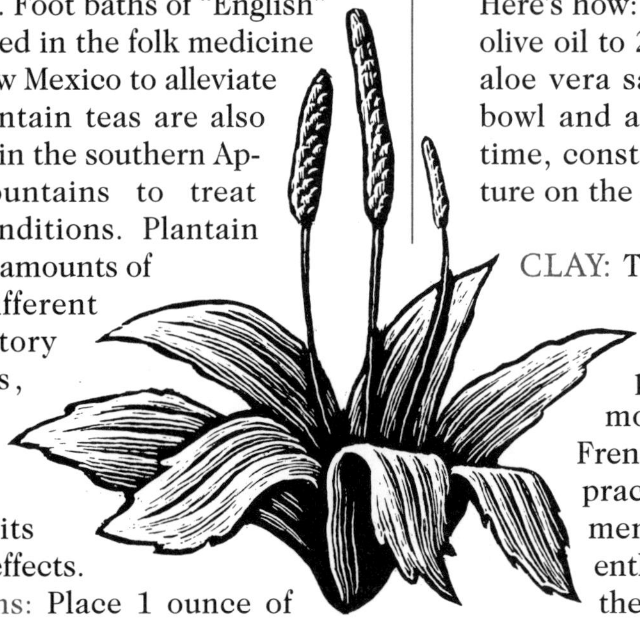

☞ Directions: Place 1 ounce of dried plantain leaf in a 1-quart jar and fill with boiling water. Cover and let cool to room temperature. Strain and apply the tea with a clean cloth to the affected areas.

ALOE VERA: Aloe vera, may be helpful for treating itchy skin as well as minor burns, according to the traditions of the Seventh Day Adventists, a religious movement that advocates natural remedies and alternative medicine. The plant's anti-inflammatory constituents that reduce blistering and inflammation in burns may also reduce itching (see section, "Burns and Sunburn," page 107). Avoid using yellowish sap under the aloe's green skin. This area of the plant contains antraquinones, which may irritate the skin or eyes.

☞ Directions: Break off a leaf, slice it down the middle, and rub the gel on the skin. You can also apply store-bought aloe vera gel or juice.

An alternative formula involves using olive oil to extend the aloe vera sap. Here's how: Add 8 ounces of extra virgin olive oil to 2 ounces of freshly squeezed aloe vera sap. Place the sap in a large bowl and add the oil a few drops at a time, constantly stirring. Rub the mixture on the skin.

CLAY: The American Indians commonly applied muddy clay to itchy skin areas. Clay applications were also commonly used in German and French folk medicine. Today, the practice remains highly recommended by contemporary Seventh Day Adventists for soothing the skin.

☞ Directions: For this remedy, you can use bentonite clay, French green clay, or other cosmetic clay—all of which are available in health food stores and cosmetic outlets. Mix clay into 1 cup of warm (not hot) water until it is the consistency of a thin pea soup. Apply it to the skin. Let the clay stay on for at least forty minutes, or for several hours, if possible. Wipe off the clay using water and a wash cloth. (You may need to scrub gently with the cloth to remove the clay if the clay has dried completely.) Wipe off the clay over a bowl and discard the waste in your garden or on your lawn because clay can stop up your pipes. Repeat as often as desired.

 Menses 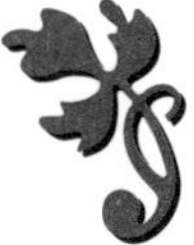

Mild to severe menstrual discomfort or other disorders of the menstrual cycle are among the most common minor medical conditions in North America

Menstruation is the monthly breakdown and discharge of portions of the endometrial tissue that lines the uterus. The normal menstrual cycle can vary from 21 to 35 days, with the flow lasting from 2 to 9 days. A 30 to 60 milliliter blood loss (1 to 2 ounces) is expected. Disorders of the cycle can be due to the length of the cycle, length (or lack of) menstrual flow, and the amount of the flow. Here are some medical terms and definitions for some abnormal menstrual conditions.

Dysmenorrhea: *painful menstruation with cramping*

Menorrhagia: *excessive menstrual bleeding lasting longer than 7 days or blood loss exceeding 80 ml (2½ ounces)*

Hypomenorrhea: *scanty menstrual flow (less than 1 ounce)*

Metrorrhagia: *irregular uterine bleeding*

Polymenorrhea: *episodes of menstrual bleeding occurring at less than 21-day intervals*

Oligomenorrhea: *menstrual cycles at greater than 35 day intervals*

Folk remedies abound for painful menstruation (dysmenorrhea) and excessive menstrual bleeding (menorrhagia), but treatments for the other conditions above do not appear in most folk literature.

A common topic in folk medicine is "delayed menstruation," often discussed hand-in-hand with painful menstruation. Delayed menstruation refers to a brief delay of the normal period, within the normal limits above, in a woman who knows that she is not pregnant. If you experience menstrual irregularity outside the normal limits above, be sure to seek a gynecologist's advice before using folk remedies. And before treating mildly-delayed menstruation be sure that you are not pregnant.

As many as 75 percent of women have pain during menstruation at some time in their lives, and 5 to 6 percent experience incapacitating pain. The conventional treatment is pain-relieving medications, and sometimes, birth control pills to prevent ovulation. The Chinese, Ayurvedic (from India), and Arabic alternative systems of medicine believe that menstruation may be painful or slightly delayed due to a condition described as "stagnant blood." An equivalent description in modern physiology would be deficient circulation of blood to the uterus. The chief causes of stagnation, when described by traditional systems, are lack of exercise and exposure to cold weather.

The Eclectic and Physiomedicalist schools of medicine, two groups of 19th century physicians, described the same condition and treated it the same way the traditional systems did—with circulatory stimulants. Circulatory stimulants are usually hot, spicy herbs that may produce flushing of the skin and sweating, and according to traditional theories, stimulate or increase the flow of menstrual blood. These herbs are called emmenagogue herbs or foods, meaning that they stimulate the flow of the menses. These plants have not been tested in clinical trials for either pain-relieving or menstrual-promoting effects, but many of them contain antispasmodic and anti-inflammatory constituents. Use of emmenagogues is contraindicated in pregnancy, although the risk of inducing abortion with the normal amounts found in herbal teas are slight.

The Risk of Miscarriage

The menstruation-promoting herbs in this section are all contraindicated in pregnancy, though the actual risk of inducing miscarriage by drinking normal amounts of teas containing these herbs is probably slight. In fact, according to MEDLINE, a database of the National Library of Medicine in Bethesda, Maryland, there are no recorded accidental miscarriages from herb consumption.

Miscarriages, injury to the mother, and even death *are* recorded for women taking concentrated essential oils of plants in attempts to induce abortion, however. Folk traditions, as well as contemporary texts of medical herbalism, include some herbs, such as blue cohosh and pennyroyal, that may induce abortion. Contemporary North American medical herbalists report that successful herbal abortions are rare, however. This may be the reason why population control in traditional societies that rely on herbal abortives is ineffective.

Women seeking to induce abortion with herbs are far more likely to make themselves ill—or even kill themselves—than to abort the fetus. If a woman seeking to induce miscarriage cannot do so by intentionally taking large amounts of strong herbs, then it is not likely that normal beverage amounts of the herbs included below will induce abortion accidentally. It is prudent, however, to avoid these herbs completely during pregnancy, especially in the first trimester, in fragile pregnancies, or when there has been a history of miscarriage.

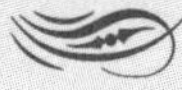

For any disorder of the menstrual cycle, also consider a visit to the chiropractor (D.C.) or osteopath (D.O.) to see if physical misalignment of the spine or conditions of the internal organs may be contributing to your health problem.

Remedies

GINGER: Ginger *(Zingiber officinale)* is perhaps one of the most popular—and relatively safe—menstrual cramp relievers. It is used either for delayed menstruation or for menstrual cramps in the folk medicine of the eastern United States. Ginger is used for these conditions in the folk traditions of New England, New York, and Indiana, and it is also used among the Amish in Michigan. Ginger is used for the same purposes in the traditional medical systems of China, India, and Arabia.

Ginger contains a number of anti-inflammatory constituents, including some that specifically suppress prostaglandins, which are thought to be responsible for menstrual cramping (see sidebar, "Calming Menstrual Pain," page 281). Ginger also contains four antispasmodic constituents. These actions may help menstruation to occur more naturally.

☞ Directions: Place ½ teaspoon of ginger powder in a cup. Fill with boiling water and let stand, covered, for five minutes. Strain. Drink a cup, hot, two or three times a day, as needed.

CINNAMON: A Chinese folk remedy uses cinnamon *(Cinnamomum verum)* to stimulate delayed menses or to treat cramps. Cinnamon was used in the same way by the Eclectic physicians of the 19th and early 20th centuries. Cinnamon contains a mixture of both anti-inflammatory and antispasmodic constituents.

☞ Directions: Place ¼ teaspoon of cinnamon powder in a cup. Fill with boiling water and let stand, covered, for five minutes. Strain. Drink a cup, hot, two or three times a day as needed.

FENNEL: Fennel seed tea *(Foeniculum vulgare)* is a treatment for menstrual cramps in Chinese folklore. Fennel, a warming spice, promotes circulation in the same manner as the other emmenagogues in this section. Fennel also contains seven different antispasmodic constituents.

☞ Directions: Grind 1 teaspoon of fennel seeds in a coffee grinder or with a mortar and pestle. Place the fennel powder in a cup. Fill with boiling water and let stand, covered, for five minutes. Strain. Drink 1 cup of the tea, hot, three times a day.

JUNIPER BERRIES: In *American Folk Medicine*, folklorist Clarence Meyer suggests drinking a tea of juniper berries to bring on delayed menstruation. This remedy was also used in ancient Egypt, although the Egyptians made the tea with milk instead of water. (The Egyptians also used juniper berries to embalm the dead). Juniper berries contain at least nine antispasmodic constituents.

☞ Directions: Crush 1 teaspoon of juniper berries in a coffee grinder or with a mortar and pestle. Place 1 teaspoon of the powder in a cup and fill with boiling water. Let steep for five to ten minutes, covered. Strain. Take ¼-cup doses every three or four hours. Don't take juniper if you have kidney disease, and don't take it daily for more than three weeks. Berries are abortifacient. Avoid excessive consumption.

continued on page 280

The Bond Among Women

Folk medicine is unofficial medicine, and the official institutions of Western culture—including Western medicine—have been dominated by men for many centuries. Yet, in the home, women have always had a great deal of responsibility for the health of their families. As a result, women have long played a central role in folk medicine. Even in recent times women have been instrumental in developing alternative medical techniques, especially those regarding their own health and the health of their children. For example, in 1992, medical researchers found that yogurt consumption can be a good treatment for vaginal yeast infections. And, in 1994, researchers for the first time stated that cranberry juice is a good treatment for urinary tract infections. Most women have suffered from yeast or urinary tract infections at some point, and these two treatments have been part of women's folk knowledge for generations. Yet it was only after many years of treating both conditions with prescription medications that are expensive and have side effects that modern medicine decided to inquire into what women themselves already knew!

THE BIRTHING PROCESS: Even before the development of modern medicine, most women knew a great deal about their bodies. Experts in female health called midwives had an extensive wealth of folk knowledge and experience as well. Midwives specialized in the delivery and care of babies, birth control, and women's health in general. Before modern medicine, midwives were readily used, and as a result, women experienced what is referred to as a social birth. When labor approached, a woman would be surrounded by female relatives, friends, and a midwife. This gathering of women accomplished several things: It provided the mother with emotional support, and it supplied many able hands for the work needed (from delivery through recovery, cooking for the family, and minding the older children). It did something else, too—it provided the women in attendance, including the laboring woman's young daughters, with a rich and intense learning experience. By the time a woman was pregnant for the first time, she would usually have attended many births and received a great deal of informal instruction.

Hospital births attended by male obstetricians didn't become common until the early 20th century. This change was encouraged by the invention of forceps, and it was promoted to ensure sterile conditions and the use of anesthetics. Although sanitary conditions in hospitals were actually very poor when this process got started, anesthetics were definitely available and used. Women, however, paid a steep price for admission to this modern birth setting. Midwives were outlawed in many places, daughters and mothers were excluded, and the laboring mother herself was rendered unconscious. As a result, within a few generations, most American women had never seen a birth, including the births of their own children! The tradition of passing on women's knowledge during social birth had ended. The resulting ignorance and fear gave official medicine the power to discourage home births and the midwives who attended them. Only after the women's health movement gathered power in the 1960s and natural childbirth again became popular, did women begin to reassert control of this aspect of their lives and recover some of their lost knowledge. Certified nurse-midwives were recognized by ACOG (American College of Obstetrics & Gynecology) in 1971, and now nurse-midwifery training programs are found in many nursing schools. Although many certified nurse-midwives have thriving practices and hospital admitting privileges, a great many births take place outside hospitals in birthing centers, where births are attended by midwives. These centers provide general women's health care. Women's health care, and the role of women in that care, has changed tremendously since the 1950s, and that has been a direct result of the demands of women themselves.

BREASTFEEDING: Another part of women's lore is the high value placed on breastfeeding, including the knowledge of how to go about it and how to deal with common problems associated with it. Just as birth was medicalized in the 20th century, so was infant feeding. Doctors supported the move away from breastfeeding and to the use of infant formula in the United States and around the world. Again, it was in the 1960s when American women began to reassert their traditional authority in this area. The skills needed for successful breastfeeding are not all instinctive, so as with birthing, a supportive and knowledgeable community is very important. This change back to breastfeeding has been a slow process resisted by the medical establishment. In the 1980s and 1990s, however, official pronouncements by the medical community once again endorsed this ancient knowledge that was once part of all women's folklore.

PLANTS AND MAGICAL CHARMS: Much folk knowledge about women's health has involved diet and the use of plants. For example, ginger, yarrow (also called "squaw-weed"), and raspberry leaves were very common treatments for menstrual problems. (Conventional medicine, for the most part, has treated menstrual and premenstrual discomforts as psychosomatic problems—a mistake no midwife would have been likely to make!) Magical and religious measures were also well known and widely used. For example, in most parts of the United States, folk tradition urged that during labor all doors be kept open and all stoppers be removed from bottles. At one point, in the 16th century, such "opening charms," which were found all over the world and even included the untying of knots, were expressly forbidden by church authorities. Anyone who continued to practice the charms would be charged with witchcraft!

The way that women's folk medicine is presented in many published collections makes it sound rather strange and old-fashioned, but in fact, these remedies are a vital body of knowledge and values, constantly growing and adapting. The remedies created by women represent their struggle to maintain the authority of their experience and the right to know about—and take care of—their own bodies.

MOTHERWORT: The use of motherwort *(Leonurus cardiaca)* as a medicine has its roots in both American Indian and European history. The Delaware, Mohegan, Micmac, and Shinnecock tribes all used the plant as a medicine for gynecological conditions. Whether or not the plant was native to the northeastern areas of the country, where the tribes lived, is not known. The Indians may have adopted the use of the plant after it arrived with the European colonists. Because of its folk use in Britain for menstrual cramps and delayed menstruation, motherwort was a household folk medicine among British colonists in the early American colonies. It was later used in the medicine of the Eclectic and Physiomedicalist physicians during the 1800s and early 1900s.

The Europeans used motherwort as an emmenagogue and a heart medicine. In describing motherwort, the 17th century British herbalist Nicholas Culpepper wrote, "there is no better herb to drive melancholy vapours from the heart, to strengthen it and keep the mind cheerful, blithe and merry."

Motherwort is approved by the German government as a sedative for "nervous" heart symptoms, such as palpitations that accompany anxiety or stress. Chinese physicians also use the herb; they have used their native species of motherwort since at least A.D. 100 for treating menstrual disorders.

☞ Directions: Place ½ ounce of motherwort herb (the dried flowering tops) in a 1-pint jar and cover with boiling water. Let stand twenty minutes. Strain and rebottle. Take 1 to 2 ounces of the tea every two to four hours for up to three days. Don't take motherwort if you are also taking medication to treat a thyroid or heart condition.

BLUE COHOSH: Blue cohosh *(Caullophyllum thalactroides)* is a native North American plant widely used by American Indians in the eastern areas of the country where it grows. The Cherokee, Fox, Menimonee, Ojibwa, and Potawatomi tribes all used it either to facilitate childbirth or to treat painful or delayed menstruation. Cohosh is an Algonquin word meaning "rough with hairs"; the word was applied to several native American plants. Today we still use this original native word when referring to both blue cohosh and black cohosh *(Cimicifuga racemosa).*

Blue cohosh was listed in the first botany books of North American plants in the 1700s and 1800s. It was introduced into medical practice in 1813 by an Indian doctor in Cincinnati named Peter Smith. From about 1850 until the early 1900s, both the Eclectic and Physiomedicalist schools of medicine considered it to be one of the most important women's medicines. The women took the plant for several weeks before childbirth to strengthen uterine contractions (it is now contraindicated for self-medication during pregnancy). Doctors also prescribed it for menstrual cramps or delayed menstruation.

Constituents in blue cohosh have been identified as uterine stimulants, or promoting contractions. Despite rumors to the contrary, blue cohosh is not a reliable

Calming Menstrual Pain

Medical researchers today think that an imbalance of prostaglandins—powerful hormonelike chemicals in the body—are responsible for menstrual pain. Prostaglandins are in all tissues, but certain varieties are concentrated in the lining of the uterus and may be responsible for the cramping of the uterine muscles. Aspirin, acetaminophen, ibuprofen, and many other pain-relieving medications inhibit prostaglandins, and this could explain why they also relieve some cases of menstrual cramps.

Many herbs traditionally used for cramps contain constituents that also inhibit prostaglandins. Ginger, perhaps the most popular emmenagogue listed here, contains four such constituents. Fennel, pennyroyal, tansy, juniper, rosemary, basil, thyme, chamomile, cinnamon, and yarrow contain such constituents as well. Although the plants themselves have not been tested for pain-relieving activity, it is possible that their constituents are responsible for some of the pain-relieving effects observed in folk medicine.

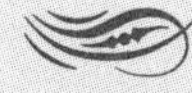

abortive herb. Most likely, it will just make you feel sick.

☞ Directions: Place ½ ounce of blue cohosh root in a pot. Cover with a pint of water. Bring to a boil and then simmer, covered, on low heat for twenty minutes. Let cool to room temperature. Strain and bottle.

GERMAN CHAMOMILE: Chamomile *(Matricaria recutita)* is considered in German medicine to be one of the most reliable herbal medicines for menstrual cramps. Chamomile is also mentioned as a cramp remedy in folk traditions throughout North America. The Latin name *matricaria* comes from the word "mater," meaning both mother and womb. The use of the plant for relieving cramps is probably ancient.

☞ Directions: Place ½ ounce of chamomile in a 1-quart jar and fill with boiling water. Let stand for one hour. Strain and drink a cup every hour or two for cramps.

BASIL: Basil *(Ocimum basilicum)* is mentioned as a remedy for painful or delayed menstruation in the folk medicine of China. It is also included in the folk traditions of Hispanics in the Southwest, where it is called "albacar." Basil contains unusually large quantities of the constituent caffeic acid, which has analgesic, anti-inflammatory, antispasmodic, and anti-prostaglandin activity (see sidebar, "Calming Menstrual Pain," above). If you don't have basil on hand, you might try thyme *(Thymus vulgaris)*, which also contains a high amount of caffeic acid and is included in American folk traditions.

☞ Directions: Place 2 tablespoons of thyme or basil leaves in a 1-pint jar and fill with boiling water. Cover tightly and let cool to room temperature. Drink ½ to 1 cup each hour for painful menstruation.

RASPBERRY: The Chippewa, Cherokee, Iroquois, Kwakiutl, and Quinalt Indians have all used raspberry leaf *(Rubus spp.)* as a gynecological medicine. In contemporary folk medicine in the United States, raspberry is probably the most famous "women's" herb. No pharmacological activities have been identified to account for the beneficial effects of this herb, but the leaf is highly nutritious, it is especially rich in minerals.

For cramps, raspberry is traditionally taken throughout the month as a beverage; cumulative mineral nutrition may account for any beneficial effects on the health. One ounce of raspberry leaf contains 408 milligrams of calcium, 446 milligrams of potassium, 106 milligrams of magnesium, 3.3 milligrams of iron, and 4.0 milligrams of manganese. The manganese concentration—which is about equal to the recommended daily allowance for women—is unusually high for an herbal source. In fact, in a sampling of 15 common herbal teas, raspberry contained about 20 times the average manganese content of the other drinks. Manganese deficiency has been associated with reproductive disorders, but not specifically with menstrual pain.

☞ Directions: Place 1 ounce of raspberry leaf in 1 quart of water. Bring to a boil, cover, and simmer on the lowest heat for thirty to forty minutes. Let cool. Stir, strain, and bottle. Sweeten as desired. Drink the tea for two to three months.

LEMON BALM: Lemon balm *(Melissa officinalis)* is used by the Amish for delayed menstruation or cramping. In the Hispanic folk tradition of the Southwest, it is used for the same purpose. The plant, which is native

continued on page 284

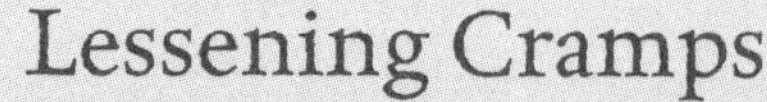

Lessening Cramps

A computer search of a U.S. Department of Agriculture database of medicinal plants for antispasmodic (cramp-relieving) activity turns up a number of traditional emmenagogue herbs. A cluster of constituents responsible for the antispasmodic activity—borneol, bornylacetate, limonene, and caryophyllene—appear in most of the plants included there.

Ginger, pennyroyal, tansy, juniper, rosemary, basil, thyme, cinnamon, and yarrow all have either three or four of these constituents. Chamomile has two such constituents, and fennel has one. The plants themselves have not been tested in trials for menstrual cramps and should not be used in excessive amounts.

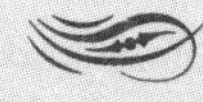

How Weather Affects Illness

Bad weather and bad health are often believed to be related. Many people believe that certain physical changes or plain ol' aches and pains—such as arthritis in the joints—can predict changes in the weather. And frequent or severe changes in the weather are believed to actually cause some people to get sick.

One common belief in North America is that a warm winter is likely to result in an increase in disease in the spring and summer. As one old saying puts it:

"A White Christmas,
a lean graveyard.
A green Christmas,
a fat graveyard."

Settlers in the upper Midwest noticed this phenomenon over a century ago. Warm winters were usually followed by epidemics of fevers that were associated with swampy environments. A similar belief is that winters with repeated freezing and thawing make some people more susceptible to disease.

Sunstroke is a very real risk in many areas of the country, especially for those individuals who work outdoors. Some people believe that you can avoid getting sunstroke by carrying charms, such as elder leaves or the rattle from a rattlesnake, in your clothes. Traditional remedies for sunstroke include using wet cloths and mustard plasters to draw the heat out of the body. A cure that uses horseradish plasters comes from the idea that the hot herb will attract the heat to itself.

Wind and night air can also be seen as dangerous, especially to children. Children, particularly babies, may be considered to be unusually susceptible to catching colds and other ailments. New parents are often cautioned not to take a young child out at night because the night air is bad for the infant. Colic is sometimes said to have been caused by taking a child out on a windy day. Some Pennsylvania Germans think that children are more likely to get sick in the spring than in any other time of the year. They believe that the March winds bring diseases that children are very likely to catch. Another belief is that sleeping with the east wind blowing on you will cause you to go insane!

Weather Benefits

All over the world people believe that the days around the changes of the seasons have tremendous power. In parts of the United States, the weather on Easter or May 1 is considered to have special benefits. Washing your face in the dew of May Day, some say, will make you beautiful. Sending a child who is suffering from head lice out into the first rain of May is believed by some to be a good way of getting rid of the pest. In fact, some people have claimed that getting wet in that first rain in May will keep sickness away for the entire summer!

to southern Europe and northern Africa, now grows throughout North America as well. It has been used as a relaxing emmenagogue herb at least since the 12th century German mystic and healer Hildegarde von Bingen stated, "Lemon balm contains within it the virtues of a dozen other plants."

Lemon balm is used in traditional herbalism for a variety of conditions that arise from nervous tension. Menstruation that is delayed by stress and tension may respond best to this mild plant. Lemon balm is approved today by the German government as a sedative.

☞ Directions: Place 1 ounce of lemon balm in a 1-quart jar and fill with boiling water. Cover tightly and let cool to room temperature. Strain and drink half a cup per hour until the cramps are gone or your period ends.

PENNYROYAL: Pennyroyal *(Hedeoma pulegioides)*, a plant native to this country, has been used by the Cherokee and Rappahannock Indian tribes to treat menstrual pain and delayed menses. Pennyroyal (and other *Hedeoma* species) has been used by Indians as a general pain reliever. In the 1800s and early 1900s, members of the Eclectic and Physiomedicalist schools of medicine prescribed pennyroyal to treat problems associated with menstruation. Today, pennyroyal is used to treat menstrual conditions in the folk medicine of New England. In the Hispanic folk culture of the Southwest, dwarf pennyroyal *(Hedeoma nana)* is used for the same purpose.

All the above species of the plant contain salicylic acid (an aspirinlike constituent), the menstrual-promoting essential oil pulegone, and a variety of other anti-inflammatory and antispasmodic constituents. Don't ever consume the concentrated essential oil of pennyroyal, however. It contains the liver toxin pulegone, which caused the deaths of several women attempting to use it to induce abortion.

☞ Directions: Place 2 tablespoons of pennyroyal herb in a 1-pint jar and fill with boiling water. Cover and let stand for one hour. Strain and take a 2-ounce dose every one to two hours. Don't take more than 1 pint a day, and don't take it for more than three days. Although it has a mintlike flavor, don't give this tea to children.

WILLOW BARK: A New England tradition suggests taking willow bark tea *(Salix alba)*

Get Moving

In 1830, J.C. Gunn, M.D., stated that a good treatment for delayed menstruation is to keep the bowels open. Contemporary Seventh Day Adventists—members of a religious movement that advocates the use of natural remedies and alternative medicine—offer the same advice today. Physicians who practice traditional Arabic medicine and conventional German medicine follow the principle as well. Dr. Gunn also suggested moderate exercise to bring on menses, which is one of the best ways to keep bowel function healthy.

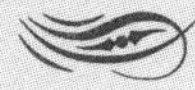

for menstrual pain. Willow bark has been used to treat arthritis, headache, and other sorts of pain in folk traditions throughout the Western world. Willow bark is approved as an analgesic by the German government. It contains salicylic acid and saligenin, compounds related to aspirin. The "sal" in the chemical name for aspirin—acetylsalicylic acid—is named after the "sal" in the plant's genus, *Salix alba.*

☞ Directions: Purchase willow bark capsules in a health food store or herb shop. Take as directed on the label. Alternatively, place 2 teaspoons of powdered willow bark in a cup, fill with boiling water, and let steep for fifteen to twenty minutes. Sweeten with honey, if desired, and drink up to four cups a day.

CRAMP BARK AND BLACK HAW: Two species of the *Viburnum* genus, cramp bark *(Viburnum opulus)* and black haw *(Viburnum prunifolium)* have been used for treating menstrual pain and other types of spasmodic pain in American Indian medicine. (The Cherokee, Delaware, Fox, and Ojibwa tribes all used cramp bark for treating pain; the Delaware in particular used it for treating menstrual pain.) In the 1800s and early 1900s, both cramp bark and black haw were used for treating menstrual pain or delayed menses by the Eclectic and Physiomedicalist physicians.

A contemporary textbook of medical herbalism called *Lehrbuch der Phytotherapie* that's used in German medical schools recommends taking between 20 and 30 drops of cramp bark tincture or as much as one teaspoon of the tincture of either plant to treat acute menstrual cramps. Both plants contain the antispasmodic and muscle-relaxing compounds esculetin and scopoletin. Black haw also contains aspirinlike compounds.

☞ Directions: Purchase 1 ounce each of cramp bark and black haw tincture in a health food store or herb shop. If both aren't available, either one will do. Mix them together, and take between 1 and 4 droppers every two or three hours for up to three days.

YARROW: Since the time of the ancient Greeks, yarrow *(Achillea millefolium)* has been used in European traditional medicine to control bleeding, whether

Water Treatments

Both the Amish and the Seventh Day Adventists use water treatments for menstrual cramps or delayed menstruation. The folk medicine of New England recommends this method as well—water treatments were common among turn-of-the-century German immigrants in New York. The method of application varies, but most common day traditions use hot water. A hot full bath, sitz bath, or foot bath are all worth trying. (You may even want to try placing a hot water bottle over the abdomen.) The heat of the baths (or water bottle) increases circulation to the uterus, accomplishing the same physiological effect as the spicy and stimulating emmenagogue herbs.

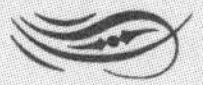

Almost Aspirin

Some of the plants traditionally used for menstrual pain contain aspirin-like compounds. Willow bark *(Salix alba)* has the most compounds, but black haw *(Viburnum prunifolium)*, pennyroyal *(Hedeoma pulegioides)*, and yarrow *(Achillea millefolium)* also contain clinically significant amounts. Raspberry leaf *(Rubus idaeus)* contains measurable amounts as well, but not enough to affect pain. The compounds in these plants are not as powerful as over-the-counter pain relievers, but if your cramps are mild, these plants may offer relief without presenting the risk of side effects that the stronger pharmaceutical pain-relievers do.

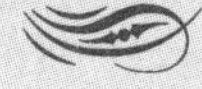

from war wounds or from excessive menstrual bleeding. Yarrow's scientific name, *Achillea,* comes from Achilles, one of the battlefield heroes of the Greek *Iliad.* Achilles reportedly used the plant to heal the wounds of his soldiers. The use of yarrow was widespread in ancient times, and names such as "military herb," "knight's millefoil," and "soldier's woundwort" survive today.

In North America, Cherokee Indian women used the plant to control heavy menstrual bleeding. Nineteenth century North American Eclectic and Physiomedicalist physicians used yarrow for treating prolonged menstrual periods. Today, yarrow is used for excessive menstrual bleeding in the folk medicine of Hispanics in the Southwest.

Besides war wounds and excessive menses, yarrow has been used by physicians of the past to reduce bleeding from hemorrhoids and intestinal ulcers. Yarrow has not been formally tested for its ability to reduce any sort of bleeding, but it contains two alkaloids—achilleine and betonicine—that have shown to reduce bleeding in animal trials.

☞ Directions: Place ½ ounce of yarrow in a 1-pint jar and fill with boiling water. Cover and let stand until the tea reaches room temperature. For heavy menstrual bleeding, drink half a cup every one to two hours for a day or two. Yarrow is not recommended during pregnancy or for epileptics.

SHEPHERD'S PURSE: Shepherd's purse *(Capsella bursa-pastoris)* is native to Europe and Asia. It became naturalized in this country in many of the areas where the early British and Spanish colonists traveled.

Shepherd's purse has been used since antiquity in Europe as a remedy for bleeding, whether from wounds or from excessive menses. The Chinese have used it to control excessive menstrual bleeding since at least A.D. 500. American Indian tribes

continued on page 288

Rootwork

Rootwork is a part of African-American folk tradition. It is a system of prevention, treatment, and causation that involves both natural and magical elements. The health aspects of rootwork are concerned with physical, mental, and emotional health—all of which are considered to be connected with one another. Like many folk belief systems, rootwork addresses itself not just to health, but to a much broader sense of well-being. It deals, for example, with such matters as job success, general happiness, success in love, peaceable family and social relations, finances, and so forth. Other names for rootwork include conjure, roots, juju, and hoodoo, which is sometimes confused with voodoo. Voodoo is actually a religion and not the same as hoodoo. African-American herbalism was sometimes historically called "root medicine," since it used the rootstock of many plants medicinally. In addition to herbs, rootwork uses plants and other substances, such as candles, oils, powders, incenses, and verbal charms and spells to provide prevention, protection, and remedies by magical means. Magical means are also used in an effort to cause certain outcomes (for oneself or others)—for example, causing the object of your affection to fall in love with you, causing an enemy to suffer or fall ill, causing an obnoxious or unfair boss to get his comeuppance, or causing your lottery number to be picked as the winner.

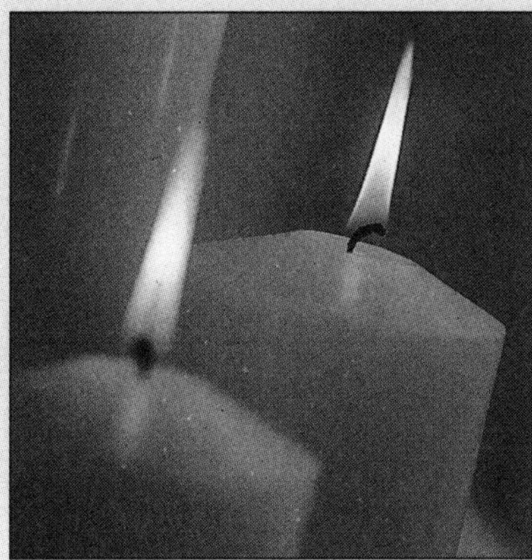

Some aspects of rootwork, such as burning special candles for desired outcomes, or "dressing" candles with special oils before burning to make them more powerful, can be done by anyone. The basic materials can be bought in any number of occult or spiritual supplies stores, and explanations of how to use them can usually be given by the store personnel. For more complicated or high-consequence outcomes, though, a special practitioner—called a "rootworker," "root man (woman)," "root doctor" (which can also sometimes just mean "herbalist"), "hoodoo doctor" (man/woman), "juju lady (man)," and sometimes "voodoo doctor"—is sought. These practitioners have special knowledge, and sometimes special powers, to bring to a case. Rootwork is indicated in the treatment of any sickness or other misfortune in which sorcery or hexing is thought to be a cause. For example, sicknesses that get worse and worse in spite of treatment or that can't be diagnosed accurately suggest the possibility that rootwork or other magic may be partly responsible. Because rootwork can be used to bring about both good and bad results, rootwork is considered by many to be a little scary. Its specialized practitioners are therefore both respected and feared.

Pennyroyal Toxicity

Pulegone, a constituent of pennyroyal oil *(Hedeoma pulegioides)*, is a highly toxic substance that is responsible for the deaths of at least two women in North America. The women used pennyroyal oil in the hopes of inducing abortion. In the past few decades, at least 18 cases of pennyroyal oil toxicity have appeared in the scientific literature. All the cases involved the ingestion of at least 10 ml (about a third of an ounce) of the concentrated plant oil. Even placing the concentrated oil on the skin (as an insecticide) can be risky. One report relates the death of a dog after pennyroyal was applied to its skin as a treatment for fleas.

Most aromatic plants, such as peppermint, chamomile, or rosemary, contain volatile oils that are dangerous. Teas made of these plants seem to present no health risk, however. But a tea containing pulegone may be more dangerous: Two case reports describe the deaths of infants who were given pennyroyal tea in the attempt to treat infant colic. If you use pennyroyal, be sure to keep the preparations away from young children, and avoid the essential oil like the deadly poison it is.

adopted its use once it was established in North America, using it to treat severe diarrhea. Later, shepherd's purse was used for excessive menstrual bleeding by both the Eclectic and Physiomedicalist physicians in the late 19th and early 20th centuries. Shepherd's purse is named for the appearance of its seed pods, which look like small purses.

☞ Directions: Place 1 to 2 teaspoonfuls of the dried herb in a cup and add 1 cup of boiling water. Let stand for three to five minutes. Strain and drink a cup every two to three hours just before and during the menstrual period.

FORMULA: Today, in professional medical herbalism in both Europe and North America, yarrow and shepherd's purse (included in this section) are used more often in combination than separately. The herbs act through separate mechanisms, so combining them can bring about a more effective treatment of excessive menstrual bleeding.

☞ Directions: Place 1 tablespoon each of yarrow and shepherd's purse in a 1-pint jar and fill with boiling water. Cover and let steep for five minutes. Strain and drink half a cup every one to two hours while bleeding.

Mouth, Gums, and Teeth

Most oral health problems are preventable. Professional care and the prevention practices in this section are key to keeping a healthy mouth intact

Dental problems are perhaps the oldest known conditions to afflict humanity. Prehistoric skulls from 25,000 years ago show signs of tooth decay. Folk remedies for tooth, mouth, and gum problems have probably existed at least since that time. By 3700 B.C., the Egyptians were using tiny drills to make a hole in the jaw to drain an infected tooth. By 2700 B.C., the Chinese had begun to treat tooth pain with acupuncture. The Greek physician Aesculapius introduced the pulling of diseased teeth in Greece sometime around 1200 B.C. It was the barbers who pulled teeth in 17th century England. Reliable dental anesthetics only became available in the United States during the 1800s; anesthetics were still not available in some isolated areas of this country as late as the early 1970s, however. Understandably, then, many folk remedies for toothache, mouth pain, and gum disease survive into present day in spite of more reliable professional dental care.

The best medicine for dental problems is prevention, which means regular cleaning of the teeth. Diet also has a strong impact on dental health, and, unfortunately, our modern processed foods promote tooth decay. During the 1930s, dentist and researcher Weston Price, D.D.S., visited more than 20 traditional cultures, including peoples in Europe, Africa, North America, South America, Australia, and the South Sea Islands. In each place, he examined the teeth of the inhabitants who ate a traditional diet and the teeth of those who ate modern foods, which were just being introduced into their villages at that time. The people eating the traditional diets averaged from 1 to 4 percent dental cavities, while those eating the modern foods averaged from 20 to 40 percent. The culprits among the foods were sugar and white flour. Price documented his research with photographs. You can see them for yourself in his book *Nutrition and Physical Degeneration,* which is still in print today.

The chief risk of unattended dental cavities is a dental abscess—an infection at the roots of the tooth within the jaw bone. An abscess can sometimes be "silent"and cause no pain. But it may cause systemic infection and health problems far beyond the site of the infection. An abscess may require removal of the tooth. Sometimes a root canal operation is performed. In that procedure, the nerves and vascular tissue (pulp) within the tooth are removed, a disinfectant is put into the root canal, and the tooth is filled. Teeth can be "saved" in this manner and last for many decades, or even for life.

Most of the remedies in this section are for treating gum disease or sores in the mouth. If you suffer from gum disease, remember to regularly clean your teeth—you also need to floss and go for a periodic cleaning at your dentist's office. The remedies here, including the ones for dental pain, may still come in handy, though, if you are traveling in a Third World country, camping in the wilderness, or are otherwise prevented from getting immediate dental help.

Remedies

CLOVE: Clove *(Eugenia caryophyllata)* has been used as a toothache remedy in Asia since antiquity. Later, it moved along trade routes from Europe to the Mediterranean. By 3 B.C., clove had become a universal folk remedy for dental pain in the Mediterranean. Nineteenth century dentists in both Europe and North America also used clove oil to relieve dental pain. Today, dentists use eugenol, a major ingredient in oil of clove, to relieve dental pain and to disinfect dental abscesses. Eugenol also has local anesthetic properties. Clove is still used for dental pain today in the folk medicine of New Englanders, the Amish, and Hispanics in the Southwest.

☞ Directions: Blend up 1 teaspoon of clove into a powder in a coffee grinder. Moisten the powder with some olive oil and pack into a cavity or area where a filling has been lost. Alternately, you can purchase clove oil at a pharmacy or health food store. Soak a cotton ball with the oil and place on the gums next to an aching tooth. Be sure to visit your dentist promptly to prevent further tooth decay.

GOLDENSEAL: Goldenseal *(Hydrastis canadensis)* was a famous dental remedy of the early American colonists. It was used for mouth ulcers and infected gums. The related plants goldthread *(Coptis trifolia)* and Oregon grape root *(Mahonia aquifolium, Berberis aquifolium)* were used by the American Indians for the same purpose. Like goldenseal, goldthread and Oregon grape root contain the antimicrobial constituent berberine. Of the three plants, goldenseal is probably best for treating sore and swollen gums because it also contains strong astringent constituents that may help to firm up swollen gum tissues.

☞ Directions: In a cup, pour 1 cup of boiling water over 1 teaspoon of goldenseal root. Let steep until the water reaches room temperature. Take 1-ounce doses. Swish around the mouth thoroughly before swallowing. Do this three times a day as needed.

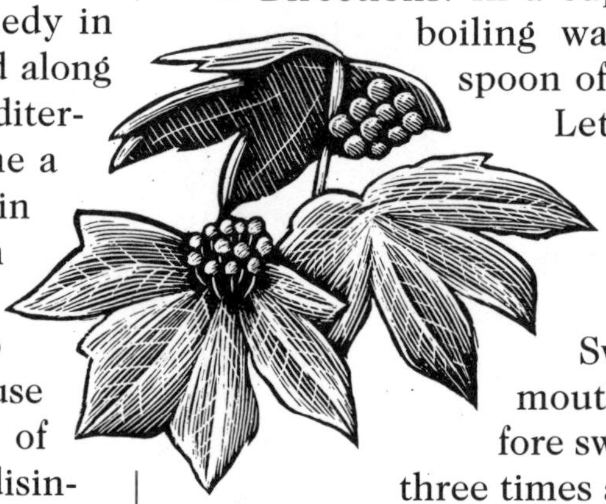

MYRRH GUM: Myrrh gum *(Commiphora myrrha)* has been used to treat mouth problems in the Middle East and North Africa since antiquity. The use of myrrh gum later spread to India, China, and Europe along Arab trade routes. Myrrh gum, like goldenseal, is astringent and tightens up loose

continued on page 292

Sties: Poor Behavior?

A Simple Cure

If a person thought his or her sty was a badge of bad behavior—or they knew that others believed so—they might have been willing to try this recipe, which was recorded in Ohio in 1960: Grind seven bedbugs with seven beans, cook, and apply to the eye in the form of a poultice.

The number of folk cures for sties are practically equal to those for warts. But there are no traditional "specialists" for the removal of sties, as there are in the case of warts. Historically, this may be because sties were believed to be self-inflicted, the punishment for some social mistake. (The painful swelling that appears at the base of an eyelash is actually the result of an infected follicle.) The most common transgressions included urinating in a walking path, in a public place, or in bed. In Germany, there were even names for those who defiled a public thoroughfare—"padepissers" and "wekschissers"—and they, too, were subject to sties.

Another alleged cause of sties was that the sty-sufferer had observed something sexually unseemly, such as dogs coupling. Or perhaps the sty resulted after the sufferer had been selfish. In light of such negative associations, it is understandable that people might resort to desperate measures to clear their eyes!

There was an abundance of remedies that used natural substances to cure sties. Among the agents that could be applied to the eye were poultices of bread and milk or potatoes, mineral spring water, tea leaves, egg whites, oats, pokeberry juice, mare's urine, or the yellow part of a lightning bug. The point of the remedies seems to have been to keep the sty moist; some would even let a dog lick the area. Other recommended moisturizers came from the human body: saliva, urine, ear wax, and breast milk.

No wonder people preferred magic! The most common magical cure for a sty was rubbing it with a gold ring or wedding band. The sty could also be touched with a cat's tail, combs, stockings, and the finger of a dead man. A few painful-sounding cures called for stabbing the sty with thorns, pins, or feathers, which were then discarded in some ritual fashion. More hygienic were the procedures that didn't involve the eye itself, such as wrapping a black thread around the middle finger of the left hand or looking through a keyhole. These remedies were sometimes combined with verbal charms such as:

Sty, sty, come off my eye,
Catch the next one who
passes by.

The patient then turned around three times and walked away, in hopes of leaving the affliction behind for someone else.

gums. It is also antimicrobial. (The Egyptians used it in their mummification process to prevent the bacterial degradation of the corpse.) The following toothache remedy comes from an 1846 herbal of the Thomsonian tradition.

☞ Directions: Combine 1½ ounces of myrrh gum and 1 teaspoon of cayenne pepper *(Capsicum annum)* in a jar containing a pint of brandy. Cover the jar, and shake it several times a day for a week. Strain and save the brandy. You now have a tincture. To treat a toothache, dip a cotton ball in the tincture and place it on the cavity. Be sure to see a dentist at the first opportunity to prevent further tooth decay.

To treat swollen and inflamed gums, make a mouthwash by combining a 1-ounce shot glass of the tincture with 3 ounces of water. Rinse the mouth frequently during the day.

WILLOW: The bark of various species of the willow tree *(Salix spp.)* have been used to treat mouth and gum infections by American Indian tribes throughout North America. Eskimo groups also used it to treat mouth infections. Although willow bark is famous for its aspirin-like constituents, it has antimicrobial constituents as well. The bark is also astringent, which can tone swollen gum tissues.

☞ Directions: Place 1 ounce of willow bark in 1 quart of water. Bring to a boil, cover, and simmer on the lowest heat for twenty minutes. Remove from heat and let stand until the water reaches room temperature. Refrigerate and use as a mouthwash up to eight times a day.

ECHINACEA: Echinacea was a universal toothache and gum disease remedy among the American Indians of the Great Plains region. Although it formerly grew in abundance in that area, echinacea is rapidly disappearing in that region due to overharvesting for worldwide medicinal use.

Applied topically, whether to skin or gums, echinacea can promote the healing of wounds and ulcers. Constituents in *Echinacea angustifolia,* the echinacea species used by the Plains Indians, are chemically related to the constituents in prickly ash (page 293) that produce a tingling sensation and act as a local anesthetic. These constituents are not present in *Echinacea purpurea,* however, which is the species most often available in health food stores and herb shops, and the one most likely to be found in your garden.

☞ Directions: Obtain a whole or chopped *Echinacea angustifolia* root at a health food store or herb shop. Grind a small amount in a coffee grinder. Pack the powder like snuff between your cheek and the tooth next to a sore area, or pack the powder directly into a cavity. Be sure to see your dentist at the first opportunity so that tooth decay does not progress.

GOLDENSEAL AND MYRRH GUM: A folk remedy from contemporary Kentucky for sore and swollen gums calls for equal parts of goldenseal *(Hydrastis canadensis)* and myrrh gum *(Commiphora myrrha).* The combination also appears today in the folk medicine of Utah. This remedy has its

Bad Breath

Many people use mouthwashes to treat bad breath, but, more often than not, the odor of bad breath is due to indigestion, not mouth infection. (For persistent bad breath, see the sections on "Digestion," page 175, and "Indigestion and Heartburn," page 252.)

If your bad breath is caused by a mouth infection, try any of the remedies in this section. Aromatics, such as clove, will also freshen the breath while disinfecting the mouth. In fact, in South Asia and the Middle East, it is a custom to chew on the seeds of aromatic spices such as clove, cardamom, or fennel after meals. These seeds contain antimicrobial substances as well as constituents that freshen the breath. Often times, the constituents that give an herb its smell and good taste are the same ones that fight infection and reduce inflammation.

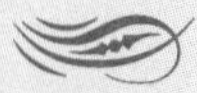

roots in Thomsonian herbalism and Physiomedicalist medicine of the 19th century.

☞ Directions: Purchase goldenseal tincture and myrrh gum tincture at a health food store or herb shop. Take 1 ounce of each tincture and place in an 8-ounce jar. Fill the jar with water. Cover the jar and shake well. Store the jar in the refrigerator. Use once a day as a mouthwash, or up to eight times a day for active gum disease.

YERBA MANSA: What goldenseal was to the American Indians of the eastern forests (and echinacea was to the Plains Indians), yerba mansa *(Anemopsis californica)* was to the American Southwest. All three herbs were used as panaceas for a wide variety of illnesses. Spanish settlers learned the uses of yerba mansa from the Maricopa, Pima, Tewa, and Yaqui Indian tribes. ("Yerba mansa" is short for "yerba del indio manso," or "herb of the tamed Indians.") The Eclectic school of medicine later used yerba mansa as a mucous membrane remedy.

Yerba mansa contains the volatile constituents thymol and methyl eugenol, both of which have demonstrated antimicrobial properties. Its other constituents, which are similar to those in goldenseal and myrrh gum, are astringent. Use yerba mansa for treating sores in the mouth.

☞ Directions: Place 1 ounce of yerba mansa in 1 quart of water, bring to a boil, and simmer for twenty to thirty minutes. Let stand until cool. Refrigerate. Use as a mouthwash for gum disease or mouth sores as often as eight times a day.

PRICKLY ASH: Prickly ash bark *(Zanthoxylum americanum)* has been used as a toothache remedy by various Indian tribes in the eastern United States; it was the most common tooth-pain remedy of the Iroquois Indians. Prickly ash is still used today in the folk medicine of the southern Appalachians and by some rural Louisiana blacks. (These two groups are sometimes beyond the reach of dental care—economically, if not geographically.) Prickly ash

continued on page 296

Baldness: Looking for a Cure

Baldness (known medically as *alopecia)* is partial or complete loss of hair on the head. A loss of hair can be caused by an inherited tendency or by aging, fever, therapeutic drugs, radiation, or disease.

Male-pattern baldness is the most common form. There seems to be an inherited tendency to it, and androgen (a male hormone) contributes to it. However, the exact mechanism by which it occurs is not known. In male-pattern baldness, hair loss is gradual, occurring at the forehead on either side of the front (sometimes leaving a center tuft, or "widow's peak"), and on top of the head. It can begin as early as age 15 or 16, in which case it may indicate that considerable baldness is likely later. However, male-pattern baldness does not usually advance at a steady or predictable rate.

Female-pattern baldness is fairly common in menopausal women. It usually involves only the area around the crown of the head. Like male-pattern baldness, it is believed to have hormonal causes.

There is no totally satisfactory medical treatment at this time to cure or prevent baldness. However, hair transplants can be effective. Scalp plugs containing active hair follicles are taken from the back of the head, which is not affected by male-pattern baldness. The transplanted follicles continue to produce hair just as before, despite the new location.

A topical form of the antihypertensive drug minoxidil is also available for use in treating baldness. This preparation has been shown to stimulate hair growth in some individuals; however, it must be applied on a continuous basis. An oral pill to combat baldness has also recently become available.

For such a common—and unwelcome—condition, traditional cures for baldness are surprisingly few. Most treatments involved the application of plant or animal materials to the scalp. Among the possibilities listed by one American compendium are chicken grease, bear's grease, cow's urine (warm), sage or thistle tea, dried mullein mixed with lard, chicken manure and honey, or fertilizer rinsed with vinegar. (The last two remedies seem to view hair as a crop in need of feeding!) Most treatments involved rubbing or massage. At the

Desperate Measures

A 20th century Irish physician, Patrick Logan, once wrote a magazine article in which he described some cures for baldness. (He found these remedies in a medieval Irish medical manuscript that was written in the year 1305.) One of the cures required that an earthen pot full of mice be buried by the fire, dug up a year later, and applied to the head. It cautioned that the user wear gloves lest he sprout hair on his fingertips! Dr. Logan actually received several calls from readers who wanted to try the remedy.

very least, this action increased circulation to the scalp and it felt good—despite some of the remedies' strange odors.

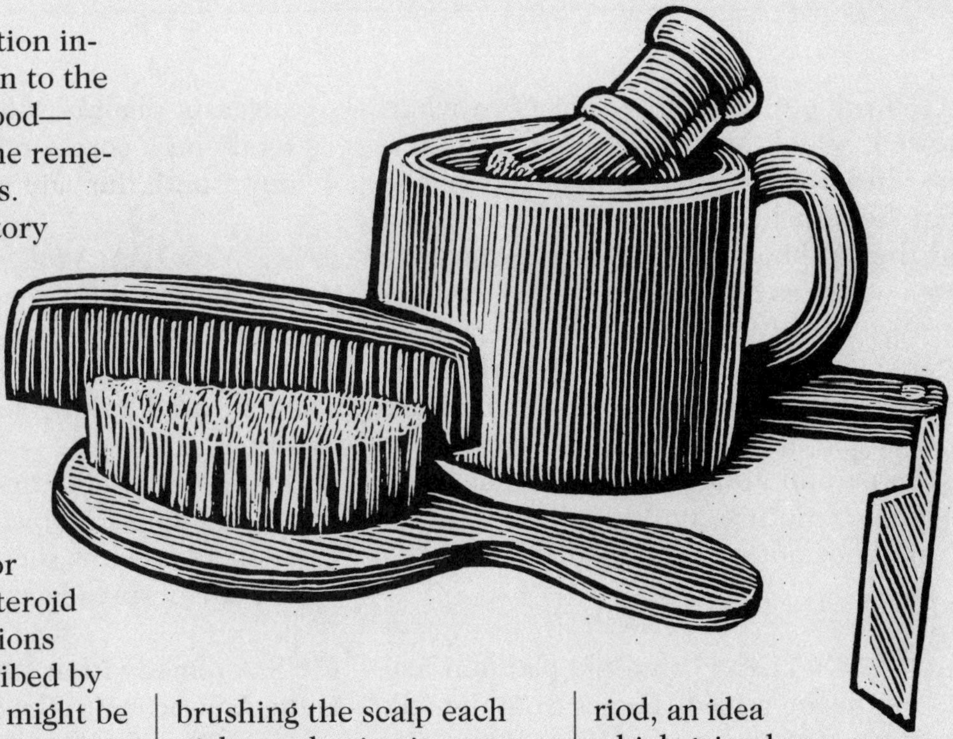

Perhaps laboratory analysis could identify chemical similarities between some of these folk substances and modern pharmaceutical treatments (like minoxidol) or the hormone or steroid lotions and injections sometimes prescribed by dermatologists. It might be hard to find participants for a clinical trial of folk remedies though. After all, who would be willing to wear an onion in a stocking cap for three months?

Magical cures, which often offer a tidier alternative to organic remedies, are almost nonexistent for baldness. Perhaps this is because most hair loss is accepted as normal, unless it's due to some other physical problem, such as a thyroid or autoimmune disorder. At present, so-called male-pattern baldness is taken as a bare fact of life. This seems to have been the case in the past as well, judging from the scarcity of magical cures for the condition. Baldness remedies that seem most closely related to magic are brushing the scalp each night or shaving it every day. Both practices seem to act as though the hair is still there, so these actions might represent a sort of sympathetic magic (see "Magical Transference," page 58). On the other hand, many who use these remedies probably think of them as natural—brushing might stimulate circulation and make hair grow. It is also widely (though falsely) believed that shaving makes hair grow back thicker than ever—which is one reason women are told to pluck facial hair instead of shaving it.

It seems it may be much better to prevent baldness in the first place. Folk tradition warns against wearing tight hats or wearing hats for too long a period, an idea which gained renewed interest in the 1960s when it was widely noted that the late President John F. Kennedy went hatless. Medical science concurs that "traction alopecia" can be caused by constant pressure, such as a ponytail. It also agrees with the traditional caution against excessive worry, because stress can cause hair loss—either all at once or gradually over time.

No matter. After all, bald(ing) men have always been able to comfort themselves with the idea that they are more virile than their hairier-headed counterparts. Some claim a scientific basis on the grounds that abundant testosterone is responsible for their lack of locks.

bark produces a tingling sensation when chewed, which soon gives way to numbness. In Louisiana, where blacks call the plant "toothache tree," the bark is crushed and then rubbed on the gums or inserted into a cavity as an anesthetic.

☞ Directions: Prickly ash is often available in health food stores or herb shops only in tincture form. Using the tincture dropper, apply the tincture directly to the painful area. Alternately, put some of the tincture, undiluted, on a small piece of cotton and hold next to the gums.

PLANTAIN LEAF: Using the plantain leaf as a toothache remedy comes from the folk medicine of Mexico and of Hispanics in the American Southwest. Plantain leaf is rich in antimicrobial and anti-inflammatory substances. The following recipe comes from Hispanic folk tradition in Los Angeles.

☞ Directions: Take a small amount of lard or other oil solid. (The lard or oil should be room temperature.) "Wash" the lard first in salt water, then in vinegar water, and finally in 100 proof spirits such as vodka. Crush a plantain leaf, spread the lard on it, and then place the leaf between your cheek and sore tooth.

SALT WATER: A remedy from New England for bleeding gums, canker sores, or toothache is to rinse the mouth with salt water. The same remedy is mentioned in the folklore of North Carolina. Salt, like many of the plant remedies above, is both antimicrobial and astringent so it can shrink swollen gum tissues.

☞ Directions: Place 1 teaspoon of salt in a cup of warm water. Rinse the mouth every two to three hours when treating an infection. North Carolina tradition suggests placing 1 teaspoon of salt directly on a sore tooth and gently biting down until the pain is relieved.

BAKING SODA: A folk remedy from North Carolina for treating toothache pain is baking soda. The same suggestion comes from the Hispanic folk traditions of Los Angeles. Concentrated baking soda acts as a disinfectant.

☞ Directions: Fill the hollow of the cavity in a sore tooth with baking soda. Go to the dentist as soon as possible before the decay spreads.

FIGS: A remedy from Mexico and Hispanics in the American Southwest requires cutting a fig in half and laying one half of it lengthwise between your cheek and the aching tooth. The same treatment is used in Arabic medicine. The Arab remedy calls for green figs, not ripe ones, however. The remedy may have been the result of a mixing of Spanish and Arabic customs. (The Muslims controlled Spain for 800 years, starting in the 7th century A.D.)

☞ Directions: If you have access to a fig tree, grab a fig and cut it in half. Set one half of the fig between your cheek and tooth, with the open side facing the sore tooth.

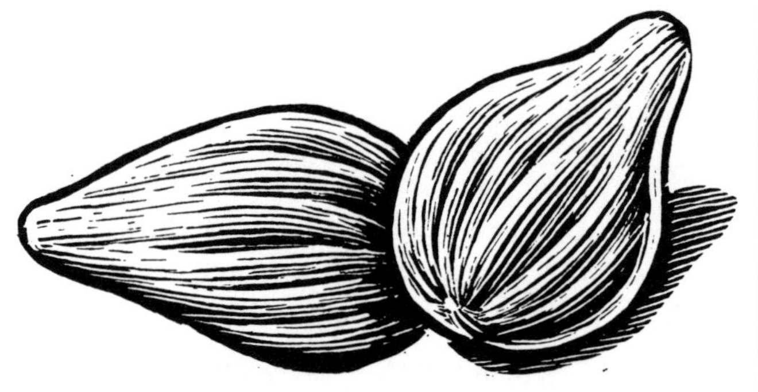

Muscle Strains and Sprains

Folk traditions throughout North America use irritating liniments and plasters to treat muscle injuries. For your muscle aches, try one of these "hot" remedies below

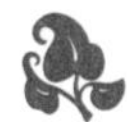

When the body's tissues are injured, the body initiates the process of inflammation to heal them. Blood flow increases to the area, causing redness. Lymph floods the tissues, causing swelling. (The initial flooding of lymph to the area can cause severe pain as the tissues are stretched.) Chemicals that cause pain are secreted to the damaged tissues. The net effect of all this swelling and pain is to immobilize the area to prevent further injury.

Next, some of the body's white blood cells migrate to the area to clear away damaged tissue. Good circulation is necessary at this stage to bring in the nutrients necessary to build new tissue and to carry away the debris of the injury.

You can decrease the pain in the area by reducing the swelling. Soak the affected part in cool water. After the first day, however, it is important to increase circulation to the injured part. To do this, treat the area with hot soaks and massage.

Folk traditions throughout North America and other parts of the world make use of irritating liniments and plasters to treat muscle injuries. These treatments are applied externally to irritate the skin at the site of the pain—a process called *counterirritation.* Experiments show that counterirritation not only increases blood flow to the skin by as much as four times, but also increases blood flow and temperature to the muscles underneath the injured area. Other folk remedies for strains and sprains are taken internally and have pharmacological effects similar to aspirin.

Remedies

CAYENNE PEPPER: In the folk medicine of Utah, Indiana, Illinois, Ohio, and China, cayenne pepper *(Capsicum spp.)* is used in liniments and plasters. Hispanics in the Southwest use cayenne pepper in their liniments as well. Cayenne became a popular folk remedy thanks to Thomsonian herbalism, which was a well-known herbal movement throughout rural New England and the

Homeopathic Arnica

One of the most popular homeopathic remedies in United States health food stores is arnica, which is used for bruises, strains, sprains, and other painful traumas. Homeopathic remedies are highly diluted substances and are a subject of controversy in science because they often contain no traces of the original substance.

Clinical trials show that some homeopathic remedies have a medicinal effect, but conventional scientists cannot explain why they work. Homeopathic arnica supposedly will relieve traumatic pain that is accompanied by bruising and has been used this way by homeopaths for several centuries. However, at least five modern clinical trials have shown that arnica works no better than a placebo. It was tested for pain accompanying abdominal surgery, tooth extraction, and heavy exercise.

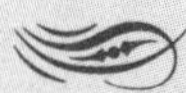

Midwest in the early 1800s. A constituent of cayenne, called capsaicin, which is also used in police "pepper spray," stimulates pain receptors without actually burning the tissues. Thus, cayenne is one of the safest items to use for counterirritation. Below is a simple cayenne liniment.

☞ Directions: Place 1 ounce of cayenne pepper in a quart of rubbing alcohol. Let the solution stand for two to three weeks, shaking the bottle each day. (You'll need to make this one in advance!) Then, apply to the affected area. (This remedy is not for internal use.)

A faster alternative is to place 1 ounce of cayenne pepper in 1 pint of boiling water. Simmer for half an hour. Do not strain, but add 1 pint of rubbing alcohol. Let cool to room temperature. Apply as desired.

Probably the fastest method, from contemporary North American Chinese folklore, is to gently melt 5 teaspoons of Vaseline in a pan and add to it 1 teaspoon of cayenne pepper. Stir well and allow to cool to room temperature. Apply as desired.

MUSTARD PLASTER: The mustard plaster, used since the dawn of history, remains today in the folk literature of Appalachia, China, and Europe. The irritating substance in mustard is not activated until the seeds are crushed and mixed with liquid.

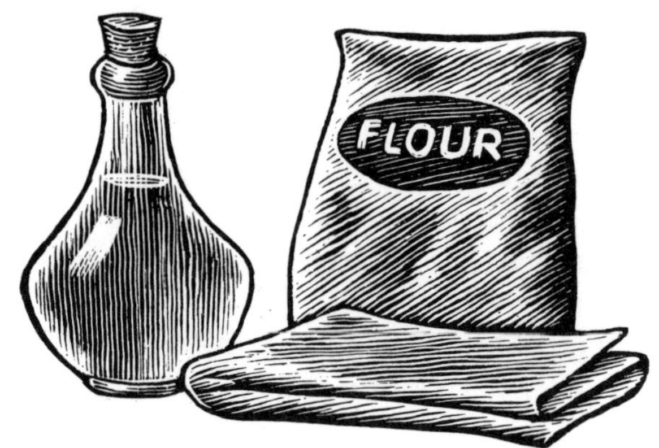

☞ Directions: Crush the seeds of white mustard *(Brassica alba)* or brown mustard *(Brassica juncea)* or grind them in a seed grinder. Moisten the mixture with vinegar and sprinkle with flour. Spread the mixture on a cloth. Cover with a second cloth. Lay the moist side across the painful area. Leave on about twenty minutes. Remove if the poultice becomes uncomfortable. Wash the affected area.

ROSEMARY: Rosemary *(Rosmarinus officinalis)* was used to relieve pain and spasm by doctors of the Physiomedicalist school in the last century. Today, rosemary is used (both externally and internally) in the folk medicine of Mexico and the Southwest for treating the pain of pulled muscles. Rosemary contains four anti-inflammatory substances, including rosmarinic acid, which has a biochemical action similar to aspirin. Rosmarinic acid is also easily absorbed through the skin and is approved as a topical analgesic by the German government.

☞ Directions: Put 1 ounce of rosemary leaves in a 1-pint canning jar and fill with boiling water. Cover tightly and let stand for thirty minutes. Apply as a wash over the painful area two to three times a day. Each time you apply the wash, drink a 2-ounce dose of the wash as well.

WINTERGREEN OIL: Wintergreen *(Gaultheria procumbens)* has been used to treat muscle pain by the Delaware, Menominee, Ojibwa, Potawatomi, and Iroquois Indian tribes. It entered into official United States medicine for this purpose in 1820 and remains, in the form of wintergreen oil, a medicine included in the *United States Pharmacopoeia.* Wintergreen and wintergreen oil also appear as treatments for muscle pain in the folk medicine of New England.

The active pain-relieving constituent in wintergreen is methyl-salicylate, a chemical relative of aspirin. The concentrated oil has been used as a pain-relieving medicine since the 1800s, but it can be toxic, even when applied to the skin. (Aspirin was discovered during the search for safer pain-relieving drugs.) If you want to use this plant, stick with the dried herb.

☞ Directions: Pour 1 pint of boiling water over 1 ounce of dried wintergreen leaves in a cup. Let stand until it reaches room temperature. Apply as a wash over the affected area, and, simultaneously, take 2-ounce doses of the tea three to four times a day.

WITCH HAZEL: Witch hazel is a tree native to North America. It contains both astringent and anti-inflammatory properties. Settlers learned the use of witch hazel for treating pain from the Indians of the Oneida tribe in New York. In the 1840s, the use of the plant spread throughout the United States in the form of various over-the-counter products. The use of witch hazel later spread to Europe, where its extract became popular. Witch hazel extract remains in use today in professional British herbalism and in conventional German medicine. The German government has approved the use of witch hazel for treating minor inflammations, especially of the skin and mucous membranes. Witch hazel is also used in the folk medicine of New England as an external application for sprains.

continued on page 302

Italian-American Folk Medicine

Most Italian Americans in the United States today are descendants of those who left southern Italy and Sicily in the late 19th and early 20th centuries. The majority of immigrants were farmers or artisans whose lives centered around agricultural cycles, their villages, and the religious festivals and holy places of their village saints. Most Italians were Roman Catholic, but their faith was comprised of a spirituality that combined church doctrine with supernatural beliefs and magical rituals stemming from ancient Greek, Roman, and Islamic beliefs.

Because God was too distant to be appealed to directly, Italian immigrants viewed the Holy Family and the saints as real individuals with whom they could bargain and request favors—the safe and healthy birth of a child, a full recovery from illness, or a good harvest. Certain saints were believed to have specific healing powers. For example, Saint Biagio was said to cure a sore throat, Saint Lucy corrected eye problems, Saint Anne alleviated the pains and dangers of childbirth, and Saint Jude provided hope in hopeless situations.

Belief in magical religious healing was central to the Italian folk healing system. This belief went hand in hand with dependence on herbs and other folk healing practices to cure disease. The two approaches were often used in combination. Italian immigrants did not view the natural and supernatural worlds as separate spheres; they believed illness could be caused by both.

An interesting case illustrating this tandem approach to healing was reported in a New York newspaper in 1892. Pasquale Siessone requested the services of the brothers Joseph and Vincenzo Libertino to cure his pneumonia. The Libertino brothers proceeded to strip him, blow in his face, and make cuts on his legs and toes. Then they wet their hands in Siessone's blood and rubbed it over his body. Finally, four times in succession, they cut off a lock of Siessone's hair, put it in an envelope that they addressed to the Devil, and threw it into a fire. The Libertinos were attempting to rid Siessone's body of the pneumonia through both folk healing practices and the supernatural practice of invoking Satan through a counter spell. When the brothers tried to bill Siessone for what he must have felt was an exorbitant fee ($120 increased to $380 if cured), he charged the Libertino brothers with fraudulent medical practice and fined them.

> **In Italian-American folk medicine, malevolent forces were often believed to be the source of illness, especially in children. The most common sources of such evil were witches and the "evil eye."**

In Italian-American folk medicine, malevolent forces were often believed to be the source of illness,

Bleeding and Cupping

Bleeding and cupping are based on the idea that some illnesses are caused by an imbalance of bodily fluids. Bleeding was a common practice in Italian folk medicine, as illustrated earlier in the Libertino case. Bleeding is the practice of making cuts, allowing a patient to bleed, and even deliberately creating scars to get rid of the evil spirits causing the illness.

Cupping originated in folk tradition and was later used and then abandoned by medical doctors. Cupping involves pressing a small cup against the skin, often on the chest or back, and burning a small bit of alcohol-soaked cotton (or other fast-burning substance) inside the cup. The fire is too brief to cause burns. It consumes the oxygen in the cup and is extinguished in a brief moment. The burning of oxygen creates a vacuum. As a result, the flesh under the cup is pulled up and the cup adheres. The cup is left on long enough to make a welt where the bodily fluid is drawn to the surface by the vacuum. This procedure brings blood to the skin surface underneath the cup. It is another method of bringing up and expelling evils causing illness. Cupping is often combined with bleeding.

especially in children. The most common sources of such evil were witches and the "evil eye." Malocchio, or the evil eye, is an illness unintentionally caused when a person who is cursed with this unwelcome power looks enviously at someone else. This belief is found in many cultures around the world. One of the most common afflictions caused by the evil eye is an unexplained headache. Common protections against the evil eye found in Italian-American folk tradition are representations of a beast's horns (cornu), claws, or teeth, or a copy of "The Only True Letter of Jesus Christ," which is said to be the original letter found in Christ's sepulcher. (This letter of prayer is believed to have miraculous powers for anyone who purchases a copy.) Similarly, protection against witches also involves religious objects and prayers.

Today, for the many generations of Italian Americans now living in the United States, many of the traditional folk beliefs and healing practices of the Italians have been abandoned, forgotten, or altered. Instead, Italians sometimes interact with other ethnic groups, exchanging or borrowing healing practices. For instance, when Italians who settled in the Pennsylvania German area of Pennsylvania could not locate an Italian practitioner to remove the evil eye, they sometimes sought a Powwow doctor to perform the function (see "Powwow and the Pennsylvania Dutch," page 102).

A few customs, such as wearing a cornu, continue, but the significance has altered. Now, this amulet against the evil eye is often worn to bring good luck or to display an Italian American identity.

Chinese "Hit" Medicine

One branch of traditional Chinese herbal medicine, called "hit medicine," deals with the treatment of traumatic injuries. In any North American Asian market that sells herbal remedies, you can find these internal and external medicines for strains, sprains, and bruises. Liniments and plasters that stick to your skin, and other formulas, are all available. Some formulas to look for are Yunnan Pi Yao, an internal formula shown in clinical trials to reduce internal bleeding and bruising; White Flower Analgesic Balm, an external liniment; and Po Sum On medicated oil, which is also for external use.

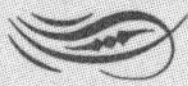

☞ Directions: Purchase a witch hazel liniment at your pharmacy. Apply the liniment externally over the painful area three to four times a day. Do this as often as desired.

ARNICA: Arnica has long been used in European folk medicine to treat injuries. The use of arnica entered into regular medical practice by the time of the colonization of North America; European physicians and folk healers brought the knowledge with them. Some American Indian groups used arnica for strains and sprains—much like the Europeans did. The herb is indigenous to Europe and Siberia, but it has been naturalized in southwestern Canada and the western United States. Do not use arnica ointments and liniments on broken skin, however. Arnica acts as a counterirritant and can sometimes irritate the skin.

☞ Directions: Pick arnica flowers (if they grow in your area) and place them in a jar. Cover the flowers with rubbing alcohol and allow to soak for two to three weeks. Shake the jar daily. Then, use as a liniment for sore muscles, bruises, and backaches.

Alternately, you can try this Gypsy remedy: Purchase an arnica tincture. Use 2 tablespoons of tincture per pint of water. Apply the diluted tincture with a piece of gauze to the affected area. Tape the gauze in place. Reapply every half an hour. (Note: Arnica is poisonous. It is not for internal use. Keep out of reach of children.)

EPSOM SALT BATHS: Folk traditions in both New England and Indiana call for Epsom salt baths to relieve the pain of strains and sprains. The salt is composed mainly of magnesium sulfate. The heat of an Epsom salt bath can increase circulation and promote the healing of strains and sprains. The magnesium of the salt is absorbed through the skin. Magnesium is one of the most important minerals in the body, participating in at least 300 enzyme systems. It also has anti-inflammatory properties. Epsom salts have been used medicinally in Europe for more than three hundred years.

☞ Directions: Fill a bathtub with water as hot as can be tolerated. Add 2 cups of Epsom salts. Bathe for thirty minutes, adding hot water if necessary to keep the water warm.

Nausea and Vomiting

Nausea and vomiting are symptoms of a wide variety of illnesses, conditions, and reactions to physical irritants. Settle your stomach with one of the remedies below

Nausea is an extremely uncomfortable or queasy feeling in the stomach area, often accompanied by an urge to vomit. Vomiting is the forceful ejection of the contents of the stomach through the mouth.

The sensation of nausea and the urge to vomit originate in an area of the brain called the vomiting center. In response to certain messages from nerves in the digestive system or in the inner ear (part of which controls balance) or to direct stimulation by certain drugs, the vomiting center can trigger the muscular actions that result in vomiting.

Nausea most often follows food poisoning or bacterial or viral infections of the intestinal tract. The nausea center can also be stimulated by ear infections, head trauma, or other neurological conditions in the brain such as migraine headache. Poisons in the bloodstream, such as alcohol, can also trigger nausea and induce vomiting. Severe vomiting, vomiting with pain as a predominant symptom, vomiting after a head injury, or chronic nausea all require medical diagnosis and treatment. Other common causes of nausea or vomiting are prescription drugs and pregnancy.

Nausea and vomiting are usually temporary conditions that can be beneficial if they result in the expulsion of something potentially harmful to the body. However, persistent or recurring vomiting can lead to a dangerous loss of fluids and salts (called *dehydration*) and nutrients. This risk of dehydration is most serious in infants and the elderly, but it is also a threat in individuals with bulimia, a condition in which vomiting is induced in order to control weight gain.

Conventional treatment for simple nausea is to drink clear fluids and, if vomiting has subsided, eat dry or bland foods such as soda crackers. Pediatric electrolyte replacement fluids, available in most supermarkets and pharmacies, may be the best treatment for children and the elderly. Conventional physicians can also prescribe a variety of drugs that can successfully control the urge to vomit.

Herbal folk remedies may work in several ways. Most of the herbs are aromatic and contain volatile oils with anti-inflammatory, antispasmodic, anesthetic, and antimicrobial properties. Their ability to relieve nausea is due to the herb's gastrointestinal local "anesthetic" effect, according to R.F. Weiss, M.D., author of *Lehrbuch der Phytotherapie* (translation: *Herbal Medicine*), the standard textbook of medical herbalism used in German schools of medicine and pharmacy. When ingested, says Weiss, the herbs work by numbing the nerve endings of the stomach, thereby reducing the gag reflex.

Remedies

MINT: Mints such as peppermint *(Mentha piperita)* and spearmint *(Mentha spicata)* are used throughout North America and Europe for soothing nausea. The Cherokee, Micmac, and Cheyenne Indians all used mints for this purpose. Today, mints are recommended for nausea in the folk traditions of Indiana and in the Hispanic folklore of the Southwest. Mints are also used to soothe nausea in contemporary Arabic medicine.

Peppermint was used medicinally by the ancient Egyptians and was also valued by the Greeks and Romans. The 17th century British herbalist Nicholas Culpepper wrote that "few remedies are of greater efficacy" for nausea than peppermint. Peppermint is approved in Germany as a medicine for weak digestion, and, according to a German textbook on medical herbalism, nausea is one of the top indications for using peppermint. According to the text, the plant reduces the gag reflex by anesthetizing the stomach lining.

☞ Directions: Place 1 tablespoon of mint leaves in a 1-pint jar and fill with boiling water. Let stand twenty to thirty minutes, shaking the bottle from time to time to mix its contents. Strain and sip as desired.

Herbs and Pregnancy

Some traditions suggest drinking coffee or black or green tea for nausea. However, all caffeine-containing drinks should be avoided during pregnancy. And, although it is still a matter of scientific debate, some trials show increased risk of miscarriage and lower birth weight for babies of mothers who consume as little as a single cup of coffee a day.

Many of the herbs in this section are contraindicated in pregnancy, especially during early pregnancy when morning sickness is most common. However, mint, ginger (doses less than 5 grams per day), chamomile, raspberry, and fennel are safe for use in the dosages recommended here, according to standard texts on botanical safety. The use of herbs such as catnip, cinnamon, clove, ginger (doses greater than 5 grams per day), thyme, and yarrow, especially in medicinal doses, should be avoided during pregnancy. Normal amounts of cinnamon, ginger, or thyme that are present in spiced foods probably present no problem, however.

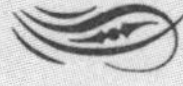

POPCORN: A nausea remedy from Indiana folk medicine calls for eating popcorn. The popcorn should be popped without oil, and then covered with boiling water. The result: a bland mush. The recommendation is consistent with the orthodox medical advice to eat bland food such as soda crackers for nausea.

☞ Directions: Pop the popcorn in a skillet with a lid, without using oil. Place the dry popcorn in a bowl. Cover with boiling water and let stand for fifteen minutes. Eat a teaspoon of the soggy popcorn every ten minutes.

YARROW: Yarrow *(Achillea spp.)* has been used as an antiemetic by American Indians of the Iroquois, Cheyenne, and Shoshone tribes. It is used for the same purpose in European folk tradition. Yarrow contains anti-inflammatory and anesthetic constituents. These constituents probably account for any effectiveness that the herb has for treating nausea.

☞ Directions: Place 1 tablespoon of dried yarrow leaves in a 1-pint jar and fill with boiling water. Cover and let stand for twenty to thirty minutes, turning or shaking the bottle from time to time. Strain and take sips of the warm tea. Don't take yarrow during pregnancy.

GINGER: Ginger *(Zingiber officinale)* is used for treating nausea in the folk traditions of New England and China. It is also approved for treating nausea by the German government. Scientific trials have shown that ginger may reduce nausea caused by several conditions, including motion sickness, morning sickness, and the nausea that accompanies chemotherapy. Doses as low as one gram have shown this effect. Ginger contains a variety of anti-inflammatory and local gastrointestinal anesthetic constituents.

☞ Directions: Place ½ teaspoon of powdered ginger spice in a cup. Fill with boiling water. Cover and let stand for ten minutes. Strain the tea and drink in sips. Don't drink more than three cups of ginger tea per day during pregnancy. And don't drink ginger tea without consulting your doctor if you have gallstones.

GERMAN CHAMOMILE: Chamomile tea *(Matricaria recutita)* has been used as a nausea remedy by the Cherokee Indians. It continues to be used in the folk traditions of New England. Chamomile contains powerful anti-inflammatory and analgesic substances that may reduce the gag reflex. Chamomile is approved as a digestive remedy by the German government, although not specifically for nausea.

☞ Directions: Place 2 tablespoons of chamomile flowers in a 1-pint jar and fill with boiling water. Let stand twenty to thirty minutes, shaking the bottle from time to time to mix its contents. Strain and sip as desired.

CHAMOMILE AND MINT: An antinausea formula found in the folk traditions of the Kentucky Appalachian mountains is a combination of chamomile and peppermint. (See the descriptions of these herbs above.) The two herbs are more often used together than separately.

☞ Directions: Place 1 tablespoon each of chamomile flowers and peppermint leaves in a 1-pint jar and fill with boiling water. Let stand twenty to thirty minutes, shaking the bottle from time to time to mix its contents. Strain and sip as desired.

RASPBERRY LEAF TEA: The Amish suggest a tea of raspberry leaves *(Rubus idaeus)* for treating nausea. The Thompson and Kwakiutl Indians used the leaves of related members of the *Rubus* genus in the same manner. No specific antinauseant or anesthetic properties have been identified in raspberry leaf constituents, but the tannin constituents in the leaves may have an anti-inflammatory or soothing effect on the digestive tract wall.

☞ Directions: Place 1 ounce of raspberry leaves in a 1-quart jar. Fill with boiling water. Place a lid on the jar and let the tea stand until it reaches room temperature. Shake the bottle from time to time to mix its contents. Drink freely.

CINNAMON: A nausea remedy from the folk traditions of Hispanics in the Southwest, and also from China, is cinnamon *(Cinnamomum verum)*. Called "canela" in

continued on page 308

Electrolyte Replacement Therapy

The main health hazard of excessive vomiting is dehydration and the loss of electrolyte salts. Replacement drinks are available in supermarkets and pharmacies, or you can make your own. The World Health Organization formula for an electrolyte replacement beverage after excessive diarrhea or vomiting is:

3.5 grams sodium chloride (table salt)
2.5 grams sodium bicarbonate (baking soda)
1.5 grams potassium chloride (must be obtained from a pharmacy)
20 grams of glucose (also available from a pharmacy)
1 liter of water (1 quart and 2 ounces)

A German medical text suggests the following formula, which includes peppermint *(Mentha piperita)* and fennel *(Foeniculum vulgare)*, two folk herbs often used in treating nausea: Make a tea by simmering 1 tablespoon each of peppermint leaves and fennel seed in 1 quart of water for 15 minutes in a covered pot. Strain and allow to cool to room temperature. To this add ½ teaspoon salt, ¼ teaspoon of baking soda, ¼ teaspoon potassium chloride, and 2 tablespoons of glucose. Drink freely.

Stopping Blood

Bleeding can be both frightening and dangerous. Even without a full understanding of the circulatory system, you can easily figure out that uncontrolled bleeding can be serious, even life threatening. Every culture has ways of stopping bleeding.

Putting substances on a cut to stop bleeding is a universal practice. Possibly the most widespread practice is washing minor cuts in cold water, or its ruder cousin, spit. A common practice in the United States is putting spiderwebs over cuts or wounds. The spiderwebs may be reinforced with soot or ashes, which must come from a wood-burning fire. This remedy is believed, however, to cause black scars.

Other widely used materials for treating wounds are axle grease and even fresh horse manure! Putting any of these substances on a cut or wound, except clean water, of course, increases your risk of infection and scarring. One good way to avoid scarring, according to the principles of sympathetic magic (see "Magical Transference," page 58), is to clean and grease the knife or ax that cut you and then promptly bury it!

Many remedies to stop bleeding focus on nosebleeds. Some claim that tying a piece of metal on a string and letting it hang down your back is a good way to stop a nosebleed. Another suggested way to stop the bleeding is to chew on a piece of paper or fold it and place it under your upper lip. Still another method is to wear a piece of red yarn or silk thread around your neck. Similar to that remedy is the practice of wearing red colored beads or red stones.

Of course, there are more technical ways to stop nosebleeds. Pressing a blood vessel behind your ear is one way, for example. A more widespread remedy requires the application of cold water to the top (or back) of the head and the back of the neck. In fact, some people have claimed that applying anything cold to the back of the neck will quickly stop a nosebleed.

Magical Means

There are two interesting practices that have been used to stop more severe bleeding. The first practice requires an individual (or the patient) to recite a verse from the Bible (often Ezekiel 16:6) three times—as fast as possible. The second practice is used by some Pennsylvania Germans, who claim that there are gifted people, "brauchers," who can stop blood in another way. The brauchers work their magic by saying the true name of the patient and then they say a prayer that calls on three roses that "grew on Jesus' grave." This, it is said, can stop bleeding in a patient no matter where the patient is located. The braucher doesn't even need to have met or seen him!

the Southwest, cinnamon contains anti-inflammatory, anesthetic, and pain-relieving constituents. Cinnamon is approved as a digestive aid in Germany, although not specifically for nausea.

☞ Directions: Place ½ teaspoon of cinnamon powder in a cup and fill with boiling water. Cover and let steep for five minutes. Strain and drink sips of the tea as desired for nausea. Don't take cinnamon during pregnancy—other than in the small amounts used to season foods.

CLOVE: Clove *(Syzygium aromaticum)* is used for nausea in the Hispanic folk traditions of the Southwest. The spice is also used throughout Southeast Asia, South Asia, the Middle East, North Africa, and Spain for the same purpose. Clove is one of the most important herbal remedies for treating nausea in traditional Indian and Arabic medicine as well. Eugenol, the main constituent of the aromatic clove oil, is used by dentists for its powerful antiseptic and anesthetic properties.

☞ Directions: Place 1 teaspoon of clove powder in a cup and fill with boiling water. Cover and let steep for five minutes. Strain and drink sips of the tea as desired for nausea. Don't use clove during pregnancy—other than in the small amounts used to season foods.

CATNIP: Catnip, a nausea remedy and sedative in European folk traditions, came to North America with the European colonists and quickly became naturalized here. The Iroquois Indians adopted its use both as a sedative, especially for children, and a digestive remedy. Catnip, like most of the other plants in this section, contains aromatic anti-inflammatory and anesthetic constituents.

☞ Directions: Place 2 tablespoons of catnip leaves in a 1-pint jar and fill with boiling water. Cover and allow to stand for twenty to thirty minutes. Strain and drink by the sip for nausea. Don't use catnip as a medicine during pregnancy.

FENNEL SEED: Fennel seed *(Foeniculum vulgare)* is a nausea remedy from the folk medicine of China. It is used in traditional medicine throughout Chinatowns in North America, usually in combination with other plants. Fennel contains anesthetic constituents that may reduce the stomach's gag reflex. Also, its constituent anethole has antiseptic and antispasmodic properties.

☞ Directions: Crush 1 tablespoon of fennel seeds in a coffee grinder or with a mortar and pestle. Place the crushed seeds in a cup and fill with boiling water. Cover and let steep for ten minutes. Drink the tea in sips for nausea.

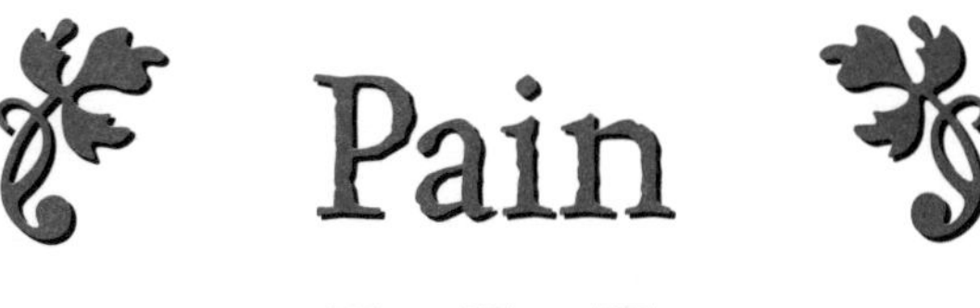

Pain

Pain is a signal—it is often a sign of disease, injury, or abnormal changes in the body

Pain is an unpleasant or uncomfortable sensation that can range from mild irritation to excruciating agony. It is probably the most commonly reported symptom and is linked to innumerable disorders and diseases.

Pain occurs when specialized nerve endings are stimulated; within a fraction of a second this pain "signal" travels through a network of nerves to the brain. Pain can be a warning sign, indicating impending damage to the body, or it can be a protective mechanism, causing the person feeling pain to remove the cause or reflexively draw away from the source.

Most healthy people have occasional, brief twinges of pain that have no specific cause and are usually harmless. However, bothersome, recurring, or persistent pain can be caused by thousands of factors. Most commonly, pain is a symptom of disease, injury, or abnormal changes in the body.

There are many types of pain. Pain can be dull and constant, sharp and sudden, crushing, burning, piercing, or aching. When it is felt in areas other than the location of the disorder (for example, when the pain of heart attack is felt in the arm), it is called *referred pain*. Unexplainable pain should be reported promptly to a doctor for investigation and possible treatment.

Using plants to quiet pain goes back before the dawn of recorded medical history, but none of these plants proved particularly effective. That is why this century brought about newer and better pain drugs and why pain medications are among the most popular over-the-counter drugs. Many of the modern drugs, such as aspirin, acetaminophen, ibuprofen, and corticosteroids, suppress the formation of prostaglandins, a class of chemicals in the local tissues that trigger pain. There are other, more potent painkillers, such as the opiates morphine and codeine, but these must be prescribed by a doctor.

Many of the plants used in folk medicine for pain relief use the same biochemical pathways as the non-opiate pain-relieving drugs, but they are not as effective. On the other hand, many of these plants have multiple effects. Their antispasmodic and circulation-promoting constituents may make up for what these plants lack in prostaglandin-suppressing strength. Comparative trials of these plants with drugs have not been performed, but the plants' persistent use in folk medicine (even with the availability of inexpensive over-the-counter drugs) indicates that they must have at least some beneficial effect. Herbal formulas that combine prostaglandin-suppressing, antispasmodic, sedative, and antidepressant plants are commonly prescribed by professional herbalists in North America, Great Britain, and Australia (see sidebar, "Formulas for Chronic Pain").

Folk traditions throughout North America and other parts of the world also make use of irritating liniments and plasters to treat muscle and joint pain. These remedies are applied externally to irritate the skin over the site of the pain. Physiological tests show that such treatments increase blood flow to the skin by as much as four times and also increase blood flow and temperature in the muscles underneath the skin. Any relief from such treatments is due to this increased circulation to the area, which ensures a healthy flow of oxygen to the tissues and relieves the swelling of stagnant lymph in the area. This method, called *counterirritation,* may also increase local or systemic levels of endorphins, the body's natural pain-killing substances that are more potent than opiates.

Formulas for Chronic Pain

Although acute pain may be best treated with pharmaceutical drugs, medical herbalists of countries such as Great Britain, North America, Australia, and New Zealand often use combinations of herbs and hydrotherapy to treat chronic pain. Chronic pain often creates a constellation of problems—besides the pain itself, tension, spasm, insomnia, or depression can often result. And while conventional pain medications may remedy one or two of these side effects, some formulas of herbs can address them all. A pain-reliever, an antispasmodic, a sedative, and an antidepressant may all be in included in a typical herbal formula created by a medical herbalist. For example, one herbal combination may include equal parts of willow bark (for pain), cramp bark (for spasm), valerian (a sedative), and St. John's wort (an antidepressant).

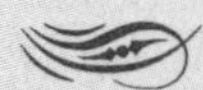

Remedies

HOT PEPPERS: Cayenne pepper *(Capsicum spp.)* is used in formulas for liniments and plasters in the folk medicine of China, the American Southwest, Utah, and throughout Ohio, Indiana, and Illinois. External and internal use of cayenne pepper to stimulate circulation was a key element of Thomsonian herbalism throughout rural New England and the Midwest in the early 1800s. (The Thomsonian movement of folk herbalism was introduced into practice in the early 19th century by Samuel Thomson, an influential New England herbalist. Thomsonian herbalism has been a powerful influence on American folk herbal traditions for the last 190 years.) Capsaicin, a constituent of cayenne, stimulates pain receptors without actually burning the tissues. Cayenne is thus one of the safest items to use for counterirritation. Below is a simple cayenne liniment.

☞ Directions: Place 1 ounce of cayenne pepper in a quart of rubbing alcohol. Let the mixture stand for three weeks, shaking the bottle each day. Then, apply to the affected part during acute attacks.

Alternately, if you can't wait three weeks for relief, try this method: Place 1 ounce of cayenne pepper in a pint of boiling water. Simmer for half an hour. Do not strain, but add a pint of rubbing alcohol. Let cool to room temperature. Apply as desired to the affected part. (Do not ingest either of these remedies.)

CRAMP BARK AND BLACK HAW: For the treatment of spasmodic pain, both cramp bark *(Viburnum opulus)* and black haw *(Viburnum prunifolium)* have been used in American Indian medicine. The Cherokee, Delaware, Fox, and Ojibwa tribes all used cramp bark to treat both menstrual pain and muscle spasm. Cramp bark and black haw were used for arthritic or menstrual pain in Physiomedicalist and Eclectic medicine. The plants contain the antispasmodic and muscle-relaxing compounds esculetin and scopoletin. The antispasmodic constituents are best extracted with alcohol (rather than water), so tinctures may be more effective than teas. Black haw also contains aspirin-like compounds.

☞ Directions: Purchase 1 ounce each of cramp bark and black haw tincture in a health food store or herb shop. If both aren't available, either one will do. Mix them together, and take between 1 and 4 droppers every two or three hours for up to three days.

WILLOW BARK: Willow bark *(Salix alba)* was used for treating pain by the ancient Greeks more than 2,400 years ago. American Indians throughout North America, from the Houma in Louisiana and Alabama to the Ninivak Eskimos in the Arctic, used it as a pain reliever even before the arrival of

continued on page 315

Compresses, Poultices, and Liniments

You can use compresses to treat headache, sore muscles, itching, and swollen glands, among other conditions. To make a compress, soak a cloth in a strong herbal tea, wring it out, and place it on the skin.

To make a poultice or plaster, mash herbs with enough water to form a paste. Place the herb mash directly on the affected body part and cover with a clean white cloth or gauze.

A liniment is a topical preparation that contains alcohol or oil and stimulating warming herbs such as cayenne. Sometimes isopropyl, or rubbing, alcohol is used instead of grain alcohol. Do not take products made with rubbing alcohol internally. Historically, liniments have been the treatment of choice for aching rheumatic joints and chronic lung congestion.

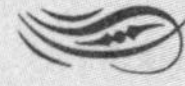

Saints & Holy People

The word saint comes from the Latin word *sanctus*, meaning sacred, holy, or belonging to Divine power. Most religions include the concept of saints. In some religions, such as Buddhism, a saint refers to anyone who has led a pure and holy life. In Christian culture, beliefs about sainthood are complex and have been a matter of debate for centuries.

At the dawn of Christianity all believers were considered saints. The Apostle Paul used the term to address all Christians in his epistles. But, by the 2nd century after Christ's death, admiration for holy living persons had changed to a veneration for martyrs—those who had died for the faith. Eventually saints came to be viewed as those in Heaven. In the 11th and 12th centuries the Catholic Church developed formal ways of recognizing those certain deceased people who were known to be in Heaven and therefore deserved public recognition. This process, called canonization, involves looking at evidence of a person's holiness in life as well as the person's supernatural help to the living after death. This help was proven with miraculous healings of the sick—giving saints a very natural role in folk medicine.

The Protestant Reformation rejected the idea of canonization, along with prayers to deceased people. But Protestants did retain the term "saint" for those in Heaven. Protestant theologians and clergy wanted to end the role of saints in folk medicine, but they could not. Instead, the idea of the intercession of the saints became a hidden, underground idea in Protestant folk medi-

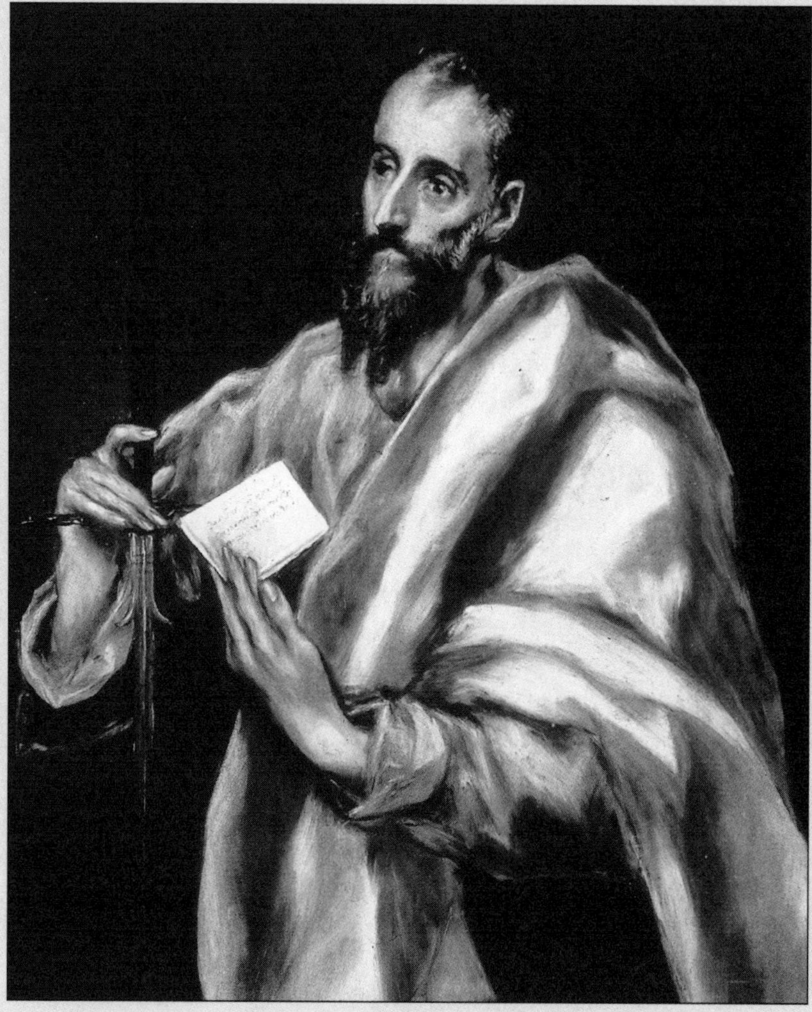

The Apostle Paul addressed all Christians as "saints."

cine, while it remained a much more publicly acceptable idea in Catholic areas.

FOLK SAINTS

To Catholics, the saints are friends, and prayers to them are like asking friends to pray for you. The belief is that saints are holy people and, because they live in Heaven, their prayers can be especially effective. The process of canonization, although sanctioned and structured by the official Church, actually begins as a folk activity. The cause for a deceased person's canonization begins with his or her reputation for holiness, but soon involves accounts of prayers answered. What saint will be asked for help, how the prayers will be offered, and how the saint's responses will be evaluated all become the responsibility of the Catholic community. This means that, in addition to those who eventually are canonized, there are others whose popular reputations for holiness and for answering prayers make them into a kind of "folk saint," even after their official cause for canonization is not successful.

One such folk saint is Don Pedro Jaramillo, who is also called Don Pedrito or "The Faith Healer of Los Olmos." Don Pedro was born into poverty near Guadalajara, Mexico, in 1829. It is said that one day as he was riding his horse a branch struck his nose, causing a very painful cut. That night, unable to sleep because of the pain, Don Pedro went into the woods where he found a pool of water and covered his injured nose with cool mud. This remedy provided so much relief that he continued the application for three nights in a row. On the third night he fell asleep and was awakened by the voice of God, telling him that he had been chosen for a Divine calling. At the same time he heard God tell him that he should go and heal the man for whom he worked, who was ill at the time. Don Pedrito obeyed. He went to the sick man and prescribed the first remedy that came into his mind: A tepid bath each day for three days. The remedy worked, and this was the beginning of Don Pedrito's healing career, and he always healed in the same way: Prescribing the first thing that came to his mind. By the time he moved to Los Olmos, years later, in 1881, Don Pedrito's reputation as a curandero (see "Curanderismo," page 260) was such that on his travels police sometimes had to provide crowd control. He charged nothing for his healing work, but he accepted free will offerings. He lived frugally and used his income to help the poor. During that time he fed so many that it was said that he took care of the whole northern part of Starr Country where he lived. He remained at Los Olmos until his death in 1907, and his grave has since become a shrine and pilgrimage site. It features a well-kept chapel with an altar and candles, a well-tended small cemetery, and a shop where candles, booklets, holy cards, and other religious objects can be purchased. The holy cards bear Don Pedro's photograph and the following prayer:

Oh, Lord of infinite goodness and mercy, Don Pedrito Jaramillo, come in these anguished moments, attend to my illness and pain, that I may be restored to good health. Come close to me and help me in my many problems.

Bring me your blessings for good fortune, success and happiness.

Similar folk saints can be found in other parts of the United States. For example, in Pennsylvania there was Mountain Mary, a German immigrant named Maria Jung who came to Pennsylvania before the American Revolution. History and legend differ on the exact circumstances, but she lived a mostly secluded existence in the woods of Berks County. She became widely known for her charitable nature and her skill as a healer, both in herbal medicine and in the Pennsylvania German folk religious tradition of powwow (see "Powwow and the Pennsylvania Dutch," page 102). Famous during her life, her acclaim has increased in the years since her death. A marker was erected in her memory in 1934 and, between 1945 and 1962, annual pilgrimages to her grave were organized.

Since folk traditions and official religious teachings often mingle, folk medicine also abounds with prayers, relics, vows, and pilgrimages involving officially recognized saints. For example, hundreds of thousands of people each year travel to Ste. Anne de Beaupré, the major North American shrine to St. Ann (the name of the mother of Mary, according to the Old Testament). Many of the pilgrims make the trip in response to their prayers being fulfilled by St. Ann. Thousands of the pilgrims are also sick people, many not even Catholic, coming to the shrine to pray for healing, on stretchers and in wheelchairs. On St. Ann's feast day, July 26, the shrine is filled with all sorts of offerings, ranging from floral arrangements to letters written to the saint and left in her chapel to crutches and bottles of medicine left by those who believe they have been healed through her intercession.

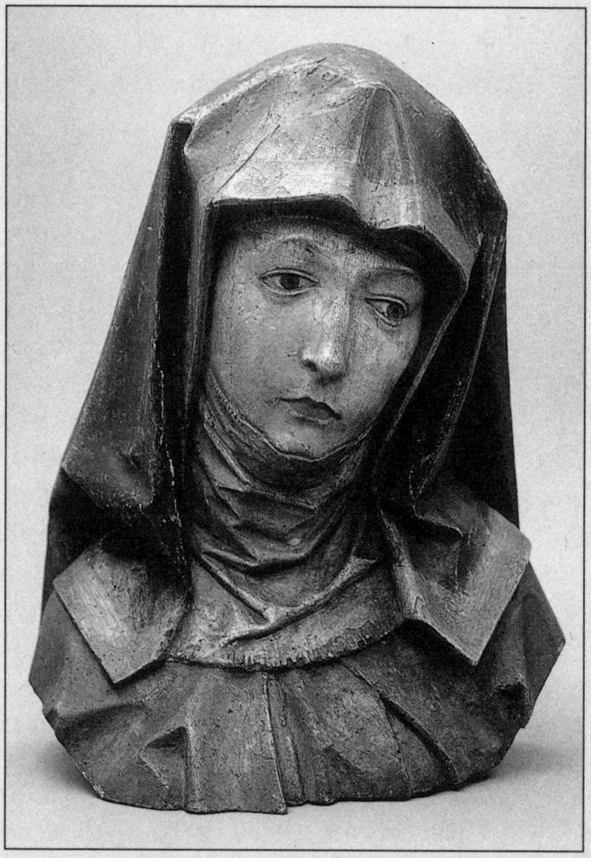

Every year, people travel to St. Ann's shrine to pray for healing.

At such pilgrimage sites it is easy to see the love and close relationships people have with saints and the faith they have that their "friends" in Heaven can help them. As official Christian ideas about the saints continue to change, folk tradition maintains a very close and loving connection with these sacred individuals.

the European colonists. Investigation of salicin, a pain-relieving constituent in willow bark, led to the discovery of aspirin in 1899. Although aspirin is now the top-selling pain-relieving drug in the world, willow bark is still used for treating pain in the folk medicine of Indiana, New England, and the Southwest, as well as by professional medical herbalists throughout the English-speaking world. The German government has approved the use of willow bark by conventional physicians for pain and fever. The most important active constituent is salicin, but other anti-inflammatory constituents also appear in the willow bark.

☞ Directions: Purchase willow bark capsules in a health food store or herb shop. Take as directed on the label. Also, you can place 2 teaspoons of powdered willow bark in a cup, fill with boiling water, and let steep for fifteen to twenty minutes. Sweeten with honey if desired, and drink up to four cups a day for five to seven days, as desired.

GINGER: Ginger is used to treat various sorts of pain in the folk medicine of China. It is also used for pain or spasm in the folk medicine of New England, Appalachia, North Carolina, and Indiana. It is an important pain medication in contemporary Arabic medicine; reports of its use there in treating migraine headache and arthritis show its effectiveness. Ginger contains 12 different aromatic anti-inflammatory compounds, including some with mild aspirin-like effects.

☞ Directions: Cut a fresh ginger root (about the size of your thumb) into thin slices. Place the slices in a quart of water. Bring to a boil, and then simmer on the lowest possible heat for thirty minutes in a covered pot. Let cool for thirty more minutes. Strain and drink ½ to 1 cup, sweetened with honey, as desired.

ROSEMARY: Drinking rosemary tea for pain is a remedy used in the contemporary Hispanic folk medicine of Mexico and the Southwest. Rosemary has not been tested in clinical trials, but it was used to relieve pain and spasm by doctors of the Physiomedicalist school in the last century. Its leaf also contains four anti-inflammatory substances—carnosol, oleanolic acid, rosmarinic acid, and ursolic acid. Carnosol acts on the same anti-inflammatory pathways as both steroids and aspirin; rosmarinic acid acts through at least two separate anti-inflammatory biochemical pathways; and ursolic acid, which makes up about 4 percent of the plant by weight, has been shown in animal trials to have anti-arthritic effects.

☞ Directions: Put ½ ounce of rosemary leaves in a 1-quart canning jar and fill the jar with boiling water. Cover tightly and let stand for thirty minutes. Drink a cup as hot as possible before going to bed, and have another cupful in the morning before breakfast.

EPSOM SALT BATHS: Folk traditions in both New England and Indiana call for Epsom salt baths to relieve pain. Epsom salt was named after a salt found in abundance in spring water near the town of Epsom, England, in 1618. The salt was reputed to have magical healing properties. Epsom salt is now produced industrially and not from the springs in England. Epsom salt is primarily magnesium sulfate and has been used medicinally in Europe for more than three hundred years. The heat of an Epsom salt bath can increase circulation and reduce the swelling of arthritis, and the magnesium can be absorbed through the skin. Magnesium is one of the most important minerals in the body, participating in at least 300 enzyme systems. Magnesium has both anti-inflammatory and anti-arthritic properties.

Homeopathic Remedies

Homeopathic medicine is based on the principle of similars, the idea that "like cures like." Homeopathic medicine holds that a substance that causes certain symptoms when given in large doses to a healthy person can cure an ill person with the same symptoms when given in very small doses. This idea that the same substance that can cause symptoms can also be used to heal is often met with skepticism.

Homeopathic remedies are highly diluted substances and are thus a subject of controversy in science. In fact, some are so diluted that they contain no traces of the original substance. Although clinical trials have shown that some homeopathic remedies do have a medicinal effect, conventional scientists have yet to prove how they work.

Perhaps the most popular homeopathic remedy sold in United States health food stores for treating pain is arnica, though it has not withstood the validity tests of clinical trials. Undiluted arnica contains various anti-inflammatory and wound-healing substances and has been used as a pain medication in the past. Users of homeopathic arnica claim the herb relieves traumatic pain that is accompanied by bruising. However, at least five clinical trials have shown that it works no better than a placebo. It was tested for the pain accompanying abdominal surgery, tooth extraction, and heavy exercise. Tests of homeopathic arnica for surgical or dental trauma have also shown the herb to be no better than a placebo for treating pain from those conditions.

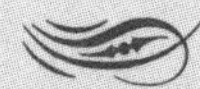

Hydrotherapy for Pain

During the 19th century in the United States, hydrotherapy was a popular form of medical treatment, especially for pain. The practice survives today mainly in the Appalachians and among the Seventh Day Adventists. (Hydrotherapy is also taught in naturopathic medical schools.)

Cold water or ice is recommended for acute pain; the cold suppresses inflammation and swelling. Hot water or alternating hot and cold water (ending with cold) is the prescription for chronic pain. Hot water or alternating hot and cold water increases local circulation and has the same benefits as counterirritation. Also, research shows that full body immersion (up to the neck) reduces swelling in inflamed joints.

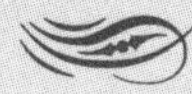

☞ Directions: Fill a bathtub with water as hot as can be tolerated. Add 2 cups of Epsom salts. Bathe for thirty minutes, adding hot water if necessary to keep the bath water warm.

ANGELICA: Various species of angelica have been used to quiet pain by American Indians throughout North America. The European species *(Angelica archangelica)* and the Chinese species *(Angelica sinensis)* have been used in the same way in the folk medicine of Europe and China respectively. The Chinese species is sometimes sold in North America under the names *dang gui* or *dong quai.* All species contain anti-inflammatory, antispasmodic, and anodyne (pain-relieving) properties. The European species of angelica has been used in European folk medicine since antiquity, as has the Chinese species in Chinese medicine.

☞ Directions: Place 1 tablespoon of the cut roots of either species of angelica in a pint of water and bring to a boil for two minutes in a covered pot. Remove from heat and let stand, covered, until the tea cools to room temperature. Drink the pint in 3 doses during the day.

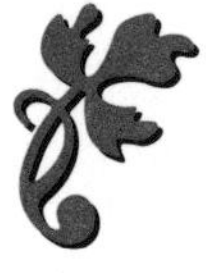

Poison Ivy and Poison Oak

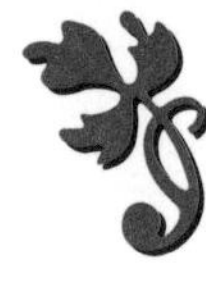

Getting a rash from poison ivy or poison oak can be very irritating. Look for relief in the folk remedies below

A rash from poison ivy or poison oak is caused by an allergic reaction to the oil, or sap, found inside the plant. This oil, which is clear to slightly yellow, is called *urushiol.* It oozes from any crushed or cut part of the leaves and stem, so just brushing against a plant may not elicit a reaction. Oil content in the plants runs highest in the spring and summer, but cases are reported even in the winter.

The first exposure to the plant does not usually cause a reaction, but it does start the process of preparing the immune system to react to subsequent exposures. That preparation can take two weeks or more, and during that time, you may seem to be immune to the plants' poisons. Once the sensitization of the immune system is complete, however, severe rashes may occur. This sudden appearance of sensitivity to the plants, after seeming immunity, can be confusing to victims, but it is the result of the normal processes of the immune system. Further adding to the confusion, urushiol is actually a mixture of related compounds, and it may be more or less allergenic depending on the mix, which may vary from plant to plant, climate to climate, and season to season. Urushiol is a resinous substance that can survive burning of its plant host, so beware of smoke from weed-burning fires, which can transport the poisonous resin in the smoke.

Common anti-allergic drugs such as antihistamines are ineffective against the type of allergic reaction these plants cause. Instead, steroid drug administration is the conventional treatment. Another important treatment for urushiol allergy is a thorough washing of the affected area with soap and water to remove the poison from the skin.

The folk remedies in this section fall into three categories: Some are astringent, which helps reduce the swelling of the allergic rashes. Some have anti-inflammatory properties that work similarly to steroid drugs. And some work by washing the plant poisons from the skin.

Remedies

JEWELWEED: Jewelweed *(Impatiens pallida, Impatiens fulva, Impatiens biflora)* is probably the most famous of the folk remedies for treating rashes caused by poison ivy. Jewelweed grows in the same sort of soil and climates as poison ivy, and can often be located near poison ivy in the eastern parts of the United States. Also called "touch-me-not," jewelweed is native to North America. It was a common remedy for poison ivy rash among the eastern American Indians, including the Cherokee and Iroquois. The Indians taught the colonists how to use jewelweed. Its use persists today in the folk medicine of New England, the Appalachians, and Indiana.

The physicians of the Eclectic and Physiomedicalist schools of the 19th and early 20th centuries also used jewelweed as a poison ivy remedy and anti-inflammatory treatment for other allergic swellings of the skin. A report in the *Physio-Medicalist Dispensatory*, a medical text published by Dr. William Cook , M.D., in 1869, relates a medical case in which jewelweed sap was spread on the severely swollen leg of a young man bitten by a snake. Although the man's life had been at risk, his recovery began immediately after the jewelweed was applied. Thirty years later, Eclectic physicians were using poultices of the plant that were boiled in milk to treat skin conditions. The *King's American Dispensatory,* an Eclectic text from 1898, stated that when the juice of the plant is applied to poison ivy, it "gives prompt relief." Dr. Harvey Felter's *The Eclectic Materia Medica, Pharmacology, and Therapeutics* (1922) states that, when jewelweed is applied to poison ivy, "The relief is almost magical." Felter, a leading Eclectic educator, was a conservative physician best known for removing many ineffectual herbal remedies from Eclectic use. Thus, his positive statement about jewelweed was all the more significant.

Modern scientific testing of jewelweed has yielded mixed results. A 1950 study found jewelweed to be of no medicinal value. Another study in 1957 found that 108 of 115 patients were completely relieved of their rash symptoms in 2 to 3 days. A 1997 study found jewelweed to be of no value in preventing poison ivy. These variable results may be due to the experiments' designs. The traditional use is to place the sap from a fresh-picked plant directly on the blisters as soon as they appear. This method was not followed in the 1997 study, but, instead, an unspecified extract of the plant was applied to artificially produced poison ivy.

continued on page 321

Trying Astringents

Probably the most famous over-the-counter treatment for poison ivy or poison oak in North America is calamine lotion, which is composed of zinc oxide. (Calamine is a term of the medieval alchemists for zinc oxide; the word is derived from the older Latin and Greek words for zinc.) Calamine lotion acts as a drying astringent to reduce the swelling of the rash. It is also slightly disinfectant, which helps prevent infection from setting in. There are several folk remedies in this section that also have astringent properties, including coffee, gumweed, clay, charcoal, and vinegar.

Poison Ivy

The rash and blisters that result from contact with either poison ivy or poison sumac are caused by a plant resin called urushiol. For those who are sensitive to urushiol, contact with these plants can be a source of great misery, and, along with those terribly itchy blisters, severe cases can bring on headache and fatigue. As is true of many sensitivities, reaction to urushiol can change (increase or decrease) over time and with exposure.

Poison ivy remedies, unlike any other set of folk cures, are practically never magical. Instead they employ herbs and common household substances such as soap and vinegar. Many of these remedies are effective, at least for symptomatic relief, though most have never been scientifically studied. A well-known treatment and preventive involves washing with old fashioned, brown laundry soap. (Actually, because urushiol is soluble in water, washing promptly with anything that includes water will help.) Another recommended wash is bleach mixed with horse urine, but soap and water are just as effective.

Prevention, of course, is better than treatment, and folk medicine offers plenty of ideas. In the Ozarks, it is said that large doses of sulfur and molasses, with a pinch of saltpeter (sodium nitrate), taken for a few weeks will confer immunity. A tea made from jewelweed is commonly applied to poison ivy rashes, but it is also said to give immunity if consumed regularly throughout the spring and summer.

Folk tradition states that the poison ivy rash is spread by the contents of the blisters. This is not true, however, since the liquid in the poison ivy blister is the same liquid found in any blister. The idea originated from two facts. First, symptoms of poison ivy can appear hours to days after exposure, partly depending on the amount of resin involved. Second, the urushiol resin easily spreads from affected areas of the skin and from clothing, shoes, and even pet fur. Thus, people often develop more and more symptoms after the days of the attack, even without new exposure to the plant. For these reasons, they are given the impression that the weeping blisters are responsible. The best way to prevent continuing misery is to wash all skin and clothing that may have been exposed to the plants.

Digesting Poison

Folk medicine tradition shows an awareness of the idea that tolerance to poisons is increased by exposure. This is true of a great many toxic substances, from alcohol to arsenic. Based on this notion, which has a superficial similarity to the medical idea of allergic desensitization, there is a widespread claim that eating small amounts of poison ivy will gradually produce immunity. This is a very dangerous practice, though, because certain individuals could develop life-threatening reactions.

☞ Directions: At the first appearance of poison ivy rash or poison oak blisters, pick some jewelweed. Crush the plant and apply the juicy sap directly to the poison ivy rash. Alternately, you can cut the plant a few inches above the ground and slit the stem lengthwise with a knife. This may expose the juicy sap more efficiently than when crushing the plant. Leave the juice in place for several hours. Reapply continuously for several days.

VINEGAR WASH: A vinegar wash to relieve the rash of poison ivy is reported in the folklore of Indiana and also in the southern Appalachian mountains. Vinegar washes are popular in many areas of the country for treating itching from various causes, including insect bites and allergic rashes. No scientific reason for the reduction of itching is apparent. It is recommended that the affected area is first washed with soap. Washing with soap and then vinegar may help to completely remove any plant poison from the skin.

☞ Directions: Wash the affected area well with soap and water. Then apply vinegar, scrub lightly, and rinse.

GUMWEED: Gumweed *(Grindelia camporum, Grindelia squarrosa)*, a species of grindelia, is an American Indian remedy that was eventually adopted by the medical profession as a treatment for rashes caused by poison ivy and poison oak. Native to the American Southwest and Mexico, the gumweed plant was used as a cough medicine and treatment of skin afflictions—including poison oak—by Indians in those areas. Its use entered into the folk medicine of nearby colonists and settlers, and, in the last century, it was adopted into use by conventional physicians. Gumweed was an official medicine in the *United States Pharmacopoeia* from 1882 until 1926. It remains an official remedy in German medicine—it is used as an expectorant for coughs. The resin contains anti-inflammatory and expectorant constituents.

☞ Directions: Apply the sticky sap from the leaves or flowers of gumweed to the affected areas. Reapply every few hours. Alternately, you can purchase tincture of grindelia and use it as a wash. Reapply the wash every few hours as well.

PLANTAIN: Plantain leaf *(Plantago major)*, used either as a wash or a poultice, is used to treat poison ivy in the folk medicine of New England and the southern Appalachians. Plantain's common names include "White Man's Footprint" and "Englishman's Footprint," names that reflect its arrival on the continent with the English-speaking immigrants and its subsequent spread wherever they moved.

According to *Herbal Medicine Past and Present* (Volume II), by John K. Crellin and Jane Philpott, Tommie Bass, a folk herbalist from northern Georgia, recommends making a tea of plantain leaf for treating the poison ivy rash. The leaf can be boiled in either water or milk and then used as a wash on the affected part. New England folklore calls for shredding the leaves, crushing them until they become juicy with plant sap, and then applying the crushed leaves to the skin.

Plantain, which is used throughout North America as a remedy for various skin inflammations and infections, contains several different anti-inflammatory compounds, including caffeic acid, chlorogenic acid, cinnamic acid, and p-coumaric acid. In laboratory trials, these four compounds act to inhibit an enzyme in the cells called *lipoxygenase.* Corticosteroid drugs also inhibit this enzyme, giving these drugs their anti-inflammatory effects. Plantain itself has not been tested in clinical trials, but these and its other anti-inflammatory compounds may account for the plant's effectiveness in suppressing the inflammation caused by poison ivy or poison oak.

☞ Directions: Pick some fresh plantain leaves. (Dried leaves probably won't work.) Shred them with your fingers, crush them until they become juicy, and press them into a poultice. Cover the affected area with the poultice and wrap with a bandage for twenty-four hours to hold the poultice in place.

MILKWEED SAP: A remedy from Indiana folklore is to squeeze the milky sap of milkweed *(Asclepias syriaca)* on the poison ivy rash. Milkweed was used by American Indians for various skin conditions, including warts and bee stings, but not specifically for poison ivy or poison oak.

☞ Directions: Squeeze the milky juice of milkweed directly onto the area affected by the poison ivy. Repeat every few hours until itching subsides and the rash goes away.

ALOE VERA: Aloe vera, more famously known for treating burns, may also be helpful for treating rashes caused by poison ivy or poison oak, according to the traditions of the Seventh Day Adventists. Aloe vera's anti-inflammatory constituents, which reduce blistering and inflammation in burns, may also reduce the inflammation of the skin caused by the plant poisons.

☞ Directions: Break off a piece of a leaf of an aloe vera plant. Apply the juicy sap to the affected itchy area. (For a large area, juice some leaves in a juicer and spread the juice over the skin.) Allow the sap to dry. Gently wash off the sap and reapply every two hours. Alternately, you can purchase aloe vera gel at a health food store.

COFFEE: According to *Herbal Medicine Past and Present* (Volume II), by John K. Crellin and Jane Philpott, Appalachian folk herbalist Tommie Bass suggests washing a poison ivy rash with black coffee. Coffee beans contain

Eating Poison

In both North Carolina and Indiana, it is believed that eating poison ivy leaves prevents contraction of the poison ivy rash. And although the mucous membranes of the mouth and digestive tract would not produce the same kind of allergic reactions that cause the rash, this is still a risky practice. Certain sensitive individuals could have other, severe reactions. Carelessness while eating the leaves could also result in a poison ivy rash on the hands or lips. In sensitive individuals, life-threatening allergic shock could occur.

5 to 10 percent chlorogenic acid, an anti-inflammatory constituent that acts in the same way as steroid drugs. Neither coffee nor chlorogenic acid has been tested as a treatment for poison ivy or poison oak.

☞ Directions: Brew a pot of strong black coffee. Allow it to cool to a tolerable temperature. Use it to wash the affected area as often as desired.

CLAY APPLICATIONS: Physicians of the Seventh Day Adventist tradition use clay packs to treat rashes from poison ivy or poison oak. (The same method is widespread throughout the world for treating various types of skin conditions.) Clay binds to different types of poisons; thus, it may bind to the poison ivy resins in a similar manner and remove them from the skin. And, even after the clay has been applied to the skin and the resin has been removed, the clay continues to work, helping to relieve itching. In conventional medicine, clay is sometimes used internally as a treatment for some types of poisoning.

☞ Directions: Mix bentonite clay or cosmetic grade clay with water to make a thin paste. Paint this onto the affected area. Let the clay dry. Flake the dry clay off the skin and dispose of it in a wastebasket. (Do not put the clay down your drain because it can clog the pipes.) Reapply as often as desired.

CHARCOAL: A charcoal poultice is a medical treatment of the Seventh Day Adventists for treating rashes resulting from poison ivy and poison oak. Charcoal has powerful drying and drawing properties and may help to remove any of the plant poison still on the skin.

☞ Directions: Grind up 3 tablespoons of flaxseed in a coffee grinder or blender. Mix with an equal amount of crushed charcoal. (The oily flaxseed acts to hold the mixture together.) Let stand for ten to thirty minutes, mixing occasionally. Apply to the affected area and secure with a bandage. Leave in place for six to ten hours. Remove and wash the area with a cold cloth. Repeat every day until the rash is gone.

BAKING SODA: Baking soda, either made into a paste or directly added to bathwater, is a poison ivy remedy from New England and Indiana. Physicians of the Seventh Day Adventist tradition also recommend the baking soda bath. This method, which cures all types of itching, appears throughout North American folk medicine, although no scientific reason for its effectiveness is evident. A thick paste of baking soda applied to skin affected by poison ivy or poison oak may remove any traces of the plant poison.

☞ Directions: Make a paste of baking soda and apply it to the affected areas. Change the application every two hours, for a total of three applications each day. Then take a baking soda bath each day until the rash is gone.

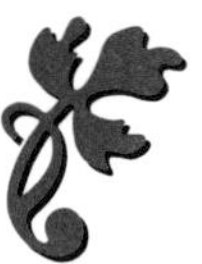

Pregnancy

Even today, the many folk traditions regarding both pregnancy and childbirth remain very useful

Until the 12th century, almost every birth in North America was a home birth, and most of these births were attended by midwives or folk healers rather than physicians. Because of this, there are many folk traditions regarding both pregnancy and childbirth. But most of these remedies are no longer appropriate in our modern society. Because of the risks inherent in childbirth, many women died giving birth in the era when folk remedies were the only assistance available. Maternal death was greatly reduced with the introduction of hospital births. Even home birth is safer today, because midwives are trained to screen for problem pregnancies and to transfer the mother to a hospital if complications develop. Midwives may still use some folk remedies, and they may work, but individuals should not try using them on their own. Some remedies that traditionally are used to "prepare for childbirth" and are given to the mother in the last month of pregnancy can actually cause prolonged labor or cause more painful contractions if taken incorrectly.

The herbs in this section fall into two categories: mineral-rich nourishing herbs and plants that help with morning sickness. Follow your doctor's or midwife's advice if you want to try these remedies.

Remedies

RASPBERRY LEAF: Raspberry leaf *(Rubus idaeus, Rubus strigosus)* is probably the most famous folk remedy for use during pregnancy. It has been used in Europe since ancient times to prepare for pregnancy and to nourish the mother during pregnancy. The use of raspberry is still mentioned in the folk medicine of New York and Michigan and in the Hispanic folklore of the Southwest. It is frequently prescribed as a nourishing beverage for pregnant women by contemporary professional herbalists in North America and Europe.

Raspberry leaf is highly nutritious, especially in the extra minerals and trace elements required during pregnancy. An ounce of the leaf contains 408 milligrams of calcium, 446 milligrams of potassium, 106 mil-

ligrams of magnesium, 3.3 milligrams of iron, and 4.0 milligrams of manganese. The concentration of manganese, an essential trace element, is about equal to the recommended dietary allowance for women. Deficiency of manganese has been associated with reproductive disorders in animals. (Neither manganese nor raspberry leaf have been tested in clinical trials of pregnancy outcomes.)

A published review of world literature on herbal safety indicates that raspberry leaf is safe for use during pregnancy. Raspberry leaf can also be taken to settle the stomach in morning sickness. It may relieve nausea through the action of its astringent constituents on the stomach lining.

☞ Directions: Place 1 ounce of raspberry leaf in 1 quart of water. Bring to a boil, cover, and simmer for thirty minutes. Strain and drink the quart during the day. Drink as a beverage during the last two trimesters of pregnancy.

EXERCISE: Exercise is the best tonic for easy delivery, according to the Amish. In William R. McGrath's *Amish Folk Remedies for Plain and Fancy Ailments,* one Amish source said: "Active farm mothers who keep working at home generally have an easier delivery than those who give up all activity and grow fat and flabby."

☞ Directions: Engage in moderate daily exercise.

STINGING NETTLE LEAF: Leaves of the stinging nettle *(Urtica dioica, Urtica urens)*

continued on page 328

Herbs in Pregnancy

The guiding principle for taking herbs during pregnancy is not to take any substance that could cause miscarriage or harm the fetus. Although no accidental miscarriages due to the use of herbs or folk remedies appear in the scientific literature, prudent advice is to avoid the use of herbs that traditionally have been used to induce abortion or to promote menstruation (see "Menses," page 275).

Many herbs that are normally beneficial to women should also be avoided during pregnancy. These include stimulating laxatives (see "Constipation," page 141) and some popular herbs that contain steroidal or alkaloid components (such as comfrey leaf, coltsfoot, goldenseal, dong quai, ginseng, and hop). In general, the rule is not to take any herb unless you know it is regarded as safe. The herbs in this section have all been classified as safe in pregnancy in the *Botanical Safety Handbook*, published by the American Herbal Products Association, which reviews the world's literature on herbal safety and contraindications.

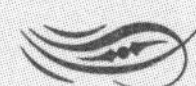

In Hopes of Fertility

Folk traditions for fertility fall into two categories. There are customs that are designed to insure fertility and there are practices to deal with the problem of infertility.

Many hopeful symbols of growth and abundance cluster around the marriage ceremony and the early days of a marriage. Throwing rice, corn, or wheat at the wedding, for instance, represents the guests' wishes for a fertile union. It is good luck to include small children in the wedding party; the presence of infants and children is representative of "sympathetic" magic (like attracting like). Plants and flowers reflect the desire for growth, so the wedding location is sometimes decorated with evergreen boughs as well.

The bride's attire has long been a focus of fertility: There was often a hair from her mother's head taped behind her ear, a wheat pattern sewn on her dress, and bread crumbs placed in her bosom.

A three-part custom says that the couple should eat rice at the wedding for fertility, drink wine for the pleasures of life, and sip vinegar so they will share all of life's bitterness and trouble together. A variation of that custom is for the couple to bring salt, bread, and wine into their new house to insure that they will be fertile and never lack for food or drink. Also to promote fertility, besides being carried by the groom, the bride can carry a baby over the threshold. The couple can also have their mothers make the bed, or they can put a leafy branch or a baby on it. Then they can toast each other and throw the glasses in the fire.

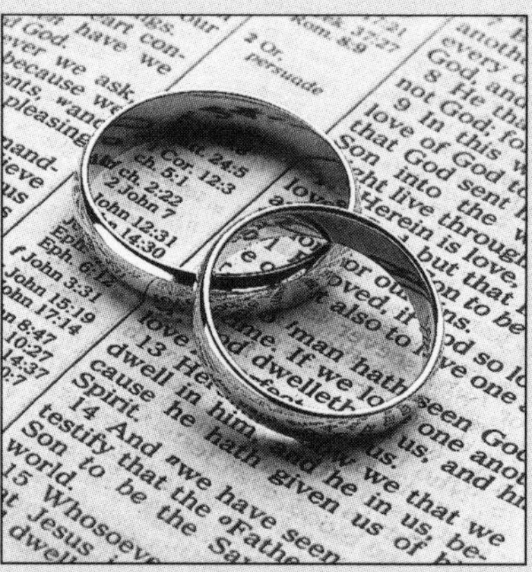

Many wedding traditions promote fertility.

If all these practices failed and the couple was not soon expecting, there were a number of things they could do. The couple could maximize their chances of getting pregnant by making love during a full moon. Also, there were several patent medicines of the past that promised "a baby in every bottle." Or, a sister of the would-be mother could lay her baby on their bed. (It was even luckier if the baby urinated there.) The couple could try putting salt in their bed or garlic under the pillow. Or they could eat the garlic, which is believed to be second only to eggs in promoting fertility. Other recommended foods include oysters (a well-known aphrodisiac), olives, onions, fish, mistletoe juice, cornflower tea, mandrake root, pomegranates, or any many-seeded plant. The wife might try eating three pickled plums a day after sex for one week; the husband could devour a wildcat.

The couple also could turn to magic or religion, such as tying a red ribbon around the finger of a deceased relative to remind him to intercede on their behalf when he appeared before God. One elaborate ritual suggested that the

Predicting Baby

Once a child is conceived, there is usually much speculation about its gender. Divination rituals such as a thread-and-needle pendulum over the mother's belly (which is believed to move in a circle for a girl or a straight line for a boy) are standard baby shower games. Physical signs noted in the mother are also considered—whether she "carries" high or low, whether her stomach is round or pointed, whether she is big or small, and so on.

Ideas about the baby's gender are often linked to the circumstances of its conception. For example, if the father's desire for a child was strongest, it would be a boy; if the mother's desire was great, a girl. Conception just before menstruation could result in a boy; just after, a girl. An ax placed under the bed could lead to a boy; scissors were used in hopes of a girl. If the weather was dry, look for a boy; if it was rainy, it might be a girl. As is typical of folk tradition, these elements are often reversed in differing cultures. There is one exception to this reversal, however: There's a notion that claims a woman is prettier when she's carrying a boy—because she has to give all of her good looks to a girl!

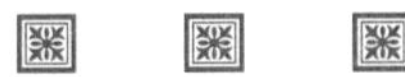

couple learn alternating verses of the story of Genesis in the Bible and repeat them to one other, a verse at a time, on alternate days, just before intercourse. A very common magical belief was that if a childless couple adopted a child, biological children would follow.

This lore demonstrates the well-known anthropological theory that people resort to magical thinking when events seem beyond their control. It also reveals the deep emotional investment in the idea of children, and how the human imagination works with this universal concern.

Sometimes, of course, it wasn't fertility that was the problem. It was that offspring could grow too numerous. "A poor man will always have many children," goes one saying, which was used to console him for his poverty (or perhaps explain it!). Folk methods of contraception did not seem to offer much for the overburdened pair, since it is often at odds with biological science: cola or vinegar douches, and coitus while standing, sitting, or with the woman on top. Some women still believe that they are more likely to get pregnant during their period than the rest of the month. This is because they envision their wombs as "open" to let out menstrual flow and "closed" the rest of the month. Of course, the exact opposite, timing-wise, is true.

A pregnant woman can become a source of further fecundity. Perfect strangers may ask to touch her stomach for luck. And, whereas menstruating women, being temporarily "sterile," were supposed to avoid tasks like planting or baking, a pregnant woman might be asked to lend her hand to these types of endeavors where increase was desired.

are a common nutritive herb prescribed by midwives in the New England area and upstate New York. Nettle is one of the most mineral-rich herbs available for common consumption. An ounce of nettle contains more than the minimum daily requirement of calcium, two thirds of the requirement of magnesium, and more than one third of the requirement of potassium.

☞ Directions: Place 1 ounce of dried nettle leaf in 1 quart of water and simmer until one third of the liquid is evaporated. Cool and strain. Drink the remaining liquid during the day in 3 doses every other day in pregnancy.

GINGER: Ginger *(Zingiber officinale)* is used for treating nausea caused by morning sickness in the folk remedies of New England and the Pacific Northwest. One scientific trial demonstrated that ginger is effective against severe morning sickness in doses as low as one gram, or the amount found in two average-sized gelatin capsules. Other clinical trials have shown that ginger may also reduce nausea caused by motion sickness or chemotherapy.

Ginger contains a variety of anti-inflammatory and anesthetic constituents. Huge doses of ginger, such as the ⅓-ounce doses common in traditional Chinese medicine, are contraindicated during pregnancy because of their possible emmenagogue effect (stimulating the flow of menses). The U.S. Food and Drug Administration considers ginger safe for human consumption in doses less than five grams. Take it in the form of tea rather than large amounts of powder, however.

☞ Directions: Place ½ teaspoon of powdered ginger spice in a cup. Fill with boiling water. Cover and let stand for ten minutes. Strain and take in sips, as desired. Don't repeat this more than three times a day during pregnancy. Don't take ginger tea without consulting your doctor if you have gallstones.

Morning Sickness

If you are experiencing morning sickness and are looking for an herbal treatment, be careful not to use an antinausea herb that might also promote miscarriage. Many herbs traditionally used for nausea, including catnip, cinnamon, clove, thyme, and yarrow, are also emmenagogues, meaning that they promote menstruation. Other traditional antinausea herbs, such as mint, ginger, and raspberry are safe herbs for morning sickness when taken in the quantities directed. Sip the teas you take and don't drink large quantities. If the sips don't work, the large quantities probably won't either.

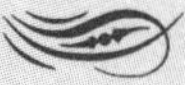

Bad Advice

Many contemporary herbalists adopt a romantic attitude towards herbs and promote the idea that plant medicines are perfectly safe and present no risks to the user. The result: Poor information in many popular contemporary herbals on the safety of herbs and pregnancy. Most of these books mention no contraindications for herbs at all, much less contraindications during pregnancy. Several best-selling herbals actually list some plants that have traditionally been used to induce abortion as "good for pregnancy." These herbs may be used by midwives during the last part of pregnancy to strengthen uterine contractions, but they are contraindicated during early pregnancy when they may cause miscarriage, a distinction missing from some of today's books.

As a rule, do not rely on popular herbals for advice on the safety of herbs during pregnancy. The herbs in this section are generally considered by both midwives and by modern governmental regulatory agencies in North America and Europe to be safe during pregnancy.

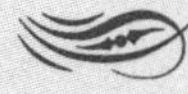

MINTS: Mints such as peppermint *(Mentha piperita)* and spearmint *(Mentha spicata)* are used throughout North America and Europe for treating nausea. Peppermint was used medicinally by the ancient Egyptians and was valued by the Greeks and Romans. The 16th century British herbalist Nicholas Culpeper claimed that it is one of the best herbal treatments for nausea. German medical texts also list nausea as an indication for the use of mint. Hispanic folklore of the Southwest recommends these herbs specifically for morning sickness. Anesthetic constituents in the mint may reduce nausea by reducing the stomach's gag reflex.

☞ Directions: Place 1 tablespoon of mint leaves in a 1-pint jar and fill with boiling water. Let stand twenty to thirty minutes, shaking the bottle from time to time to mix its contents. Strain and sip as often as desired for nausea.

Prenatal Influences

Modern medicine and folk tradition agree that the health of a pregnant woman directly affects the unborn child. Folk tradition, however, goes much further than the standard clinical advice of a balanced diet and exercise. It asserts that the fetus can be influenced not only by physical health, but by actions, emotions, and events in the life of the mother, and sometimes even the father.

The idea of "marking" a child is the most direct expression of this symbiotic relationship. According to this theory, the baby may be born with some unusual physical or mental trait as a result of something the mother did or didn't do. Food cravings are the most common cause of a child's peculiarity or condition. If a mother craves strawberries and doesn't get them, for instance, the baby might be born with a strawberry birthmark. If she happens to touch herself while thinking of what she wants, the birthmark will be on the same spot on the child. For example, if she touches her shoulder while thinking of chocolate, the child will have a brown mark on his shoulder.

The anthropologist Loudell Snow reports that, in her observation in Michigan prenatal clinics, this belief is so strong that mothers eat food they know isn't good for them (by the clinicians' standards) because they feared that to withhold it would mark the child. One young woman told Dr. Snow that, if a woman craved chicken and didn't get it, the child might have skin like a chicken. Too much of a food, however, can have the same effect—if the mother eats a lot of bananas, the child will have a banana mark, or perhaps a loathing for that fruit.

Another common cause of marking is said to be the result of a shock or fright: A child whose mother is frightened by a cat during pregnancy might look like a cat. (Or, the child will have a lifelong fear of cats.) Any strong emotion or preoccupation has the potential to inflict a mark.

Because of the belief in marking, pregnant women have been advised to use care in what they see and do. Some of the recommendations are strangely specific: "A pregnant woman should never clean fish or her baby will have a fish mouth." More typically, they suggest avoiding potentially upsetting situations such as funerals or horror movies. Instead, to produce a beautiful baby, a pregnant woman should dwell on beautiful things. She should listen to music to produce a musician, study art for an artist, and so on. The father, too, must be careful of his conduct: "If a man calls his pregnant wife a rat, the child will look like a rat."

It should not be surprising that these beliefs are so prevalent in folklore. They were part of official medical doctrine in the United States well into the 20th century. These ideas were discarded slightly earlier in Europe, after centuries of acceptance. Hippocrates was said to have saved the day for a white princess who gave birth to a black baby by explaining that there was a picture of a black man in her room.

The idea of parental marking takes on a darker cast in the suggestion that a child may be born with

Devil Babies

Stories of "devil babies" born as the result of their parents' wickedness are the most dramatic manifestation of the idea of "marking." The medieval legend of Robert the Devil set the pattern for a long line of diabolical infants. During Robert's conception, which occurred after years of childlessness, his mother vowed that if only she would get a child she would give it to the devil. The infant Robert grew at a preternatural rate, but was most distinguished by his evil disposition.

In North America, devil babies continued to be born in the popular imagination; reports have come from at least a dozen Canadian provinces and American states. The offenses leading to the demonic birth are usually uncharitableness (a woman refuses food to a beggar) or blasphemy (a man with many daughters says he'd rather have the devil than another girl).

The most famous American demon baby is the Jersey Devil of the Pine Barrens region of southern New Jersey, born to a Mrs. Leeds in the seventeen or eighteen hundreds. In one of many versions of the legend, Mrs. Leeds, finding herself pregnant for the 13th time, shouted, "This time I hope it's a devil!" Shortly she gave birth to a creature with huge bat-like wings and a dragon's head and tail. It flew up the chimney and out to the woods and marshes, where it is believed to have lived ever since.

some peculiarity or disability as a punishment for its parents' sins. A Canadian maritime legend tells of a man who shot seagulls or small birds and all his descendants had beady bird-like eyes. The most common transgression is the result of the mother's mocking of someone less fortunate than herself. A woman who made fun of a club-footed man had a child with a clubfoot, for example. A rich woman observing a poor woman and her children remarked, "Doesn't she look like a sow with her litter?" The rich woman's child was born with a pig's hoof for a hand.

Another possible cause of abnormality was the result of a curse put on the child by an enemy of the parents. The idea that a child's abnormality was the result of wrong-doing must have engendered terrible feelings of guilt in parents and a sad legacy for the child. Some children were even hidden from society out of a sense of shame.

Some ideas about prenatal influences were of a purely physical nature. Reaching above the head—to hang clothes or get something from a cupboard, for instance—was feared to cause the umbilical cord to wrap around the baby's neck. Repetitive motions, like working a treadle sewing machine, might be avoided for the same reason.

Concern for the unborn infant is at the heart of all prenatal folk belief, however farfetched it may seem. Pregnant women can hardly be blamed when they wonder about some of these older ideas.

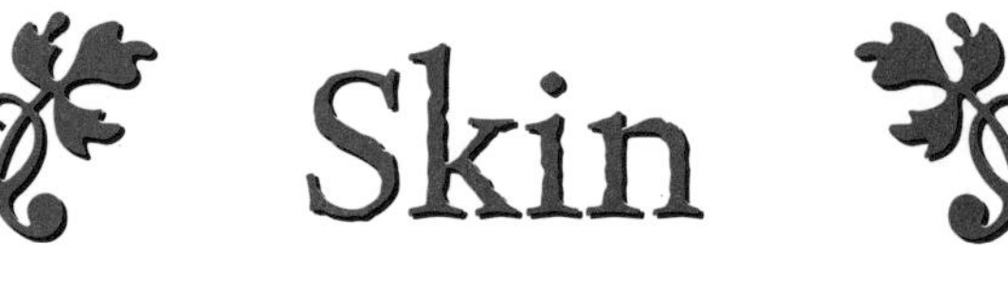

Skin

More folk remedies appear for treating skin problems than for any other type of condition

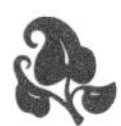

The reason why treatments for skin conditions are so plentiful is because skin ailments, although usually minor as far as health risk is concerned, are so common. But skin conditions are also visible and uncomfortable and demand our attention.

Over time, useless folk remedies for the skin were smoothly weeded out—many were topical remedies, so it was usually obvious whether they worked or not. People kept the skin remedies that worked effectively and incorporated them into folk tradition.

Elsewhere in this book we cover acne, athlete's foot, bites and stings, boils and carbuncles, burns and sunburn, eczema, itching and rashes, poison ivy and poison oak, splinters, wounds and cuts, and sores and chronic skin ulcers. In this section, we'll discuss remedies for heat rash, chapped skin, and impetigo as well as remedies designed for better overall health of the skin.

Of the conditions here, impetigo is the most serious. Impetigo is a skin condition that may be caused by *Staphylococcus* or *Streptococcus* bacteria. And, because of decades of antibiotic overuse, antibiotic-resistant strains of these bacteria are now common. It is possible, although rare, that an antibiotic-resistant strain of the bacteria might cause a systemic infection. Any infection of the skin that develops red streaks around it requires immediate medical attention.

Remedies

RED CLOVER: Red clover *(Trifolium pratense)* is a commonly used remedy for treating skin conditions (such as acne, eczema, boils, and rashes). It can be applied externally, which is recorded in the folk traditions of Indiana, or it can be taken as a tea, which is the practice in the southern Appalachian region.

Red clover tea is also one of the most often prescribed remedies for skin conditions in professional medical herbalism in North America. Red clover was used both internally and externally for skin conditions by the Eclectic physicians at the turn of the century. Harvey Felter, M.D., an Eclectic professor of medicine, said in his *King's American Dispensatory* that red clover, when applied externally, soothes inflamed skin, disinfects it, and promotes the growth of healthy tissue.

The plant contains more than 30 identified chemical constituents. Their properties support Felter's observations: Besides containing antimicrobial and anti-inflammatory chemicals, red clover also contains allantoin, which promotes the healing and growth of healthy skin tissue. Red clover has a high mineral content as well: An ounce of the flowering tops contains one half of the minimum daily requirement of calcium, one fourth of the requirement of magnesium, and one third of the requirement of potassium. Red clover should not be used simultaneously with pharmaceutical blood-thinning medications, however, including aspirin. Taken internally, red clover may thin the blood through the actions of its coumarin constituents.

☞ Directions: To treat the skin from the inside out, add 1 ounce of red clover tops to 1 quart of water. Simmer on the lowest possible heat until one third of the water is gone. Cool and strain. Drink the liquid in 3 doses during the day.

For external use, try this remedy from Indiana: Simmer whole flowering red clover plants until tender. Use just enough water to cover. Strain, press the plants into a thick mass, and sprinkle with white flour. (The flour helps add consistency to the poultice.) Place the floured poultice directly on the irritated skin. Leave on for about half an hour. You can use the red clover poultice several times a day. (The poultice can last a few days if it's kept in the refrigerator between applications.) The poultice is designed to help reduce inflammation and promote healing.

From the Inside Out

Some common folk remedies fall into the traditional category of "blood purifiers" (see "Blood Purifiers and Blood Builders," page 82). Traditional "blood tonic" herbs mentioned in the folk literature for skin conditions are red clover, burdock, boneset, sarsaparilla, and wild cherry bark. The idea of blood purifiers has a solid physiological basis because the skin receives all of its nutrients from the blood. Thus, these herbs are used to treat the skin "from the inside out." In the same way, toxins, allergens, or irritants in the blood can also cause symptoms of skin infection.

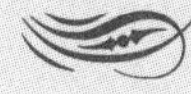

JOJOBA OIL: The Papago Indian tribe of the Southwest has used jojoba nut *(Simmondsia chinensis)* preparations to treat skin conditions such as boils and rashes. The nuts are traditionally dried and then pulverized and applied to the skin. Jojoba oil is now commercially extracted, and it is a popular addition to skin creams, oils, and ointments available in health food stores. The oil is also used today in the folk medicine of the Southwest for chapped skin.

☞ Directions: Apply commercial jojoba oil as desired to dry, chapped skin.

PLANTAIN LEAVES: Plantain leaves *(Plantago major)* are a common weed found on lawns throughout the United States. It was naturalized in North America after the arrival of the Europeans. American Indians called it "White Man's Footprint" because it seemed to follow the European colonists wherever they went. The Delaware, Mohegan, Ojibwa, Cherokee, and other American Indian tribes used plantain for treating minor wounds and insect bites.

Plantain has been used in cultures around the world to treat wounds and skin conditions. Plantain contains a pharmacy of constituents that are beneficial to the skin, including at least 15 anti-inflammatory constituents and six analgesic chemicals. Like red clover, it contains the constituent allantoin, which promotes cell proliferation and tissue healing.

☞ Directions: Crush a small handful of fresh plantain leaves and apply the juice locally to dry, chapped skin.

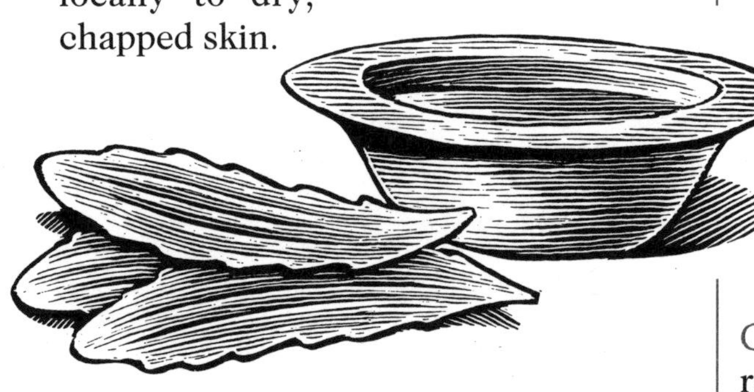

VINEGAR: Vinegar is also a remedy for chapped hands, according to folklorist Clarence Meyer's *American Folk Medicine*. The Amish use vinegar and water to treat heat rash in babies. No scientific reason for such a treatment is apparent.

☞ Directions: After washing and drying the hands thoroughly, apply vinegar, put on a pair of gloves, and go to bed.

URINE: Using your own urine as a treatment for chapped hands is part of the folklore of New England. Urine is also used for chapping in the folklore of Hispanics in the Southwest and among blacks in Louisiana. Urine therapy for cleansing wounds and treating skin infections appeared in the ancient medical systems of Mexico, Egypt, Persia, India, and China. It was used in 17th and 18th century Europe as well. Urine contains the substance urea, a disinfectant and skin moistener used in modern pharmaceutical preparations to cleanse wounds and in cosmetic products. (It is animal urine that is used in these preparations, of course.)

☞ Directions: Apply fresh warm urine to chapped hands and skin and allow skin to air dry.

OATMEAL: Oatmeal is a treatment for chapped hands in folklorist Clarence Meyer's collection of remedies called *American Folk Medicine.* In the method described below, oatmeal is used to both moisten *and* dry the skin.

☞ Directions: Use wet oatmeal instead of soap to wash chapped hands. Then, after drying hands with a towel, rub the hands with dry oatmeal.

CLAY: Clay application is a common folk remedy for treating various skin conditions throughout the world. It was common among the North American Indians even before the arrival of the European colonists. Today, the therapeutic use of clay makes up an important part of modern Seventh Day Adventist traditions. Clay is drawing and cooling. It is most effective on moist and inflamed conditions rather than on dry, chapped skin.

☞ Directions: Purchase bentonite clay or cosmetic grade clay at a health food store or drugstore. Mix the clay with water to make a paste and apply to the skin. Allow to dry, then gently flake off after a few hours. Wipe the clay off over a bowl. Discard the waste in your garden or on your lawn, because clay can stop up your pipes. Apply clay every few hours.

continued on page 336

Sweating It Out

Many folk remedies aim to provoke heavy perspiration, although it is seldom known why this is done. The implicit principle seems to be that the body leaches dangerous substances along with the sweat, which may explain why at one time sweat was thought to be poisonous. "Cleaning the blood" was a common phrase used with these cures (replaced today by "ridding the body of toxins"). A hot drink was usually the first step to getting things flowing: teas of sassafras root, bitter orange, and boneset (alias "sweatweed") were just a few of the suggested infusions. Many of the medicinal recipes included alcohol; one cure bypasses drinking the beverage altogether and suggests rubbing the person with whisky until he sweats. In Hawaii, persons with fever would lie under a blanket of ti leaves until they sweated enough to "break the fever."

Sweating it out—whatever "it" is—may or may not be a good idea in the case of fever, however. Certain organisms cannot survive in an abnormally high body temperature, and some doctors now suggest that reducing a fever may hinder the body's efforts to heal itself. By this logic, to elevate a fever even more, as the folk cures suggest, could conceivably speed the process along. A high fever can be dangerous, however, and pushing one even higher seems extreme.

The idea of sweating as a healthful and cleansing process is found in many cultures. Some even build special structures for sweatbaths: The Russian have the "bania"; the Greeks have the "laconica"; and many American-Indian groups have the "maquiq."

Sweat-bathing practices often have social and spiritual significance in addition to their hygienic function. Finnish immigrants used the sauna as a place to get clean and to meet friends each week. The sauna is considered essential to health: "If sauna, brandy, nor tar helps, the disease is of death," according to an American-Finnish proverb.

The Sweat Doctor

Samuel Thomson, a self-trained doctor born in New Hampshire in 1769, was contemptuously described by medical doctors of the area as the "sweating and steaming doctor" and "the old wizard." Condemning the standard medical treatments of the day (like bleeding), Thomson used herbal preparations (mainly lobelia) to make his patients vomit and sweat copiously to clear the body of "obstructions." He patented his "system," which consisted of mail-order medicine and a manual for its use, and his methods gained widespread currency throughout America. But, by the mid-1800s, contemporaries pronounced that "steamery was out of fashion" and "the day of the sweat doctor was over."

GOLDENSEAL: Goldenseal *(Hydrastis canadensis)* was used as an American Indian remedy for skin infections, such as impetigo, even before the European colonists arrived. Its use as a topical disinfectant and internal bitter tonic spread rapidly to the English colonists in the eastern parts of the country. It has been used in one school of American medicine or another ever since. Goldenseal contains the antimicrobial substance berberine, which kills both *Streptococcus* and *Staphylococcus* bacteria, the two most common infecting agents in impetigo. Other berberine-containing plants include Oregon grape root (*Mahonia aquifolium, Berberis aquifolium)* and barberry (*Berberis vulgaris*).

☞ Directions: Place ½ ounce of goldenseal root bark or powder in 1 pint of water. Bring to a boil, then simmer for twenty minutes. Allow the water to cool to room temperature. Stir and, without straining, apply to the affected area with a clean cloth. Cover with a clean bandage or gauze pad. Reapply the application every two hours as desired.

GUMWEED: Gumweed *(Grindelia spp.)* grows throughout the American Southwest and northwestern Mexico. It has been used as a skin remedy in those regions first by the American Indians and later by others who settled there.

Gumweed entered into the medical practice of the Eclectic physicians during the late 19th and early 20th centuries. In *The Eclectic Materia Medica, Pharmacology, and Therapeutics,* Harvey Felter, M.D., an Eclectic professor of medicine, states that gumweed was especially well-suited to treat those skin conditions characterized by "feeble circulation and a tendency to ulceration."

Gumweed was an official medicine in the *United States Pharmacopoeia* from 1882 until 1926. It remains an official medicine in Germany; it is used there as an expectorant for coughs. Little research has been performed into the constituents of

Scarred for Life?

Reduction or elimination of scars is a common human desire, and remedies to reduce scarring appear in several North American folk traditions. Scar formation results from wound healing or from inflammation. This natural process leaves the injured tissue stronger than it was before the injury, which helps to protect the area against repeat injury. Unfortunately, most agents that suppress scar formation, whether pharmaceutical or herbal, also tend to suppress healing. To be effective, treatments must be applied as soon as the wound is closed. Folk traditions emphasize the importance of being persistent when rubbing the oils into the skin. Coconut oil, cocoa butter, castor oil, and vitamin E oil are all used in folk medicine. Vitamin E, which is present in each of these oils, has been shown to reduce minor scarring while not suppressing healing.

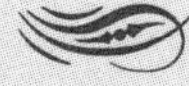

gumweed. The resin contains anti-inflammatory constituents, so it may be useful in treating infectious or inflammatory skin conditions.

☞ Directions: Apply the sticky sap from the leaves or flowers of gumweed to the affected areas. Reapply every few hours. Alternately, you can purchase some tincture of gumweed and use it as a wash. Reapply the tincture every few hours.

GARLIC PASTE: In Gypsy traditions garlic is used as a treatment for all types of skin infections, including impetigo, cuts, and wounds. When garlic is cut or crushed, it releases a substance called allicin, one of the most potent broad-spectrum antimicrobial chemicals known. This same substance, which is part of the plant's defense system against bacteria, virus, molds, and yeast, is responsible for the burning effect of fresh cut garlic.

☞ Directions: Pulverize 3 cloves of garlic in a blender or with a mortar and pestle. Add vinegar a drop at a time to make a thin paste that can be applied to the infected area. Apply twice a day, leaving in place for ten to fifteen minutes each time. This preparation can cause skin burns, including severe blistering, so don't exceed the recommended time limit. Afterward, wash the area thoroughly and cover the area with a clean dressing.

ROSEMARY: Rosemary leaf *(Rosmarinus officinalis)* is a remedy from the Southwest for treating windburn and cracked and chapped skin. It is also used in that region (and other areas as well) as a wash for infectious skin conditions. The plant's leaf contains four anti-inflammatory substances—carnosol, oleanolic acid, rosmarinic acid, and ursolic acid. Rosemary also contains more than ten antiseptic constituents.

☞ Directions: Crush some rosemary leaves and warm in a pan on low heat. Add some lard to make a salve. Simmer over low heat until the lard takes on the color and aroma of the rosemary. Let cool. Apply to the affected areas as desired.

Alternately, place 1 ounce of crushed rosemary leaf in a 1-pint jar and fill with boiling water. Cover tightly and let stand until the water reaches room temperature. Apply as a wash to the affected area, using a clean cloth, as often as desired.

CORNSTARCH AND CORNMEAL: Cornstarch and cornmeal are common agents used to treat moist skin conditions such as heat rash, according to folklorist Clarence Meyer's *American Folk Medicine.* Cornstarch and cornmeal are also used to treat chapped skin and prickly heat. Cornstarch "dusting powder" appears in the contemporary folklore of Indiana.

☞ Directions: Wash the affected area, wipe it dry, and dust with cornstarch.

VITAMIN E OIL: Vitamin E oil rubbed into scar tissue will help to reduce a scar, according to the traditions of the Amish.

Salves and Ointments

Homemade salves and ointments are commonly used throughout the folklore of the world. To make one, a medicinal plant is cooked or mixed in lard, butter, beeswax, or other oily substance that remains solid at room temperature. The oily portion of the salve helps to soften and penetrate the tissues and also serves to hold the medicinal portion in place. To make a simple salve, chop, powder, crush, or grind the medicinal material as small as possible and place in the bottom of a skillet or a crock pot. Place enough lard, butter, or beeswax in the pan or pot; it should cover the plant material when melted. Leave on very lowest heat for a while—at least ten to twenty minutes for a leafy substance, forty to sixty minutes for roots. Remove from heat. Let the ointment cool to a solid state. Store lard or butter ointments in the refrigerator. Plantain, grindelia, goldenseal, rosemary, and osha are all easy to make into salves. Combinations of the herbs may make more effective salves than single herb preparations.

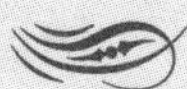

The Amish also use cocoa butter and castor oil for the same purpose. All three oils contain vitamin E, but the vitamin E oil contains higher amounts. Vitamin E has been shown to reduce scarring in a variety of scientific experiments. Treatment with vitamin E for skin grafts after severe burns did not work in one trial, however, so there may be a limit as to what can be accomplished with this simple remedy.

☞ Directions: As soon as possible after a wound is closed, rub vitamin E oil (or one of the other oils above) into the tissues for five to ten minutes twice a day. The rubbing, which increases circulation and can break up deep scars, is an important part of the application process. Continue rubbing in the oil on a daily basis for months if necessary, or at least until improvement appears.

POTATO POULTICE: According to folk traditions of the Gypsies, a potato poultice will improve puffy skin, especially those "bags" under the eyes. This same method is taught in contemporary naturopathic medical schools to reduce inflammation of the skin.

☞ Directions: Thoroughly clean 2 or 3 potatoes. Grate (including the potato skins) and press them with your hands into a paste. Apply to the affected areas of the skin. Leave in place while relaxing for fifteen minutes. Remove the poultice and clean and dry the area.

MILK: Milk is applied to the skin to relieve the irritation and discomfort of a variety of skin ailments in the folklore of the Hispanic Southwest. The remedy is also popular in the folk medicine of New England. In the southern Appalachians, it is buttermilk that's preferred. These remedies traditionally used whole

continued on page 340

Falling Out

"Falling out" is a term used in the rich and varied African-American cultural tradition to refer to fainting or losing consciousness. Falling out can happen in different ways and for different reasons, some considered good and some bad. For instance, in the Holiness and Pentecostal religions, when a person is touched by the Holy Spirit in worship, he or she may faint or "fall out," slumping to the floor or onto a pew in church. This is a good kind of falling out. No one who is familiar with this type of falling out will find this action unusual or frightening, either to see or to experience. Members of the congregation may briefly check on the person who has fallen out, however, to make sure that their modesty is preserved (i.e., skirts are not raised) and that there has been no injury (although injuries, such as head bumps or bruises, during this type of falling out are very rare). The person who has fallen will be left alone while God "works with them." When she regains ordinary consciousness she will usually feel energetic and uplifted, joyful and thankful for a blessing received.

This type of falling out may occur at any worship service, healing service, prayer meeting, or revival. At some healing services, those seeking healing may fall out when the minister lays hands on them, because the touch of the minister conveys the healing power of God to the worshiper.

The person who has fallen out will be left alone while God "works with her." When she regains ordinary consciousness, she will feel uplifted and joyful.

Some churches have congregational nurses who check on those who have fallen out, or who are "slain in the spirit." At any given service, there may be many or few who are touched in this way. This experience of having the consciousness taken over or smitten by the Holy Spirit is considered a gift and a blessing, a direct personal experience of divine contact.

Falling out can also refer to the kind of fainting or loss of consciousness that is considered a symptom of illness or even an illness in itself (like being prone to "fainting spells"). This kind of falling out is generally not welcomed because it is a sign of trouble. Problems with the state of the blood in the body, poor nutrition, serious but masked illness, and other causes—from minor to major—can cause falling out. Excessive worry can also make a person susceptible to dizziness and fainting and is considered an unnatural state for human beings, one that leads to illness. The most alarming of the possible causes for falling out—one recognized by those who accept the possibility of magical and supernatural causes for illness—is the possibility that falling out, especially if it has a sudden onset and cannot be traced to any other source, may be a sign that someone has used malign magic, sorcery, or rootwork against the fainter.

Sweating It Out

Many traditional folk remedies are called *diaphoretics*—plants or foods that make you sweat. Constituents in these plants increase the blood circulation to the skin, which, when taken internally, can be helpful in healing various skin conditions. Some diaphoretics are recommended for common skin ailments in the folklore of the southern Appalachian mountains. For example, burdock, boneset, elder flowers, and yarrow have all been used in folklore there to treat skin conditions "from the inside out" by increasing circulation to the skin.

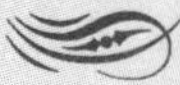

milk right from the cow, which, these days, is not usually available for sale. If you're going to try this remedy, use whole milk, not low fat milk. The short- and medium-chain fatty acids in the butterfat of whole milk may have a mild antimicrobial effect on the skin. Any beneficial effect of this remedy is more likely due to the soothing quality of the milk rather than any actual pharmaceutical activity.

☞ Directions: Wash the affected area with milk or buttermilk as desired.

MUNG BEAN PASTE: A treatment for heat rash or prickly heat from Chinese folklore is mung bean "soap," which is made from a mixture of cooked mung beans and sugar. The most important component of the formula may be the sugar, however, because by nature it is drying and cooling. Sugar has been used in various cultures to cleanse wounds. The astringent and drying properties of the beans may also have a beneficial effect on the rash.

☞ Directions: Cook mung beans until they can be mashed into the consistency of a paste. Add enough sugar so that the beans are sweet to the taste. Apply to the affected area, rubbing as if the paste were soap. Leave the paste in place for ten to fifteen minutes. Then remove, dry the area well, and dust with talcum powder or another drying agent.

WATERMELON RIND: To treat rash in babies, the Amish suggest rubbing the affected area with watermelon rind.

☞ Directions: Rub the affected area with the inside of a watermelon rind. Be sure to dry the area thoroughly and apply a talcum powder or some other drying agent.

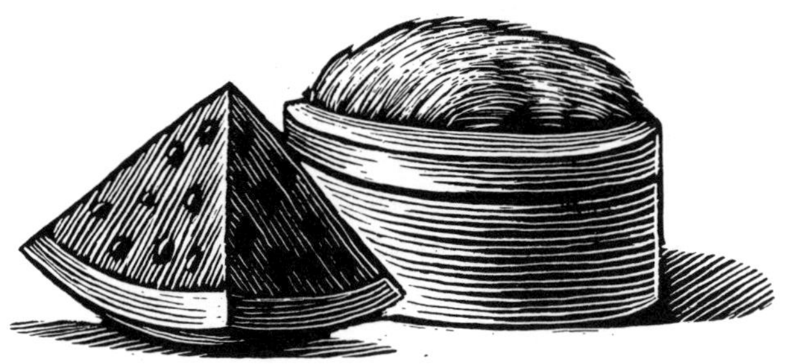

OSHA: Osha *(Ligusticum porteri)*, which is native to the Rocky Mountains, was a panacea to the American Indians in the area. The plant remains one of the most important folk remedies of the residents of the upper Rio Grande Valley. Osha is used for colds, flu, bronchitis, and also as a skin wash for superficial infections.

Very little scientific research has been performed into either the constituents or the pharmaceutical properties of the plant, but a close Chinese relative of the plant *(Ligusticum wallichi)* has been studied extensively. The main constituent of its aromatic oil is alpha-pinene, which has antimicrobial and disinfectant properties. Constituents called *ligustilides,* which are common to both the North American and Chinese species, have broad spectrum antibiotic effects as well as antiviral and antifungal properties.

☞ Directions: Using a coffee grinder, grind a piece of osha root into a powder. Spread the powder in a small skillet. Add enough lard or butter to cover the powder when melted. Put on low heat until the lard or butter is melted. Stir well and let stand at room temperature until the salve becomes solid. To treat a skin infection, apply the salve to the skin every two to three hours.

Alternately, mix the osha with enough honey to make a paste. Apply to a piece of gauze and use a bandage to hold in place over the affected area. Osha may irritate the skin. If this occurs, reduce the frequency of the treatments or try another remedy.

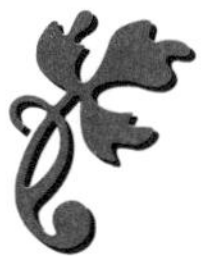

Sore Throat

A sore throat can be a minor, but annoying, ailment—or it can be a symptom of a serious illness

A sore throat is a painful irritation in the throat. A sore throat can range from mild scratchiness to severe pain and difficulty in swallowing.

A sore throat is most frequently seen as a symptom of a virus. When an individual suffers from a common cold, the nasal passages are congested and the person is forced to breathe through the mouth, leaving the throat dry and irritated. Coughing may also irritate the throat, as will the secretions that drain into the throat from the back of the nose during a cold.

A severe sore throat may be caused by a bacterial (usually *Streptococcus* bacteria, or strep) infection of the throat, middle ear, or sinuses. It is difficult to determine from the symptoms whether a sore throat is due to a virus or to strep (although a doctor can tell the difference using laboratory tests). Both infections may be accompanied by fever, headache, and fatigue, and both infections normally get better on their own. The fever subsides within a few days, the sore throat improves, and all signs of infection are usually gone within two weeks.

The complications of a strep throat begin between one and six weeks after the first appearance of the sore throat, usually after about two weeks. For this reason, any sore throat that lasts more than a week requires a visit to the doctor. A number of individuals who carry *Streptococcus* bacteria are without any symptoms at all. In fact, 15 to 20 percent of children are carriers, and most are asymptomatic. Concern for complications comes only with active inflammation, although the symptoms may seem minor.

Strep throat can have serious complications, however. A prolonged strep infection can result in damage to the heart (called *rheumatic fever)* or to the kidneys. These complications are rare, however—less than 1 percent of strep throats result in these illnesses. But the complications are common enough to warrant antibiotic prescriptions for strep infections, which is the standard treatment in modern medicine. Antibiotics for strep also reduce secondary infections, such as ear infection or pneumonia, that might accompany the sore throat. (Antibiotics are of no value in sore throats caused by viruses.)

Folk remedy treatments for sore throats fall into five categories. First, there are remedies that act as astringents, which reduce swelling of the mucous membrane tissues and thereby reduce pain. Second, there are demulcents such as slippery elm. These herbs or foods have a slimy constituency that is soothing to inflamed tissues. The third category contains plants used to treat sore throat like goldenseal or garlic that are antibacterial and antiviral. In the fourth category are the remedies such as mint and echinacea that contain local anesthetics that help numb a sore throat. Finally, many of the herbs used in folk remedies for sore throat contain anti-inflammatory constituents that may reduce pain and swelling. Most of the remedies combine more than one of these actions. For example, sage leaf is both astringent and antiseptic. Mint is both antiseptic and anesthetic. Willow bark is both astringent and anti-inflammatory. Most folk remedies call for gargling the substance, and most can be swallowed after gargling for further benefits.

Remedies

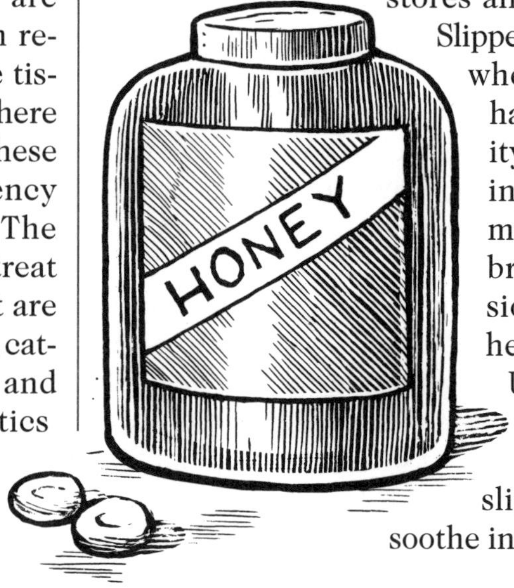

SLIPPERY ELM: Slippery elm bark *(Ulmus spp., Ulmus fulva)* was used to treat sore throats by members of at least six American Indian tribes, including the Iroquois and the Cherokee, even before the arrival of the European colonists. Slippery elm has been a folkloric treatment for sore throat in the United States at least since the early 1800s when its use was popularized by the Thomsonian herbalists. Slippery elm was an official remedy in the *United States Pharmacopoeia* from 1820 until 1930. Slippery elm throat lozenges have been sold throughout the United States since the late 1800s. They are available today in many health food stores and pharmacies. Slippery elm powder, when moistened, has a slimy quality that is soothing to inflamed mucous membranes. Professional medical herbalists in the United States, Australia, and Europe use slippery elm to soothe inflammations of the mouth, throat, and intestines. Its use continues today in the folk medicine of New England, North Carolina, and Indiana.

☞ Directions: Place 1 tablespoon of powdered slippery elm bark in a cup. Fill with boiling water. Let steep for ten minutes. Stir, without straining, and first gargle, then swallow ½-cup doses to soothe a sore throat. Do this as often as desired.

Alternately, make honey lozenges of slippery elm by mixing the slippery elm powder with hot honey. Spread the paste on a marble slab or other nonstick surface coated with sugar or cornstarch. With a rolling pin, roll the mixture flat to about the thickness of a pancake. Sprinkle with sugar and cornstarch. With a knife, cut into small, separate squares. Or pinch off pieces and roll into ¼-inch balls. Flatten the balls into round lozenges. Allow lozenges to air-dry in a well-ventilated area for twelve hours. Then store them in the refrigerator. Suck on lozenges to help heal sore throats.

Also, the most basic method, mentioned in several folk traditions, is to chew on the bark and swallow the juice or suck on the plain bark powder.

RED ROOT: Red root *(Ceanothus americanus, Ceanothus spp.)* was used for a wide variety of ailments, including colds and coughs, by American Indians living in the regions where it grows. Eclectic and Physiomedicalist physicians adopted the use of red root in the mid-19th century. A tea of the leaves was used during the Civil War as a treatment for malaria. Today, red root is used to treat sore throats in the folk medicine of Appalachia and by Hispanics in the Southwest.

Red root is astringent like black tea and was even used as a substitute for tea during the Civil War when black tea was unavailable. Some *Ceanothus* species contain a small amount of caffeine. Red root also contains anti-inflammatory and antimicrobial constituents that may help soothe and disinfect a sore throat. Its constituents ceanothic acid and ceanothetric acid have specifically shown to inhibit the growth of *Streptococcus* bacteria in laboratory experiments. (A tincture must be used, rather than a tea, to take advantage of the anti-streptococcal activity, however.) Red root has not been tested in clinical trials. The tea is a better source of the astringent constituents than the tincture and is the form used by physicians during the last century.

☞ Directions: Simmer 1 ounce of red root in 1 pint of water on low heat for twenty minutes. Let cool to room temperature. Gargle doses of 1 tablespoon and swallow, four times a day. Alternately, you can purchase a tincture of red root at a health food store or herb shop. Hold a teaspoon dose of the tincture in the mouth and swish it around. Then gargle and swallow. Do this four times a day for as long as necessary.

GOLDENSEAL: Goldenseal *(Hydrastis canadensis)* was a sore throat remedy among eastern American Indian tribes. The colonists quickly adopted the plant as a household medicine and by the 1830s physicians were using it to treat sore throats. Goldenseal was an official medicine in the *United States Pharmacopoeia* from 1840 until 1920. It is still used today to treat sore throats in the folk medicine of North Carolina.

The plant's constituent berberine is a strong antibiotic—about as potent as pharmaceutical drugs of the sulfa group. Berberine must come in direct contact with microorganisms in order to kill them, and it does not enter the bloodstream the way most pharmaceutical antibiotics do. Oregon grape root *(Mahonia aquifolium, Berberis aquifolium)* and barberry *(Berberis vulgaris)* also contain berberine. (Both plants were used for treating sore throats by American Indians in the regions where they grow.) Of the three plants, goldenseal is probably best for treating sore throats because, unlike the other two plants, it contains powerful astringents. However, goldenseal is now an endangered species and is very expensive. Oregon grape root and barberry root, on the other hand, are inexpensive and plentiful.

☞ Directions: Place 1 ounce of one of the above roots in a pint of water. Bring to a boil and simmer on the lowest heat for twenty minutes. Let cool to room temperature. Gargle and swallow doses of 1 to 2 tablespoons three to four times a day.

OAK BARK: Oak bark *(Quercus spp.)* has been used to treat sore throats since antiquity in European folk medicine. In this country, oak bark was used for the same purpose by members of the Delaware, Cherokee, Houma, Alabama, and Iroquois Indian tribes. Later, from 1820 until 1930, oak bark was an official medicine in the *United States Pharmacopoeia*.

Oak bark contains a high level of tannins—the same substances found in black tea. Oak bark is mentioned today in the folk medicine of North Carolina. It is also used by professional medical herbalists in North America and Europe.

☞ Directions: Boil 3 tablespoons of oak bark in 1 pint of water for twenty minutes. Let cool to room temperature and strain. Gargle with 1 or 2 tablespoons of the tea three to four times a day for as long as necessary.

HOREHOUND: A folk remedy for sore throats from contemporary Indiana is horehound *(Marrubium vulgare)*. Horehound has been used in European folk medicine since the time of the ancient Greeks. It was later used for treating sore throats in this country by the Mahuna and Navaho Indian tribes. Horehound became an official cough remedy in the *United States Pharmacopoeia* between 1840 and 1910. It remains an approved medicine for coughs by the German government today.

The herb is most famous as a cough medicine. Horehound cough drops are available in some health food stores and pharmacies. Besides its expectorant properties, horehound also contains astringent tannins (like those in tea) and anti-inflammatory and antimicrobial aromatic oils.

☞ Directions: Place 1 tablespoon of dried horehound in a cup and fill with boiling water. Cover and let steep for fifteen minutes. Strain and sweeten with honey. Gargle ½-cup doses as desired.

LICORICE: A folk remedy from China for sore throats is licorice tea. Licorice is used as a medicine in every major traditional medical system in the world. Extracts of licorice were originally used to make licorice candy, but the spice anise is used for that purpose today. Licorice was an official medicine in the *United States Pharmacopoeia* from 1820 until 1975; it was listed as a flavoring agent and a demulcent and expectorant for cough syrups.

Licorice root has a sweet flavor and a soothing demulcent quality. It also contains anti-inflammatory constituents similar to steroid drugs. (These constituents act systemically; that is, after the licorice has been digested. These constituents are therefore unlikely to account for any soothing topical effect of the licorice tea.) The following method of preparing the tea comes from Chinese folklore.

☞ Directions: Place ½ ounce of licorice root in 1 quart of water. Boil on low heat in an uncovered pot until half the water has evaporated. Drink the remaining pint in 2 doses during the course of a day. Repeat for up to three days. Don't take licorice if you are taking steroid drugs.

ROSE: A sore throat remedy in the Hispanic folklore of the Southwest is a tea of rose petals *(Rosa spp.)*. Rose petals have also been used by American Indians of the Costanoan, Skagut, and Snohomish tribes to treat throat problems. In addition, rose petals are among the top ten of the most often prescribed herbs in contemporary Arabic medicine.

The petals have a strong astringent action and can tone up swollen and inflamed mucous membranes, which is their chief medicinal use in Arabic medicine. The rose oil that gives the flowers their scent also contains antimicrobial and anti-inflammatory substances. The petals are considered to be "cooling" in Arabic medicine, indicating that clinical anti-inflammatory effects have been observed in their medical traditions.

☞ Directions: Pour 1 pint of boiling water over a handful of rose petals in a 1-pint jar. Cover well to retain the aromatic oils, and let stand until the water reaches room temperature. Gargle ½-cup doses as desired for sore throat. Avoid commercial roses and roses that have been sprayed with strong pesticides.

SAGE LEAF: Another sore throat remedy from Indiana is sage tea *(Salvia officinalis)*, which is made from the common kitchen spice. Sage is a strong astringent, and it also contains anti-inflammatory and antimicrobial aromatic oils. Cultivated garden sage has been used as a medicine in the Mediterranean region since the time of the ancient Egyptians. It is a common remedy for sore throat in the professional medical herbalism of Europe and North America. It is an approved medicine for sore throats in Germany.

☞ Directions: Place 1 tablespoon of sage leaf in a cup and fill with boiling water. Cover and let stand until it reaches room temperature. Gargle ¼-cup doses three to four times a day for sore throats for as long as necessary. The concentrated essential oil of sage, or the alcohol tincture, should not be taken during pregnancy.

ECHINACEA: Echinacea *(Echinacea angustifolia)* was used by the Plains Indians for a wide variety of infectious diseases. The Cheyenne, Comanche, and Kiowa all used the herb to treat sore throats. Constituents in the *angustifolia* species can offer some relief from sore throat pain by producing a tingling and numbness in the mouth and

continued on page 348

English Folk Medicine

The English colonists of North America brought with them a folk medical tradition that was little different from the "official" medicine of the time. In 17th century England, licensed physicians studied theory and classical texts, but in practice could seldom do more than good lay practitioners could. All classes of healers borrowed from one another as freely as literacy and access allowed, and collections of published remedies included contributions from professionals and nonprofessionals alike. Unlettered people depended on oral tradition, which in addition to material remedies, included many magical charms. Metaphysical ideas about healing and disease were hardly a peasant preoccupation, however. In fact, one of the reasons that medicine had such difficulty getting established was the existence of an intensely religious climate—one in which illness was seen as God's will. Almost everyone in the colonies believed in witchcraft, and the learned held astrology as an indispensable tool of the trade.

England distinguished itself among the northern European nations with the early production of medical manuscripts in the native tongue. These were the *Anglo-Saxon Leechbooks,* written in Old English. The oldest copy is from the late 9th century, but there is evidence that even earlier copies existed and were lost. ("Leeches" were physicians, probably so named for their use of leeches in blood-letting.) Some of the books included methods proved to be quite effective. Mandrake, henbane, and poppy were recommended pain relievers. Roasted buck's liver, which is high in vitamin A, was used to cure night blindness. An enlarged spleen, often the result of anemia, was treated with a drink of iron acetate, made by plunging a red-hot poker into vinegar or wine. Onion, garlic, and plantain were used as antibiotics. Between 80 and 90 percent of the early English pharmacy was based on plants.

Herbal manuscripts exist from the 11th century on and were among the earliest printed books. There were at least 20 different titles of printed herbals in the 17th century, many of which went through numerous editions. For example, there were over 100 editions of *Culpeper's Herbal* between 1652 and 1700. Nicolas Culpeper was a vocal critic of the medical profession, especially of doctors who would not treat the poor, and he translated several medical works from Latin to English to enable ordinary people to access the texts. Literate gentlewomen were perhaps his largest audience. Barred from formal education and licensing, women nevertheless often acted as physicians, drawing on published herbals and compiling their own "receipt" books as well.

The poor had a huge body of oral herb-lore, to which official remedies were often indebted. Some professional doctors denounced nonprofessionals, but others accepted their worth. In *Popular Medicine in Seventeenth-Century England,* Doreen Evenden Nagy writes that the scientist and philosopher Robert Boyle knew of "ladies and old wives" who "performed more constant and easy cures than learned physicians."

Many villages had "cunning folk" or "wise" women and men who offered advice and magical remedies for a host of ills. Some charmers had a single charm, some possessed many. Some kept them secret, others did not. There were charms for almost every ailment, although toothache, warts, and bleeding seemed to be most amenable to charms.

Because of their uncanny reputations, particularly cunning people were consulted if a malady was thought to be supernaturally caused. According to *The Elizabethan Fairies: The Fairies of Folklore and the Fairies of Shakespeare* by Minor White Latham, the physician John Webster complained in 1673 that "the common people, if they chance to have any sort of the Epilepsie, Palsie, Convulsions, or the like, do presently perswade themselves that they are bewitched, forespoken, blasted, fairy-taken, or haunted with some evil spirit, and the like."

The belief in witchcraft and magical healing was, however, found in all social classes. Magical healing was carried out by the English monarchs themselves, who were believed to heal "king's evil" with the touch of their hands. (Technically, king's evil referred to scrofula, a tubercular swelling of the lymph glands of the neck, but in practice it was applied to assorted diseases of the head, neck, and face.) Huge church assemblies were conducted by clergy who would read a verse from the Bible, while the king touched the sufferers' faces and gave them a "touch-piece" (a gold coin strung on a white ribbon) to wear home. The ceremony began in the 13th century, peaked in the 1680s, and declined shortly after that.

The Leechbooks

Some of the English-language charms of the *Anglo-Saxon Leechbooks* apparently recognized contagion and infection; they spoke of "flying venoms" and "onfliers" that carried disease from one person to another. "Elfshot" referred to a sudden pain or illness, which was possibly a dart from supernatural forces into the body. One charm commanded it: "Out, little spear, if it be herein.... If it were shot of gods, or if it were shot of elves, or if it were shot of witches, now I shall help thee." The charms were often replete with the number nine, a crucial figure in folk medicine even today.

English methods and worldview transplanted well to the New World. The long reliance on plants as medicine made the colonists eager to seek new botanical sources, even from the Indians, despite the ministers' teachings that claimed the natives were in league with the devil. According to Whitfield J. Bell, in *The Colonial Physician and Other Essays,* official medicine in the early 1700s was summed up by a New England physician as consisting uniformly of "bleeding, vomiting, blistering, purging, Anodyne & c.," prompting another to observe that "frequently there is more danger from the Physician, than from the distemper." Thus folk healers continued to play an important and innovative role in medicine.

throat that can last for more than half an hour. (These local anesthetic effects are not present in *Echinacea purpurea*, the species used in most of the commercial echinacea products, however. The root or powder of the *Echinacea angustifolia* species is sometimes available, however.) In addition, echinacea is an immune stimulant. It may help the body fight the infection that is causing the sore throat.

☞ Directions: Obtain whole or chopped *Echinacea angustifolia* root at a health food store or herb shop. Grind a small amount in a coffee grinder. Stir ½ teaspoon of the powder into 2 ounces of warm water. Gargle the water, powder and all, for as long as you can, allowing the powder to coat your throat and mouth.

MINT: Both the Chinese and the Paiute Indians used mint teas *(Mentha spp.)* when treating sore throats. Mint contains a number of anti-inflammatory, antimicrobial, and local anesthetic constituents. The eight anesthetic constituents it contains may provide immediate (but temporary) relief from the pain of sore throat.

☞ Directions: Place 1 ounce of peppermint leaves in a 1-pint jar and fill with boiling water. Cover tightly and let the tea cool to room temperature, shaking the bottle from time to time to mix the contents. Gargle ½-cup doses of the tea as desired.

HERBAL STEAM: An entry in folklorist Clarence Meyer's collection of remedies, called *American Folk Medicine*, suggests inhaling steam from an herbal tea to treat severely painful sore throats. The herbs included are sage *(Salvia officinalis),* boneset *(Eupatorium perfoliatum),* catnip *(Nepeta cataria),* hop *(Humulus lupulus),* and horehound *(Marrubium vulgare)*. The mixture contains anti-inflammatory and antiviral aromatic oils that presumably can rise with the steam and affect the throat. The steam itself may be antiviral. Most of the viruses that infect the mucous membranes cannot survive at temperatures equal to those in the body's core—about 98.6°F. Thus, the viruses remain at the cooler membranes, near the surface of the body (in the mucous membranes of the respiratory tract). Inhaling hot steam may kill the viruses on contact.

☞ Directions: Place a handful each of sage, boneset, catnip, hop, and horehound in a large bowl. Pour 1 quart of boiling water over the herbs and inhale the steam that rises, being careful not to burn yourself. If you don't have one or two of the herbs in the formula, use the ones mentioned that you do have.

WILLOW: Willow bark *(Salix spp.)* is used as an astringent gargle for sore throats in the Hispanic folk medicine of the Southwest. The same method has been used by the Cherokee and Iroquois Indians and also by the Alaskan Eskimos. Willow bark is astringent. It also contains aspirin-like compounds that may help reduce a fever.

☞ Directions: Simmer 3 tablespoons of willow bark in 1 pint of water for twenty to thirty minutes. Gargle with ½-cup doses as desired throughout the day as often as necessary.

OSHA: Osha *(Ligusticum porteri),* a Rocky Mountain plant, was used for a variety of ailments by American Indians living in that region. Osha remains one of the most important folk remedies of American Indians and Hispanic residents of the upper Rio

Grande Valley in New Mexico and Colorado. A traditional herbalist of the area, Michael Moore, recommends the tea below for sore throat. Osha contains disinfectant aromatic oils and local anesthetic aromatic oils. One of its constituents has antibacterial and antiviral properties.

☞ Directions: Grind an osha root in a coffee grinder. Place 1 teaspoon of the powder in a cup and fill with boiling water. Cover tightly and allow to stand until the water reaches room temperature. Gargle ¼- to ½-cup doses as desired.

Alternately, mix the powdered osha with enough hot honey to make a paste. Roll the paste into balls as big around as dimes. Store the balls in the refrigerator, where they will cool to a more solid consistency. Suck on the lozenges for sore throat. You can do this as often as desired.

ONION SYRUP: Here's a recipe from New England for onion syrup that is remarkably similar to a recipe from North Carolina. The New England recipe calls for sliced raw onions to be placed in a bowl and covered with sugar. Allow the onion to stand until a syrup forms. Adding water is not necessary because the sugar draws the onion juice out of the onions. (It may take a day or two for the syrup to form, however.) The method used in North Carolina is similar, but the onion-and-sugar mixture is placed in a baking pan and baked in the oven until the syrup forms. (Baking presumably speeds up the process. The onions contain antimicrobial substances, which attack the organisms that are causing the infection. These substances are the same ones that give an onion its odor, and they are also responsible for the burning sensation your eyes feel after you slice an onion.

☞ Directions: Fill a bowl or baking pan with raw onions. Pour enough sugar over them to cover. Then, either let them stand or bake them on medium heat, depending on how fast you need the syrup. Take the syrup in single tablespoon doses as often as desired.

MYRRH GUM: Myrrh gum *(Commiphora myrrha)* has been used as a disinfectant in the Mediterranean region since the time of the ancient Egyptians. Its use spread to India, China, and Europe along Arab trade routes. Its use as a disinfectant was popularized throughout the eastern United States by the Thomsonian herbalists of the early 1800s. Myrrh gum is a powerful antiseptic and it is also astringent—both properties are beneficial to a throat infection.

☞ Directions: Purchase some myrrh gum tincture at a health food store or herb shop. Add 1 teaspoon to ¼ cup of hot water and use as a gargle as often as necessary.

COLD COMPRESS: A hydrotherapy treatment from North Carolina folklore calls for applying a cold wet compress to the throat and covering it with a dry one. The method is also used in the Seventh Day Adventist healing tradition. The treatment has its roots in the nature cure and hydrotherapy traditions of Germany, brought to North America by German immigrants near the turn of the 20th century.

☞ Directions: Soak a cotton cloth in cold water. Wring it out and wrap it around the front of the neck below the ears. Be careful to avoid chilling the back of the neck. Wrap a warm wool scarf around the cold cloth and lie down. The cold cloth will supposedly attract circulation to the area, which in turn, promotes healing of the throat. The body will usually heat the cold cloth in twenty to forty minutes. Repeat the treatment two to four times each day.

GARLIC: Both the Amish and the Seventh Day Adventists, two religious groups that advocate natural remedies, suggest sucking on a garlic lozenge to treat a sore throat. Garlic, when sliced or crushed, releases the antimicrobial substance allicin. Allicin kills many bacteria, including strep, and some viruses. Seventh Day Adventists Agatha Thrash, M.D., and Calvin Thrash, M.D., in their book *Home Remedies: Hydrotherapy, Massage, Charcoal, and Other Simple Treatments*, say that sore throats sometimes disappear within a few hours of using this technique.

☞ Directions: Slice a garlic clove down the middle and place a half clove on each side of the mouth, between the teeth and cheeks. Suck on the cloves like lozenges as often as necessary.

HOT WATER GARGLE: The Seventh Day Adventists advise a hot water gargle for a sore throat. The viruses most often responsible for sore throats cannot survive at temperatures above normal body temperature. If you gargle with hot water, it will come in contact with the throat's membranes, raising the temperature there and killing the viruses. Hot water also draws blood circulation to the area, which increases the natural immune response to the infection.

☞ Directions: Gargle with water as hot as you can stand.

SALTWATER GARGLE: An Indiana sore throat remedy is the saltwater gargle. Salt is astringent and antimicrobial, so it may relieve pain while attacking the organisms causing the infection.

☞ Directions: Add 1 teaspoon of salt to a cup of hot water, mix, and use as a gargle as often as desired.

LEMON: An Indiana folk tradition for curing a sore throat suggests sucking on a lemon that has been sprinkled with salt. A Gypsy version of the same treatment calls for lemon juice and salt diluted with water. Lemon is naturally acidic. Salt increases the lemon's acidity through a chemical reaction that forms dilute hydrochloric acid, which is even more acidic than lemon juice is alone. Many microorganisms are killed by weak acids, so this strong Gypsy gargle may indeed kill infectious organisms.

☞ Directions: To use the Gypsy method, juice a whole lemon into a bowl and add a pinch of sea salt. Add 1 teaspoon of the concentrated lemon-salt mixture to 1 cup of water. Gargle some solution three to four times a day as often as necessary.

VINEGAR: To treat a sore throat, Indiana folklore advises a gargle with vinegar. Another tradition suggests alternating vinegar gargles with saltwater gargles. Most microorganisms cannot live in an acid medium. Vinegar is a weak acid, so it may kill the infectious organisms. Salt also kills some microorganisms and has astringent properties.

☞ Directions: Gargle with straight vinegar two to four times a day. Wait ten minutes after the vinegar gargle and gargle with salt water. To make the saltwater gargle, add 1 teaspoon of salt to 1 cup of hot water and mix. Gargle as often as desired.

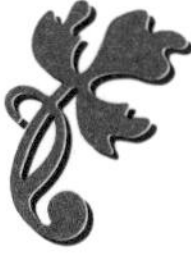

Sores and Chronic Skin Ulcers

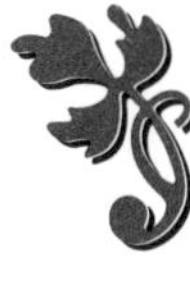

To treat sores, folk traditions often employ remedies with disinfecting and circulatory-stimulating properties. Try one of the remedies below

Sores, called *skin ulcers* in medical terminology, are localized sore spots on the body where the tissues are ruptured or abraded. These sores may result from a slow-healing wound or other trauma to the skin, acute bacterial infections, chronic bacterial and fungal infections, or rare systemic diseases. Bedsores, called *decubitus* or *trophic ulcers,* can be caused by pressure from a bed, wheelchair, or other constant source of stress on the bony parts of the body. (Bedsores tend to occur in the bedridden, paralyzed, or chronically incapacitated patients.) Poor circulation to the skin, malnutrition, chronic infection, and deficient immune response all play a part in the chronic nature of skin ulcers as well.

Most folk remedies combine disinfecting and circulatory-stimulating properties to treat sores. Others provide soothing, protective coatings for the sores. Note that sores that accompany nerve damage, such as may occur in paralysis or diabetes, must be treated only with medical supervision. Some of the herbs and remedies in this section can cause burns to the skin or skin irritation, so individuals with impaired sensory nerves should not use them; they may not realize that their skin is becoming inflamed.

Remedies

GARLIC: A remedy from contemporary Appalachia for treating sores is garlic *(Allium sativum)*. Garlic is also recorded as a treatment for skin infection in contemporary Gypsy folklore. When garlic is crushed, it releases allicin, a potent broad-spectrum antimicrobial agent. Allicin protects the plant against infection by bacteria, viruses, molds, yeast, and fungi. It will also kill these organisms in laboratory dishes or in open wounds. Allicin breaks down into other substances within a few days, so disinfectant garlic preparations should be made fresh. Fresh garlic can cause serious skin burns, however, and should never be left in contact with the skin for more than 20 to

25 minutes. The use of garlic can be especially risky for patients who have neurological conditions. Garlic can irritate the skin, and these individuals may not be able to feel the garlic's burning sensation. For this reason, they should use garlic with care or avoid using it altogether.

☞ Directions: Crush 3 cloves of garlic with a mortar and pestle, or blend the cloves in a blender. Mix with an equal volume of hot honey. Allow to stand until the honey reaches room temperature, mixing occasionally. Apply the mixture to the ulcer with a piece of gauze. Then remove and wash the area thoroughly after ten to fifteen minutes. Repeat the treatment three to four times a day.

GOLDENSEAL: In the early 1800s, American botanist Constantine Rafinesque traveled throughout the Ohio and the upper Mississippi River Valley, investigating the American Indians' use of local plants. He eventually published *Medical Flora* in 1830, one of the first books on the botany of North American plants. In the book he described a plant called "yellow puccoon," which we now know as goldenseal *(Hydrastis canadensis)*. Rafinesque noted that the American Indians made a powder of goldenseal and used it to treat ulcers and slow-healing wounds.

Goldenseal rapidly entered into medical practice in North America and has been used ever since by one medical discipline or another. Goldenseal contains the antimicrobial substance berberine, which kills a broad spectrum of bacteria, viruses, yeast, and molds. In the folklore of Appalachia, a tea of goldenseal is recommended as a wash for skin ulcers. Although some Appalachians can still find goldenseal growing underfoot, it is now an endangered species and may soon be unavailable in stores. Other berberine-containing plants such as Oregon grape root *(Mahonia aquifolium)* or barberry (*Berberis vulgaris*) make good substitutes.

☞ Directions: Place ½ ounce of goldenseal root bark or powder (or use one of the other herbs above) in a pint of water. Bring the water to a boil, then simmer for twenty minutes. Allow to cool to room temperature. Stir and, without straining, apply the tea to the affected area with a clean cloth. Do not wipe off, just cover with a clean bandage or gauze pad. Apply the tea every two hours. Simultaneously, drink 2-ounce doses of the tea two to four times a day.

HONEY: Since the dawn of medical history, honey has been used around the world as a folk remedy to disinfect wounds and burns. Honey appears today in the folk literature of the Amish, Hispanics in the Southwest, Chinese immigrants, and residents of Indiana.

Honey, because it is naturally dehydrated, attracts water. When applied to an ulcer, honey draws fluid out of the tissues, which simultaneously cleanses the sore. Thus, most infectious microorganisms cannot live in the presence of honey, because the honey literally sucks the fluid right out of them. Physicians in India experimented with honey-gauze dressings for treating burns and found that the honey applications had stronger antibiotic effects than silver

continued on page 354

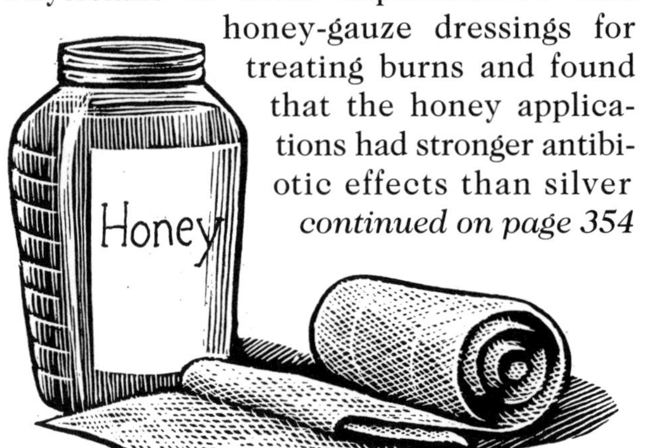

Naturally Healthy Skin

A beautiful and youthful complexion seems always to have been highly valued, so folk tradition is filled with advice on clarifying the skin, removing blackheads and pimples, and making freckles disappear. Many of these are herbal treatments that work similarly to some of our modern over-the-counter facial products. In the Midwest, for example, the "milk" of milkweed was once used for facials. Milkweed actually secretes latex, so when the dried "milk" was peeled off the skin, it may have taken oils and blackheads with it.

Many folk treatments for the complexion seem to involve the idea of bleaching, or lightening, the skin. Although other acidic substances like tomato juice are used for this purpose, lemon juice is perhaps the most common application—it is also used to gradually bleach the hair. Cucumber pulp has also been a skin lightener in folk practice, and cucumber masks and ointments are common today in drug stores. Buttermilk is another traditional facial application that remains with us in popular complexion treatments. A little beyond buttermilk is the Midwestern advice to use sour milk that has stood at least five hours. (Mix the milk with grated horseradish and apply to the skin twice daily.) But if sour milk sounds unpleasant for a facial, it is far from the worst remedy. In the Ozarks it has been reported that a face mask of cow dung will not only clarify the complexion but also remove wrinkles! (This remedy is not recommended.) And, from the same region, it has been reported that scarring from smallpox could be prevented with the application of warm blood from a freshly killed black dog.

The most frequently reported unpleasant complexion remedy uses urine. A urine soaked diaper has been claimed as a guaranteed pimple remover in many traditions—some of these remedies specify using a boy's diaper or a girl's. More extreme is the recommendation that you drink your own urine to cure acne.

Many complexion cures do not seem to have any medical relevance, grotesque or otherwise. For example, in Europe and North America, there is a very old folk tradition that says you can rid yourself of pimples and blackheads by crawling under a bramble bush on a Friday!

To judge from the number of freckle cures found in folk tradition, these markings were once almost as despised as pimples. While some treatments aim at bleaching the skin to make the freckles fade, many remedies are magical. For example, from Georgia comes the idea that you should count your freckles, then place the same number of pebbles in a paper bag and leave the package where someone else will step on it. The person who steps on the package will get the freckles.

Water has been used magically to clear the complexion. These treatments included using water from a tree stump, water from a blacksmith's tub in which red hot metal had been plunged, water gathered on the first of June, or dew collected on the first day of May.

sulfadiazine, the most common antibiotic dressing used for burns. The burns of the honey-treated patients also healed faster. What's more, the honey offered greater relief of pain and reduced scarring as well.

☞ Directions: Apply honey to a piece of sterile gauze and place directly on the ulcer. Hold in place with tape. Change the honey dressing three or four times a day.

CHAPARRAL: Chaparral *(Larrea tridentata)* is a popular remedy of the American Indians of the Southwest. It is most commonly used by tribes in that area as a wash to treat various skin conditions. Chaparral has a powerful odor, and its aromatic constituents, which include alpha-pinene, camphor, and limonene, all have antiseptic effects.

☞ Directions: Crush some chaparral leaves. (You can use fresh leaves if you live in the Southwest and can find them.) Mix the leaves with an equal amount of lard and simmer the mixture on the lowest possible heat for two to three hours. Strain and allow the salve to cool to room temperature. Apply to sores three to four times a day for as long as desired.

YERBA MANSA: Among American Indians and Hispanic settlers, yerba mansa *(Anemopsis californica)* was the most popular medicinal herb of traditional medicine in the Southwest. Spanish settlers learned the plant's uses from the Maricopa, Pima, Tewa, and Yaqui Indian tribes. "Yerba mansa" is short for "yerba del indio manso," or "herb of the tamed Indians." The plant was used both externally and internally to treat a variety of conditions, especially those affecting the mucous membranes. It may be best suited to treat ulcerations of the mouth or lips. Yerba mansa contains the volatile constituents thymol and methyl eugenol, both of which have demonstrated antimicrobial properties. Its use was adopted by the Eclectic physicians in 1877.

☞ Directions: Place 1 ounce of yerba mansa in 1 pint of water, bring to a boil, and simmer for twenty to thirty minutes. Let stand until cool. Apply the tea to the ulcer every few hours with a clean cloth. Continue doing this as long as desired.

ALOE VERA: Although aloe vera is better know as a burn remedy, the Amish also use it to treat sores and ulcers. Aloe vera, in addition to its ability to reduce pain and inflammation, also has antiseptic effects that make it useful for treating infected ulcers. In 1988 at the University of Puerto Rico, during research on the plant's effects on burns, it was discovered that not only did aloe vera gel speed the healing time of burns but it also reduced the bacterial counts in the burns. We can suppose that it has the same effect on skin ulcers.

☞ Directions: Break off a piece of an aloe vera leaf. Apply the juicy sap to the skin ulcer. Alternately, you can purchase some aloe vera gel at a health food store and use that instead of the plant's sap. Repeat the applications every few hours. Continue doing this as long as desired.

PLANTAIN LEAVES: Plantain *(Plantago major)* is a common lawn weed throughout North America. Although it arrived in North America with the English colonists, its use was rapidly adopted by the indigenous residents of the continent. The Delaware, Mohegan, Ojibwa, Cherokee, and many other Indian tribes have used plantain to disinfect and relieve the symptoms of minor wounds and other skin conditions.

The plant contains a large number of anti-inflammatory constituents and at least six antiseptic ones. Plantain also contains the constituent allantoin, which promotes cell proliferation and tissue healing. Fresh leaves must be used to derive the antiseptic benefits.

☞ Directions: Crush a small handful of fresh plantain leaves and apply the juice to the ulcer. Hold the leaves in place against the ulcer with a bandage. Renew the dressing three to four times a day. Continue doing this as long as desired.

PINE AND PINE BARK: Pine bark poultices *(Pinus spp.)* appear in the folklore of a number of American Indian tribes for treating sores. The practice, whether it was introduced by the Indians or borrowed from similar traditions in Europe, was later adopted by the colonists. The remedy is still practiced today in the folklore of North Carolina and Appalachia. Pine sap contains a variety of antimicrobial substances.

☞ Directions: Strip some bark from the branches of a white pine. Boil the bark in water for twenty to thirty minutes. Let cool. Then scrape the soft inner bark away from the hard outer bark. Moisten with liquor to make a poultice and apply to sores three to four times a day.

Alternately, purchase some White Pine Compound Syrup, a nonprescription item, at a pharmacy. Apply to the ulcer with a clean cloth three to four times a day. Be careful not to irritate the skin with the pine syrup.

ROSEMARY: A remedy for sores from the Hispanic folklore of the Southwest is rosemary leaf *(Rosmarinus officinalis)*. Rosemary contains more than ten antiseptic constituents.

☞ Directions: Crush some rosemary leaves and mix with an equal amount of hot honey. Keep the mixture warm on a hot plate or in a crock pot for half an hour. Using gauze, apply to the ulcer and use a bandage to hold the mixture in place. Change the dressing two to three times a day. Alternately, place 1 ounce of rosemary leaf in a 1-pint jar and fill with boiling water. Cover tightly and let stand until the water reaches room temperature. Strain. Apply the solution to the ulcers every hour or two, using a clean cloth.

GINGER POULTICE: Folklorist Clarence Meyer's collection of remedies, called *American Folk Medicine,* lists an 1831 entry calling for a poultice of ginger *(Zingiber officinalis)* and slippery elm *(Ulmus fulva)* to treat sores. The slippery elm is mucilaginous and forms the bulk of the poultice. The spicy oils in ginger are antibacterial and also stimulate local circulation to the skin.

☞ Directions: Boil ½ cup of water and add 1 tablespoon of ginger powder. Allow to steep for a minute or two, and then stir in slippery elm powder until a thick mass forms. Allow to cool. Apply enough of the mixture to cover the ulcer, and hold it in place with gauze and a bandage. Change the dressing two to three times a day. Continue using this remedy for as long as desired.

CALENDULA: British folk medicine records the saying "Where there is calendula, there is no need of a surgeon." But calendula (*Calendula officinalis)* is not really a miracle herb that can prevent modern surgery. The British saying was coined during a time when the most common surgery was amputation and the most common cause of amputation was infected wounds.

Calendula has been used to cleanse wounds and promote healing since ancient times. The plant's flowers contain constituents that kill bacteria, viruses, and molds, as well as other constituents that are powerfully anti-inflammatory. Still more constituents promote cell growth in wounds and ulcers. Calendula is approved in Germany today in topical preparations that are specifically designed to treat ulcers and slow-healing wounds.

A caution with calendula: Do not use it on wounds or ulcers that are oozing pus. The plant can promote cell growth so efficiently that it can cause a wound to close prematurely and form an abscess, raising the risk of systemic infection. Calendula, which is also called "pot marigold," is a different plant than the common garden marigold *(Tagetes erecta)*, which contains different constituents than calendula.

☞ Directions: Place 1 ounce of calendula flowers in a 1-pint jar and fill with boiling water. Cover the jar tightly and allow to steep until the brew reaches room temperature. Strain. Apply externally with a clean cloth to ulcers and slow-healing wounds. Allow the area to dry and then place a dressing on the sore. Re-apply three to four times a day. Also, take 1 tablespoon of the tea internally along with each external application.

Alternately, crush several handfuls of dried calendula flowers into a powder and place in a crock pot or glass pot on a hot plate. Add enough honey to cover. Allow to steep on the lowest heat for ten to fifteen minutes after the honey has melted. Let cool to room temperature. Do not strain. Apply with gauze to the wound and use a bandage to hold the gauze in place. Apply three to four times a day. Remember to clean the wound well each time to remove any plant material or honey before reapplying the remedy.

ONION: In the folk medicine of Appalachia and the Southwest, onion poultices *(Allium cepa)* are used to treat sores and ulcers. Onion, like garlic, contains antibacterial compounds, including allicin, which is also in garlic. Onion is not as irritating to the skin as garlic and it is less likely to cause skin burns. Its mild irritation, in addition to its killing microorganisms, increases local circulation.

☞ Directions: Pulverize half an onion in a blender, or crush until juicy with a mortar and pestle. Mix the onion with a little honey and apply to the ulcer. Don't leave in place for more than an hour. Then wash the ulcer and cover with a clean dressing. Do this three times a day. Don't use this treatment on patients with paralysis or other conditions that would prevent them from feeling any irritation that might be caused by the onion salve.

GUMWEED: Gumweed *(Grindelia spp.)* is a major skin remedy of the American Indians of the

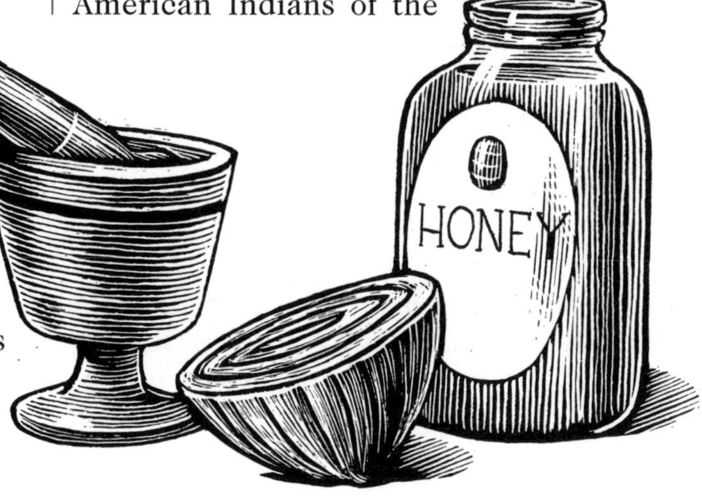

Southwest and northwestern Mexico. The plant entered into Eclectic medical practice during the late 19th century. Eclectic professor Harvey Felter, M.D., stated in *The Eclectic Materia Medica, Pharmacology, and Therapeutics* that gumweed was especially well-suited to skin conditions with poor circulation and a tendency to form ulcers. Gumweed was an official medicine in the *United States Pharmacopoeia* from 1882 until 1926. The plant's resin contains anti-inflammatory and antimicrobial constituents.

☞ Directions: Apply the sticky sap from the leaves or flowers of gumweed to the affected areas. Reapply every few hours. Cover with gauze and a clean bandage. Alternately, you can purchase some tincture of gumweed, and use it as a wash. Reapply every few hours.

GYPSY SALVE: A Gypsy salve for ulcers and poorly healing wounds combines a number of the other remedies mentioned in this section. The Spanish Gypsy herbalist Pilar, who provided the remedies published in the book *Gypsy Folk Medicine* by folklorist Wanja von Hausen, calls the ointment "Bride of the Sun Salve." The remedy is slightly modified below for ease of use.

☞ Directions: Warm 1 cup of olive oil in a pan. Mix a handful of pot marigold flowers *(Calendula officinalis)*, 9 rosemary blossoms, and 9 lavender blossoms into the oil. Simmer for three minutes, and remove from heat. Pulverize 3 cloves of garlic (not the larger bulbs) in a blender or use a mortar and pestle. Add the garlic to the oil. Let cool to room temperature, cover, and store overnight. Heat the salve again the next day on the lowest possible heat for seven minutes. Let cool to room temperature. Strain the mixture and apply to the wound. Reapply three to four times a day as often as desired.

Splinters

Most slivers aren't serious and can be treated with one simple remedy or another

Splinters under the skin are a common occurrence wherever people live or work. They were probably even more common in the past, when our ancestors used more wooden implements and worked with more rough and unfinished wood than we do today. We still get splinters, however, and they are still hard to get out.

The best method to extract a splinter is to use a pair of tweezers. Pull the splinter out gently, taking care not to leave any broken pieces behind. Then clean the wound thoroughly to prevent infection. Application of topical anti-infectives (alcohol or an antibiotic ointment) are recommended.

The folk remedies for extracting splinters and thorns generally act to soften or moisten the area around the sliver or to "draw" the object to the surface for easier extraction with the fingers or with tweezers.

A deep or stubborn splinter may require the assistance of a physician, who can use surgical instruments to remove it and can give antibiotics to prevent infection. Even modern medical treatment for splinters sometimes fails, however, because the imbedded pieces of the splinter are not visible on X ray unless they are metallic.

The chief health risk of splinters, especially those that go deep into the tissues, is tetanus, or lockjaw. In this disease, a germ that is common in animal feces, and in soil that has been exposed to animal feces, infects the wound. The germ produces a nerve toxin that can result in death. Tetanus is a rare disease in North America. In the 1990s, fewer than a hundred cases a year have been reported. Nevertheless, it is a serious illness, with about a 50 percent mortality rate, so a tetanus shot is prudent, especially if a splinter or other wound goes deep into the tissues and carries dirt or manure with it.

Remedies

BREAD AND WATER: In New England folk medicine a poultice of bread and water or bread and milk is a favorite for treating splinters. In *Country Folk Remedies: Tales of Skunk Oil, Sassafras Tea and Other Old-Time Remedies Gathered by Elisabeth Janos,* (authored by Janos), one elderly New England gentleman once said that he would refuse to eat bread pudding when he was growing up because he was afraid he would be eating a poultice. The combination of heat and the astringent action of the drying bread combine to soften the skin and draw the splinter out.

☞ Directions: Break up the bread and mix it with milk or water. Heat the mixture on the stove and apply it as hot as you can tolerate. Let it cool on the wound in order to bring the splinter closer to the surface of the skin.

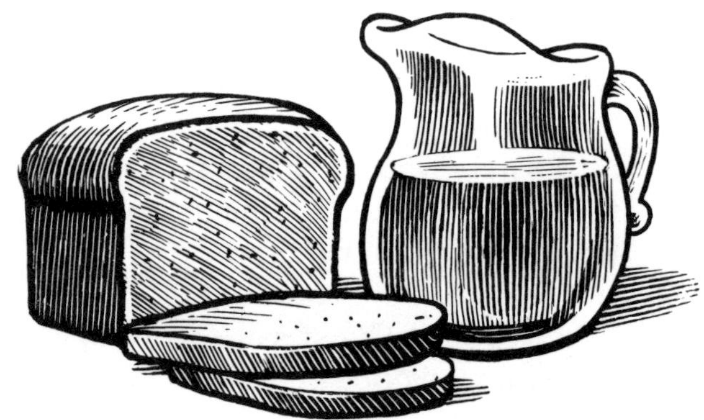

PLANTAIN LEAVES: Plantain *(Plantago major)* has been used in cultures around the world as a drawing and wound-healing agent. Applied externally, the plant stimulates and cleanses the skin and encourages wounds to heal faster. It was naturalized in North America after the arrival of the Europeans, and American Indians called it "White Man's Footprint," because it seemed to follow the European colonists wherever they went. The Delaware, Mohegan, Ojibwa, Cherokee, and many other Indian tribes used plantain to treat minor wounds and insect bites. Hardy and adaptable, plantain has made itself at home throughout the world. Often you'll see it growing along roads, in meadows, and, to the chagrin of homeowners, in lawns.

☞ Directions: Crush up plantain leaves and apply them directly to the wound.

Pork

Farmers throughout the eastern and midwestern United States have applied pork or bacon poultices to the skin to draw out splinters. Why pork? Probably because of its salt, which acts as an astringent. (Pork and bacon have traditionally been cured in salt.) You might improve on the method and avoid some of the mess by soaking the injured area in hot salt water until you can better get at the splinter with a pair of tweezers.

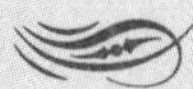

SUGAR AND SOAP: A folk remedy from early Indiana settlers calls for a mixture of sugar and soap. This poultice combines both moistening and drawing qualities.

☞ Directions: Mix equal parts of brown sugar and laundry soap. Moisten and apply to the wound for twelve to twenty-four hours.

SUCTION: Using suction is a traditional New England method for drawing out splinters. This method is closely related to "cupping," a practice that remains a part of traditional medicine throughout Europe, the Middle East, and Asia.

☞ Directions: Fill a wide-mouthed bottle with steaming hot water. Put the injured spot over the mouth of the bottle and press down. As the steam cools, it quickly forms a suction, drawing the skin lightly up into the jar. The steam softens the tissues and the suction will stretch the skin and draw the splinter to the surface.

CLAY PACKS: Clay or mud packs were favorite wound-healing and splinter-extracting poultices used by various American Indian groups as well as the German immigrants of the 18th century. Any type of clean clay soil (free from animal fecal matter or other pollutants) will do, or you can use the type of cosmetic clay that's sold for facial masks at your local drugstore.

☞ Directions: Make a poultice by mixing the clay with hot water. Apply to the wound. Let the mixture dry, then flake the residue off. If the splinter still isn't close enough to the surface of the skin to draw it out, apply another poultice.

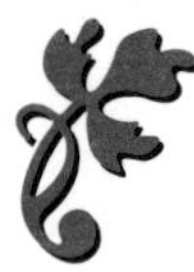 Wounds and Cuts 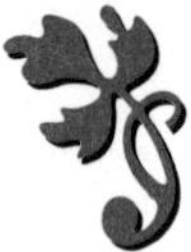

Even if you're extra careful, you can't always avoid the cuts and wounds of life. But you can learn to care for your injuries and speed their healing

Until the 20th century, serious wounds and cuts were as likely to be treated by a folk practitioner as a physician. After all, the methods of physicians were about the same as those of the folk practitioners: Stop the bleeding, clean the wound, disinfect it, and manage any infection. Both groups used simple herbs, spices, or cleaning agents such as alcohol.

The great Roman physician Galen won the appointment of doctor after devising a way to stop the bleeding of the serious sword wounds of the gladiators. (He filled the bleeding wounds with garlic-infused flour.) Later, Roman soldiers introduced into Britain the practice of dressing serious wounds with garlic-soaked moss. The moss provided a matrix for the blood to clot in, and the garlic is antimicrobial. The practice survived in the conventional medicine of Britain until the 1920s and was heavily used during World War I. (The horse soldiers of Genghis Khan practiced preventive wound care by wearing silk undershirts. An arrow penetrating their body carried the silk in with it. Not only would this keep debris out of the wound, but the arrowhead could be pulled out using the shirt.)

The advent of guns created more serious wounds and infections, because the bullet invariably carries debris from the clothing into the wound, and the small entry wound is difficult to clean. The result was the massive numbers of amputations necessary during the Civil War and World War I following gunshot wounds to the extremities. Great advances in wound care arrived during World War II and the Korean and Vietnam wars, when surgeons had plenty of opportunity to practice advanced techniques in stopping bleeding and repairing damaged tissue. Antibiotic drugs were also used during this time and greatly reduced the danger of infections.

Folk healers also paid attention to wounds. They knew that even small cuts, ruptured blisters, scratches from fish hooks, and other such minor wounds could become infected. Superficial infections can penetrate deeper into the body to form an abscess. The infection may then spread to the bloodstream and reach internal organs and other parts of the body, which results in a life-threatening condition called *septicemia.* The most important sign that a minor infection has become dangerous is the appearance of red streaks radiating from the site.

Any serious or infected wound today must be treated by a physician. Some of the remedies in this section may still be useful for disinfecting minor cuts and wounds, however, especially if you are beyond the reach of medical care.

Remedies

GARLIC: Garlic *(Allium sativum)* has been used since ancient times to prevent infection of wounds and cuts. Its use as a medicine is recorded in every major culture in the world. Galen, the most famous of the ancient Roman physicians, earned his first medical appointment after devising a way of using garlic to save the lives of seriously wounded gladiators. Garlic's properties for minor cuts and wounds were already well known, but Galen mixed freshly chopped garlic with whole grain flour and poured the mixture directly into the major wounds of the gladiators. The flour formed a matrix that allowed the blood to clot, and the garlic disinfected the wounds. Galen then covered the flour dressings with cloth and kept the entire dressing moist with garlic-infused wine. Today, garlic is still used to prevent infection in the folk medicine of blacks in Louisiana and by residents of the southern Appalachian mountains.

When a garlic clove is cut or crushed, it releases the potent antibiotic substance allicin. The allicin degrades quickly, disappearing within a few days, so fresh cut garlic must be used for disinfectant purposes. Teas of garlic cannot be used because heating destroys the allicin very quickly. Allicin is extremely irritating—it's responsible for the burning sensation of fresh garlic. Fresh cut garlic can cause third-degree burns if left in place on the skin for too long. Any preparation using garlic must dilute the allicin. Honey or wine are good carriers for the garlic in wound cleaning. With a good carrier, the allicin can kill the bacteria and other organisms of the infection but not inflame the wound or the skin around it.

☞ Directions: Using a blender, mix 3 cloves (not whole bulbs) of peeled garlic with 1 cup of wine. Allow the mixture to stand for two to three hours. Strain the garlic mixture. Clean the wound using soap and water, then apply the garlic preparation with a clean cloth. Cover the wound with gauze and tape. Apply the garlic preparation one to two times a day. If the treatment irritates the wound, try something else.

YARROW: The Latin name for yarrow *(Achillea millefolium)* is taken from Achilles, the hero of the Greek epics *The Iliad* and *The Odyssey*. Achilles used the plant to treat the wounds of his comrades. Historians believe that Homer, the author of the stories, was himself a battlefield physician who knew of the plant's wound-healing properties. Achilles (and perhaps Homer) may have packed the wounds of injured soldiers with yarrow leaves.

Yarrow has long, narrow, feather-like leaves. When made into a tightly packed poultice, the leaves make a dense matrix to aid in the clotting of a serious wound. The aromatic oils in yarrow, released by crushing the leaves, are disinfectant. Before the 20th century, yarrow had been used in Europe as a disinfectant for battle wounds since Homer's time, earning it the common names of "Soldier's Woundwort," "Knight's Milfoil," and "Herbe Militaris."

Yarrow is a universal remedy for infections among American Indian tribes throughout North America. Yarrow is also sometimes taken internally to reduce bleeding and was used in this manner by North American physicians of the Eclectic school during the last century and the first two decades of the 20th century. Yarrow has not been formally

continued on page 363

Latino Folk Illnesses

Folk illness is the name some people give to kinds of sicknesses that are recognized in one or more specific cultural groups but are not known or recognized by conventional medicine. Medically recognized or not, people within the culture know how to recognize these illnesses, what causes them, what happens when they are left untreated, and either how to treat them or who to take the patient to for treatment—usually a folk healer of some type.

It is safe to say that every culture has some of these folk illnesses. One that is commonly found in many cultures, and very prominent in Latino culture, is "nerves." Although it may have slightly different meanings in different cultures, and the causes for the condition may vary, nerves generally refers to a condition in which a person is edgy, jumpy, irritable, easily startled or upset, over-worried, and perhaps not able to eat or sleep well. The condition is usually thought to involve some kind of upset or aggravation of the nervous system, in which physical nerves become tightened up or flayed. (Modern medicine does not agree with this explanation.) The condition is considered likely to lead to more serious sickness if not treated or reversed. We make reference to this folk condition when we say he is "high strung" or "this is really getting on my nerves." In each culture, the names and types of folk illnesses vary. In Spanish, the condition of nerves is called "nervios."

A related, but very different Latino illness is "ataques (attacks) de nervios." These are episodes that come on suddenly—causing the victim to shriek or faint, to have seizures, or to tear at her hair or clothing as if in torment. The attacks may occur after suddenly receiving shocking news, by extreme grief or fear, or by spiritual disturbance.

In Latino culture, empacho is the name of a particular kind of stomachache and digestive trouble that is frequently an illness of children and older people. The condition is believed to be caused by undigested food that sticks to the lining of the stomach. The condition can be the result of eating foods that are hard to digest or by eating too much. In children, the condition can occur if they are made to eat foods they do not want. Empacho is treated with warm oil massage to the stomach area, herb teas, and laxatives.

To Latinos, "mollera caida," or fallen fontanelle, is the term describing an illness of babies. The condition is mainly identified by a sunken appearance of the soft spot on top of the baby's head. It is thought to result from handling the baby improperly or roughly or from suddenly pulling the breast or bottle away from the sucking baby's mouth. Mollera caida is treated by gentle scalp massage, pushing upward on the baby's palate, and/or sucking gently on the fontanelle to pull it up.

In Latino culture, babies are also especially vulnerable to being made sick by mal de ojo, or the "evil eye" (see "The Evil Eye," page 202). This condition has supernatural causes and is sometimes unintentionally cast upon a child as a result of another's envy.

Meat Poultices

Poultices of pork or other fat meats appear as wound treatments in the folklore of New England, Indiana, and by some blacks in Louisiana. Such treatments date to 3000 B.C. in ancient Egypt. The usual prescription is to use fat meat. Of the meats, salt pork is mentioned in folk remedies more often than any other. No rationale for any effectiveness of fat meat is apparent, but the endurance of the tradition is remarkable. In salted meats like salt pork or bacon, the salt itself may disinfect the wound. The practice seems to risk introduction of bacteria from the meat into the wound, however. A wash using clean salt water would be far more sanitary.

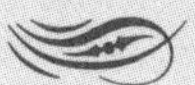

tested for its ability to reduce any sort of bleeding, but it does contain two alkaloids—achilleine and betonicine—that have shown to reduce bleeding in animal trials. The alkaloids may act by constricting the blood vessels near the surface of the body.

☞ Directions: Place 1 ounce of yarrow leaves in a 1-pint jar and fill with boiling water. Cover tightly to prevent the active constituents from escaping with the steam. Let the water cool to room temperature. Strain. Apply the solution with gauze or a clean cloth to the cut or wound and let it dry in place. Dress the wound with a clean bandage. Repeat for a total of three or four applications per day as long as desired.

YUNNAN PI YAO: An over-the-counter medicine called Yunnan Pi Yao can be found in almost any Asian market in North America. This is one of the premier wound medicines of China. The tiny bottle of Yunnan Pi Yao was a standard issue medicine to North Vietnamese troops during the Vietnam War. The wounded soldier would apply the medicine while awaiting medical attention.

Yunnan Pi Yao has shown to reduce bleeding by more than 50 percent in animal trials. Yunnan Pi Yao can also be used to reduce excessive menstrual bleeding or internal bruising after trauma. Yunnan Pi Yao contains mainly san-chi *(Panax notoginseng)*, a relative of the more famous Asian ginseng *(Panax ginseng)*. San-chi contains more than 22 identified chemical constituents, and four of them have shown to reduce bleeding in animal trials.

☞ Directions: Purchase Yunnan Pi Yao at an Asian market and keep it in your first aid kit. Follow its directions for use. Apply some immediately after dialing 911 for any wound with severe bleeding.

PLANTAIN: Plantain *(Plantago major)* is used to disinfect wounds and promote healing by the Delaware, Iroquois, Mohegan, Ojibwa, Cherokee, and other American Indian tribes and also by some of the Hispanic residents of the Southwest. Plantain contains at least five antiseptic constituents. It also contains the constituent allantoin, which promotes cell proliferation and tissue healing. Use the freshly crushed leaves to get the antiseptic benefits. You can probably find this four-leafed weed in your backyard. This plant grows in backyards all over the country.

☞ Directions: Crush a small handful of fresh plantain leaves and apply the juice to the cut or wound. Then, place the leaves on the wound and hold them there with some gauze and a bandage. Renew the dressing three to four times a day until the wound heals.

COMFREY: Comfrey *(Symphytum officinale)* is another wound-healing plant from European folk medicine. Its use continues today in Appalachia. Comfrey contains the constituent allantoin, which promotes cell growth. Do not use comfrey on wounds that are still oozing pus. The plant can promote healing so rapidly that an infection can be sealed inside the closed wound, causing an abscess and, potentially, the spread of the infection internally. Instead, use the plant on older, slow-healing wounds that are not infected. Another caution: Recent scientific research has shown that comfrey can cause serious liver disease if taken internally. The regulatory agencies of several countries have therefore restricted it to external use.

☞ Directions: Use a coffee grinder to powder some comfrey root. Moisten ½ teaspoon with 1 teaspoon of warm honey. Place in the cut or wound and cover with a clean dressing. Apply three times a day. Clean the wound before each application.

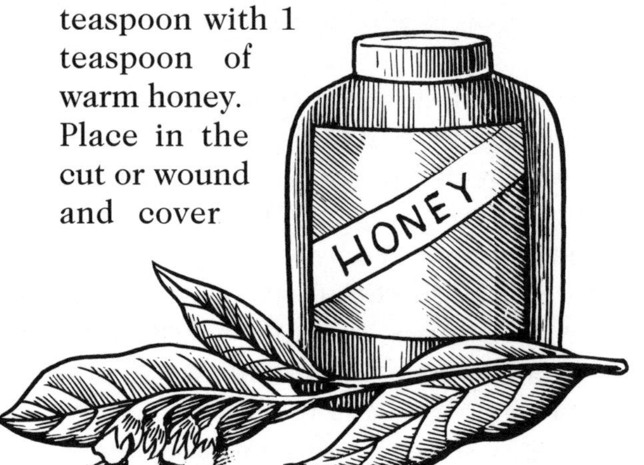

CALENDULA: Calendula flowers, or pot marigold *(Calendula officinalis)*, is an old European folk remedy for wounds. The flowers and their use came to North America with the British colonists.

The flowers contain both anti-inflammatory and antiseptic constituents. The other constituents it contains promote cell growth in wounds and ulcers. It is approved in Germany today in topical preparations for slow-healing wounds.

Do not use calendula on wounds that are oozing pus, however. The plant promotes cell growth so efficiently that it can cause a wound to close prematurely. An abscess or systemic infection can result. Pot marigold is a different plant than common garden marigolds *(Tagetes erecta)*, which contain different constituents than calendula.

☞ Directions: Place 1 ounce of calendula flowers in a 1-pint jar and fill with boiling water. Cover tightly and allow to steep until the brew reaches room temperature. Strain. Apply the tea externally with a clean cloth to the cut or wound. Allow to dry and then cover with a dressing. Apply two to three times a day until the wound heals. Take 1 tablespoon of the tea internally with each external application.

Alternately, crush several handfuls of dried calendula flowers to make a powder and put in a pot. Add enough honey to cover. Place on a burner on the lowest heat possible or on a hot plate. After the honey has melted, allow to steep on the lowest heat for ten to fifteen minutes. Let cool to room temperature. Do not strain. Apply with gauze to the wound and use a bandage to hold the gauze in place. Apply three to four times a day, cleaning the wound first to remove any old plant material or honey.

MYRRH GUM: Myrrh gum *(Commiphora myrrha)* has been used as a disinfectant in the Middle East and North Africa since antiquity. The Egyptians used myrrh gum in their mummification process to prevent the bacterial degradation of the corpse. The use of myrrh as a disinfectant spread to India, China, and Europe along Arab trade routes.

The gum is a secretion of the plant. It is discharged into the bark's cavities when the plant is wounded. The gum then hardens to a red-brown mass about the size of a walnut. Myrrh gum is a powerful antiseptic, but care must be taken not to irritate or inflame the skin. The alcohol tincture of the gum is less likely to irritate the skin.

☞ Directions: Purchase some myrrh tincture at a health food store or herb shop. Saturate a gauze pad with the tincture and apply to the wound. (Remove gauze and allow the tincture to dry in place.) Cover with a clean dressing. Change the dressing two or three times a day.

YERBA MANSA: The most popular medicinal herb of southwestern traditional medicine, among American Indians and Hispanic settlers, is yerba mansa *(Anemopsis californica)*. The Costonoan, Mahuna, and Shoshone Indians all have used it as a disinfectant; the Hispanic settlers in the region followed suit. Eclectic physicians began using yerba mansa as a medicine in 1877. The herb contains the volatile constituents thymol and methyl eugenol, both of which have antiseptic properties.

☞ Directions: Place 1 ounce of yerba mansa in a pint of water, bring to a boil, and simmer for twenty to thirty minutes. Let stand until cool. Apply the tea to the wound every few hours with a clean cloth. Allow the solution to dry in place, and cover with a clean dressing. Apply three to four times a day until the wound heals.

JUNIPER: A common disinfectant for wounds among American Indians of the West is juniper *(Juniperus communis)*. Juniper is mentioned in the folklore of the Comanche, Paiute, Shoshone, and Tewa tribes. The ancient Egyptians also used juniper berries—to embalm the dead. The plant's antimicrobial constituents can help to disinfect a wound—and retard the decay of a corpse!

☞ Directions: Purchase a commercial juniper berry tincture at a health food store or herb shop. Saturate a gauze pad or clean cloth with it and apply directly to the wound. Allow the solution to dry. Then cover the wound with a clean dressing. Change the dressing two or three times a day.

ROSEMARY: Rosemary leaf *(Rosmarinus officinalis)* is a popular remedy to disinfect cuts and wounds in the Hispanic folklore of the Southwest. Rosemary also contains at least ten antiseptic constituents.

☞ Directions: Place 1 ounce of rosemary leaf in a 1-pint jar and fill with boiling water. Cover tightly and let stand until the tea reaches room temperature. Apply as a wash to the wound three to four times a day, using a clean cloth.

LICK YOUR WOUNDS: "Spit on a wound to cure it," says a source in the *Frank C. Brown Collection of North Carolina Folklore.*

continued on page 368

New Age Folk Healing

"To get well, think of yourself as well, create mental pictures of your body defeating your disease."

"You are learning great things from this sickness (even if you don't realize it now)."

"You should try aromatherapy or crystals, something holistic that will lift and balance your energy."

Folk tradition surprises us by turning up in unexpected places and forms. The New Age, which is loaded with ideas about healing, is just one of those places! Not that New Age healing is folk medicine—by definition, much of it is not. But New Age beliefs and practices do incorporate folk medicine. Also, because being a New Ager does not involve formal membership in an organization, much of New Age culture, like folk medicine, operates on an oral and informal basis. But what is this "New Age"? What are its beliefs about healing, and where does it come from?

The New Age perspective includes ancient beliefs that come from Buddhism, Hinduism, and American Indian religions—basically, it incorporates religious beliefs from all over the world. The particular way in which New Age beliefs have come to be organized is the result of the "scientific revolution." By the 1800s many people in Europe and the United States had begun to feel that new scientific ideas—from Darwin's evolution to the discoveries of medicine and psychology—had made "old-fashioned Christianity" impossible to accept. But they also felt that science alone could not supply the spiritual needs of the people. Many well-educated persons believed it was necessary to create a new religion, one that would fit well with both science and spirituality. That effort produced many different New Age groups and movements: transcendentalism, spiritualism, Christian Science, Anthroposophy, theosophy, and later hippies and the 1960s counterculture. This pursuit of a more balanced religion was also instrumental in bringing alternative medicine to its present popularity.

The features of New Age thought have always been somewhat similar, even before the term New Age was created. Those who accept New Age ideas believe in intuition as well as intellectual knowledge. They see the world as filled with spirit. They do not reject science but try to change it—in order to harmonize science with mysticism and spirituality. They value all sorts of spiritual traditions and beliefs, but they reject the idea of evil. (They believe evil is a spiritual misunderstanding.) This very general set of ideas allows for the tremendous diversity of specific activities, goals, and healing practices—all within a common but somewhat vague framework—that is so typical of the New Age.

In some ways, the New Age is the intellectual parallel to folk tradition, a kind of re-invention or translation of the magical ideas about the world. Medicine and science once contained magical and spiritual ideas. Folk medicine retains many of those ancient beliefs and values. The New Age movement is intent on bringing back those beliefs. It is not surprising, then, that New Agers have always borrowed ideas from folk tradition, especially in connection with healing.

New Agers believe that you should be able to "think yourself well" because the material world is a reflection of the spirit, and thoughts help to shape and create physical reality. This is especially true of living things, because all living things are considered basically spiritual, and because the life force itself is conceived of spiritually. This connection of thought, spirit, and all the rest of reality makes thinking very similar to praying as a kind of spiritual act. The equation of thought and prayer is one reason that New Agers are attracted to the traditional use of magic in folk medicine. To many members of mainstream Christian denominations, magic seems either foolish or evil; the fear is that, if it works, it must do so by means of spirits other than God. Thus, it is believed that magic is false because illusory and Christian beliefs are the only true supernatural beliefs. The New Age rejects this distinction that magic is false, because New Age thought embraces all religions as having spiritual truth. But New Agers do not follow all the teachings of all religions—no one could! They feel free to adopt whatever spiritual ideas feel right to them. One of those ideas is the belief in reincarnation, which has become a hallmark idea of the New Age. The idea of being reborn again and again is used to explain sickness or other suffering. Souls are said to choose their futures between lives, selecting those experiences that will teach them and help them to evolve spiritually. Thus, reincarnation makes it possible to find positive value in suffering.

The New Age is fascinated with the idea of energies of all kinds—from physical energy to the vital energy of living things to the "subtle energies" that are felt in some healing practices, such as Therapeutic Touch. Connecting the various energies helps in harmonizing science and spirit, and this is often done through quantum physics. Quantum physics deals with subatomic particles and the fundamental connections between matter and energy. Physicists have described many strange things happening at the quantum level, including what seem to be dramatic effects of an observer on what is observed, and the fact that at this level the boundary between energy and matter seems indistinct. New Agers like to suggest that this "New Physics" will eventually clarify the reality of spirit and the ways that all sorts of energy effect life. The ways that New Agers use the physics concepts are not the way that physicists normally use them, but a few physicists have published popular works endorsing a connection between quantum physics and mystical ideas. This supports the New Age idea of bringing science and spirit together, especially in healing, and it accounts for the emphasis on manipulating and balancing energy, with crystals or acupuncture, for example, on which all New Age ideas of healing depend—from the healing of a broken body to the healing of Earth in preparation for the New Age.

Folk medicine ideas from all traditions seem comfortable to New Agers, although New Age ideas may be incomprehensible to most folk healers! And while the language is very different, and the effort to combine all spiritual ideas makes for a complicated vision, New Age healing is, in a sense, the folk medicine of the college-educated modern!

Saliva therapy has a sound physiological basis according to modern science. Saliva is a natural part of the immune system, and it contains at least seven antimicrobial substances. One antibacterial substance from saliva, called lysozyme, has been developed into a commercial drug in Europe for treating wounds and infections. Saliva also contains antibodies and can enhance the body's natural immune response to any infectious material in the wound. Other constituents in saliva—called growth factors—promote the growth of new cells. These saliva-based growth factors are currently being tested by pharmaceutical and biotechnology companies for possible use as wound-healing drugs. Wound licking is common in the animal world as well.

☞ Directions: Lick your wounds.

COBWEBS: A spiderweb poultice was an early American pioneer dressing for wounds. Throughout the world, the practice dates back to antiquity. A compressed poultice of spiderwebs can form a matrix that promotes blood clotting. Spiderwebs are also sterile, being immune to degradation by bacteria, molds, and fungi. If the web is free from other debris, it makes a sterile dressing. Cobwebs are also acidic in nature, giving mild antimicrobial properties.

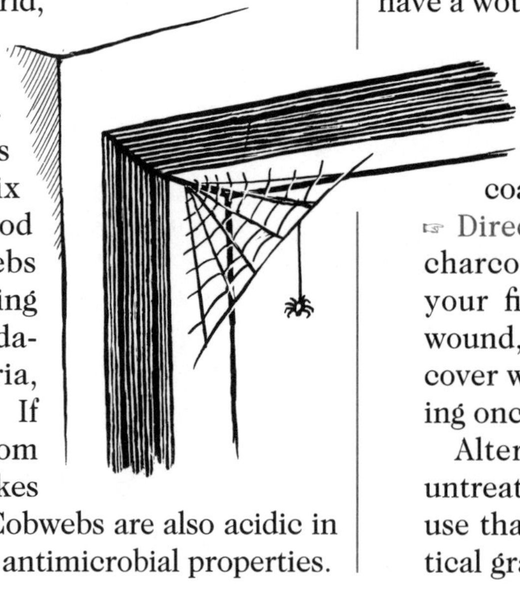

☞ Directions: Find some fresh cobwebs. Ball them up and put in (or on) the cut or wound.

CHARCOAL: Charcoal is a remedy used to cleanse wounds that are oozing pus, according to folk traditions in North Carolina. The Seventh Day Adventists recommend the same. Charcoal is possibly the most ancient of the wound remedies in this section.

Charcoal preparations are used in modern medicine to control infection in burns and in wounds that ooze pus. The charcoal readily binds substances to itself. In the case of a wound, it draws out the pus and inflammatory substances in the wound.

Sometimes the modern charcoal preparations are combined with topical antibiotics to increase their effectiveness. Charcoal-impregnated gauze-wound dressings have been shown in clinical trials to reduce healing time and reduce secondary infections. If you have a wound that is oozing pus, please consult a physician for immediate medical attention. If medical care is not available for some reason, you might try a charcoal dressing for temporary first aid.

☞ Directions: Purchase some activated charcoal at a pharmacy and keep it in your first aid kit. Clean the infected wound, apply the charcoal directly, and cover with a bandage. Change the dressing once a day.

Alternately, you can pulverize the untreated charcoal from a wood fire and use that if you do not have pharmaceutical grade-activated charcoal.

Bibliography

Web Sites

Beckstrom-Sternberg, Stephen M., and James A. Duke. "The Phytochemical Database." Http://probe.nalusda.gov:8300/cgi-bin/browse/phytochemdb (ACEDB version 4.3) Data version, July 1994.

Beckstrom-Sternberg, Stephen M.; Duke, James A.; and Wain, K.K. "The Ethnobotany Database." Http://probe.nalusda.gov:8300/cgi-bin/browse/ethnobotdb (ACEDB version 4.3) Data version, July 1994.

Books and Periodicals

Baldwin, Rahima. *Special Delivery.* Berkeley, California: Celestial Arts, 1979.

Bell, Whitfield J. *The Colonial Physician and Other Essays.* New York: Science History Publications, 1975.

Bhagvan-Dash, Vaidya. *Materia Medica of Ayurveda.* New Delhi: B. Jain Publishers, 1991.

Boyle, Wade. *Herb Doctors: Pioneers in 19th-Century American Botanical Medicine and a History of the Eclectic Medical Institute of Cincinnati.* East Palestine, Ohio: Buckeye Naturopathic Press, 1988.

Boyle, Wade. *Official Herbs: Botanical Substances in the United States Pharmacopoeias, 1820-1990.* East Palestine, Ohio: Buckeye Naturopathic Press, 1991.

Cameron, M.L. *Anglo-Saxon Medicine.* Cambridge, England: Cambridge University Press, 1993.

Casetta, Anna; Hand, Wayland D.; and Pickett, Newbell Niles. *Popular Beliefs and Superstitions: A Compendium of American Folklore.* Boston: G.K. Hall, 1981, 3 volumes. (Copyright: John G. White Department of the Cleveland Public Library, 1981.)

Castetter, Edward F., and Ruth M. Underhill. "The Ethnobiology of the Papago Indians Ethnobiological Studies in the American Southwest." *The University of New Mexico Bulletin* #275, Vol. II, 1935.

Chevallier, Andrew. *The Encyclopedia of Medicinal Plants.* New York: DK Publishing, 1996.

Chishti, Hakim G.M. *The Traditional Healer: A Comprehensive Guide to the Principles and Practice of Unani Herbal Medicine.* Rochester, Vermont: Inner Traditions International Ltd., 1988.

Classen, Constance; Howes, David; and Synnott, Anthony. *Aroma: The Cultural History of Smell.* London and New York: Routledge, 1994.

Colby, Benjamin. *A Guide to Health, Being an Exposition of the Principles of the Thomsonian System of Practice, and Their Mode of Application in the Cure of Every Form of Disease,* 3rd ed. Milford, New Hampshire: John Burns, 1846.

Cook, William H. *The Physio-Medicalist Dispensatory.* Cincinnati, Ohio: Wm. H. Cook, 1869.

Crellin, John K, and Jane Philpott. *Herbal Medicine Past and Present: Trying to Give Ease.* (Vol. I) Durham, North Carolina: Duke University Press, 1997.

Crellin, John K, and Jane Philpott. *Herbal Medicine Past and Present: A Reference Guide to Medicinal Plants.* (Vol. II) Durham, North Carolina: Duke University Press, 1997.

Culpeper, Nicholas. *Culpeper's Complete Herbal: Consisting of a Comprehensive Description of Nearly All Herbs With Their Medicinal Properties and Directions for Compounding the Medicines Extracted From Them.* London, England: Foulsham & Company Ltd., 1995.

Densmore, Frances. "Uses of Plants by the Chippewa Indians." *SI-BAE Annual Report* (1928), pp. 44: 273-379.

Der Marderosian, Ara, and Lawrence E. Liberti. *Natural Product Medicine: A Scientific Guide to Foods, Drugs, Cosmetics.* Philadelphia, Pennsylvania: Lippincott-Raven Publishers, 1988.

Edelsward, L.M. *Sauna as Symbol: Society and Culture in Finland.* New York: Peter Lang, 1991.

Ellingwood, Finley. *American Materia, Therapeutics and Pharmacology.* Portland, Oregon: Eclectic Medical Publications, 1919.

Erichsen-Brown, Charlotte. *Medicinal and other Uses of North American Plants: A Historical Survey with Special Reference to the Eastern Indian Tribes.* New York: Dover Publications, 1979.

Felter, Harvey, and John U. Lloyd. *King's American Dispensatory,* Vol. I and II. Portland, Oregon: Eclectic Medical Publications, 1898.

Felter, Harvey. *The Eclectic Materia Medica, Pharmacology, and Therapeutics.* Portland, Oregon: Eclectic Medical Publications, 1922.

Ferreira, Antonio. *Prenatal Environment.* Springfield, Illinois: Charles C. Thomas, 1969.

Firestone, Melvin M. "Sephardic Folk-Curing in Seattle." *Journal of American Folklore,* Vol. 75 (1962), pp. 301-310.

Fontenot, Wonda L. *Secret Doctors: Ethnomedicine of African Americans.* Westport, Connecticut: Bergin and Garvey, 1994.

Frankel, Barbara. *Childbirth in the Ghetto: Folk Beliefs of Negro Women in a North Philadelphia Hospital Ward.* San Francisco: R & E Research Associates, 1977.

Fried, Lewis. *Handbook of American-Jewish Literature: An Analytic Guide to Topics, Themes, and Sources.* New York: Greenwood Press, 1988.

Gilmore, Melvin R. *Some Chippewa Uses of Plants.* Ann Arbor, Michigan: University of Michigan Press, 1933.

Grieve, M. *A Modern Herbal,* Vol. I and II. New York: Dover Publications, 1978.

Grinnell, *George Bird. The Cheyenne Indians: Their History and Ways of Life,* Vol. II. Lincoln, Nebraska: University of Nebraska Press, 1972.

Grünwald, Jörg. Heilpflanzen: *Herbal Remedies.* (CD-ROM) Berlin: Thomas Brendler, 1996.

Halpert, Herbert. "Supernatural Sanctions and the Legend." *Folklore Studies in the Twentieth Century,* ed. V. Newall, Woodbridge, U.K.: D.S. Brewer, 1978.

Hamel, Paul B., and M.U. Chiltoskey. *Cherokee Plants.* Sylva, North Carolina: Herald Pub. Co., 1975.

Hand, Wayland. *American Folk Medicine: A Symposium.* Berkeley and Los Angeles, California: University of California Press, 1976.

Hand, Wayland. *Magical Medicine: The Folkloric Component of Medicine in the Folk Belief, Custom, and Ritual of the Peoples of Europe and America.* Berkeley and Los Angeles, California: University of California Press, 1980.

Hand, Wayland, ed. *The Frank C. Brown Collection of North Carolina Folklore, Vol. VI, Popular Beliefs and Superstitions from North Carolina.* Durham, North Carolina: Duke University Press, 1961.

Harding, A.R. *Ginseng and Other Medicinal Plants,* revised ed. Columbus, Ohio: A.R. Harding, 1972.

Harris, Marvin. *Culture, Man, and Nature: An Introduction to General Anthropology.* New York: Thomas Y. Crowell Company, 1971.

Hatfield, Gabrielle. *Country Remedies: Traditional East Anglian Plant Remedies in the Twentieth Century.* Woodbridge, Suffolk: Colleagues Press, 1995.

Hendrickson, Robert. *The Facts on File Encyclopedia of Word and Phrase Origins.* New York and Oxford: Facts on File Publications, 1987.

Herrick, James W., and Dean R. Snow. *Iroquois Medical Botany.* Syracuse, New York: Syracuse University Press, 1994.

Hister, Art. *Dr. Art Hister's Do-It-Yourself Guide to Good Health.* Toronto, Canada: Random House, 1978.

Hoebel, E. Adamson. *The Cheyennes: Indians of the Great Plains.* New York: Holt, Rinehart and Winston, 1960.

Hsu, Hong-Yen. *Oriental Materia Medica: A Concise Guide.* New Canaan, Connecticut: Keats Publishing, 1986.

Hufford, David J. "Contemporary Folk Medicine." *In Other Healers: Unorthodox Medicine in America,* ed. Norman Gevitz. Baltimore: Johns Hopkins University Press, 1988, pp. 228-264.

Hunter, David E. and Phillip Whitten, ed. *Encyclopedia of Anthropology.* New York: HarperCollins, 1976.

Hyatt, Harry M. *Hoodoo—Conjuration—Witchcraft—Rootwork.* Hannibal, Missouri: Western Publising Company, 1970, 4 volumes.

Janos, Elisabeth. *Country Folk Remedies: Tales of Skunk Oil, Sassafras Tea and Other Old-Time Remedies Gathered by Elisabeth Janos.* New York: Galahad Books, 1990.

Jarvis, D.C. *Folk Remedies: A Vermont Doctor's Guide to Good Health.* New York: Holt, Rinehart, and Winston, 1958.

Kelly, Isabel. *Folk Practices in North Mexico: Birth Customs, Folk Medicine, and Spiritualism in the Laguna Zone.* Austin, Texas: Institute of Latin American Studies, University of Texas Press, 1965.

Kingston, Maxine Hong. *The Woman Warrior: Memoirs of a Girlhood Among Ghosts.* New York: Vintage, 1989.

Kirchfeld, Friedhelm, and Wade Boyle. *Nature Doctors: Pioneers in Naturopathic Medicine.* Portland, Oregon: Medicina Biologica, 1994.

Kitzinger, Sheila; Jessel, Camilla; and Nancy Durrell McKenna. *The Complete Book of Pregnancy and Childbirth.* New York: Alfred A. Knopf, 1991.

Kneipp, Sebastian. *My Water Cure.* New York: Mokelumne Hill Press, 1972.

Krochmal, Arnold and Connie. *A Guide to the Medicinal Plants of the U.S.* New York: Quadrangle, 1973.

Krupat, Arnold. *For Those Who Came After: A Study of Native American Autobiography.* Chicago: University of Chicago Press, 1989.

Ladenheim, Melissa. *The Sauna in Central New York.* Ithaca, New York: DeWitt Historical Society, 1986.

Laguerre, Michel. *Afro-Caribbean Folk Medicine.* South Hadley, Massachusetts: Bergin and Garvey, 1988.

Latham, Minor White. *The Elizabethan Fairies: The Fairies of Folklore and the Fairies of Shakespeare,* 1930. (Reprint New York: Octagon, 1972.)

Leslie, Charles M., ed. *Asian Medical Systems: A Comparitive Study.* Berkeley, California: University of California Press, 1976.

Leung, Albert Y. *Chinese Herbal Remedies.* New York: Universe, 1984.

Lewis, Walter H., et al. *Medical Botany: Plants Affecting Man's Health.* New York: John Wiley & Sons, 1982.

Lindlahr, Henry. *Natural Therapeutics,* Vol. II. Saffron Walden, United Kingdom: C.W. Daniel Company, 1983.

Logan, Patrick. *Making the Cure: A Look at Irish Folk Medicine.* Dublin, Ireland: The Talbot Press, 1975.

Malpezzi, Frances M. and William M. Clements. *Italian-American Folklore.* Little Rock, Arkansas: August House Publishers, 1992.

Manniche, Lise. *An Ancient Egyptian Herbal.* Austin, Texas: University of Texas Press, 1989.

Maressa, John. *Maqiuq: The Eskimo Sweat Bath.* Hohenschaftlarn: Klaus Renner, 1986.

McBride, L.R. *Practical Folk Medicine of Hawaii.* Hilo, Hawaii: The Petroglyph Press, 1975.

McGrath, William R. *Amish Folk Remedies for Plain and Fancy Ailments.* Burr Oak, Michigan: Schupps Herbs & Vitamins, 1987.

McGuffin, Michael; Hobbs, Christopher; Upton, Roy; and Goldberg, Alicia. *American Herbal Products Association's Botanical Safety Handbook.* Boca Raton, Florida: CRC Press, 1997.

McIntyre, Anne. *Folk Remedies for Common Ailments.* Toronto, Ontario: Key Porter Books Ltd., 1994.

McMahon, William. *Pine Barrens Legends, Lore and Lies.* Wilmington, Delaware: Middle Atlantic Press, 1980.

Meyer, Clarence. *American Folk Medicine.* New York: Meyerbooks, 1985.

Meyer, George G. *Folk Medicine and Herbal Healing.* Springfield, Illinois: Charles C. Thomas, 1981.

Milinaire, Caterine. *Birth: Facts and Legends.* New York: Harmony Books, 1974.

Moerman, Daniel E. *Geraniums for the Iroquois: A Field Guide to American Indian Medicinal Plants.* Algonac, Michigan: Reference Publications, Inc., 1982.

Moore, Michael. *Medicinal Plants of the Mountain West.* Santa Fe, New Mexico: Museum of New Mexico Press, 1979.

Moore, Michael. *Medicinal Plants of the Desert and Canyon West.* Santa Fe, New Mexico: Museum of New Mexico Press, 1989.

Moore, Michael and Mimi Kamp. *Los Remedios: Traditional Herbal Remedies of the Southwest.* Santa Fe, New Mexico: Red Crane Books, 1990.

Nagy, Doreen Evenden. *Popular Medicine in Seventeenth-Century England.* Bowling Green, Ohio: Bowling Green State University Popular Press, 1988.

Naeser, Margaret A. *Outline Guide to Chinese Herbal Patent Medicines in Pill Form: An Introduction to Chinese Herbal Medicines.* Boston, Massachusetts: Boston Chinese Medicine, 1990.

Newall, Carol et al. *Herbal Medicines: A Guide for Health Care Professionals.* London, England: Rittenhouse Book Distributors, 1996.

O'Connor, Bonnie Blair. *Healing Traditions: Alternative Medicine and the Health Professions.* Philadelphia, Pennsylvania: University of Pennsylvania Press, 1995.

Ody, Penelope. *The Complete Medical Herbal.* London: Key Porter Books, 1994.

Opie, Iona and Moira Tatem, Eds. *A Dictionary of Superstitions.* Oxford, England: Oxford University Press, 1989.

Osol, Arthur, and George E. Farrar. *The Dispensatory of the United States of America,* 24th ed. Philadelphia, Pennsylvania: J.B. Lippencott Company, 1947.

Patai, Raphael. *On Jewish Folklore.* Detroit, Michigan: Wayne State University Press, 1983.

Pedersen, Mark. *Nutritional Herbology: A Reference Guide to Herbs.* Warsaw, Indiana: Wendell W. Whitman Company, 1994.

Rafinesque, C. *Medical Flora: Manual of the Medical Botany of the United States,* Vol. II. Philadelphia, Pennsylvania: Samuel C. Atkinson, 1830.

Ray, Verne F. "The Sanpoil and Nespelem: Salishan Peoples of N.E. Washington." *University of Washington Publications in Anthropology,* Vol. V, 1933.

Roeder, Beatrice A. *Chicano Folk Medicine from Los Angeles, California.* Berkeley, California: University of California Press, 1988.

Root-Bernstein, Robert S., and Michéle Root-Bernstein. *Honey, Mud, Maggots, and Other Medical Marvels: The Science Behind Folk Remedies and Old Wives' Tales.* Boston, Massachusetts: Houghton Mifflin, 1997.

Rorie, David. *Folk Tradition and Folk Medicine in Scotland: The Writings of David Rorie,* ed. David Buchan. Edinburgh, Scotland: Canongate Academic, 1994.

Sagendorph, Robb. *America and her Almanacs: Wit, Wisdom & Weather.* Brown, Massachusetts: Little, Brown, 1970.

Samuels, Mike, and Nancy Samuels. *The Well Pregnancy Book.* New York: Summit Books, 1986.

Saxon, Lyle. *Gumbo Ya-Ya: Folk Tales of Louisiana.* Boston, Massachusetts: Houghton Mifflin, 1945.

Shyrock, Richard Harris. *Medicine in America: Historical Essays.* Baltimore, Maryland: The Johns Hopkins Press, 1966.

Slater, Candace. *Dance of the Dolphin: Transformation and Disenchantment in the Amazonian Imagination.* Chicago: University of Chicago Press, 1994.

Smith, Huron H. "Ethnobotany of the Ojibwa Indians." *Bulletin of the Public Museum of Milwaukee* (1932), pp. 4: 327-525.

Snow, Loudell F. *Walkin' Over Medicine.* Boulder, Colorado: Westview Press, 1993.

Spicer, Edward H. and Eleanor Bauwens. *Ethnic Medicine in the Southwest.* Tucson, Arizona: University of Arizona Press, 1977.

Speck, Frank G. "Catawba Medicines and Curative Practices." *Publications of the Philadelphia Anthropological Society,* Vol. I, 1937.

Steedman, E.V. "The Ethnobotany of the Thompson Indians." *SI-BAE Annual Report* (1928), pp. 45: 441-522.

Stone, Eric. *Medicine Among the American Indians.* New York: Hafner Publishing, 1962.

Stowell, Marion Barber. *Early American Almanacs: The Colonial Weekday Bible.* New York: Lenox Hill Publishers, 1977.

Strehlow, Wighard and Gottfried Hertzka. *Hildegarde of Bingen's Medicine.* Santa Fe, New Mexico: Bear and Company, 1988.

Tantaquidgeon, Gladys. *A Study of Delaware Indian Medicine Practice and Folk Beliefs.* Harrisburg, Pennsylvania: Pennsylvania Historical Commission, 1942.

Terrell, Suzanne J. *This Other Kind of Doctors: Traditional Medical Systems in Black Neighborhoods in Austin, Texas.* New York: AMS Press, 1990.

Thomson, Samuel. "A Narrative of the Life & Medical Discoveries of Samuel Thomson, Containing an Account of His System and the Manner of Curing." *Twelve Works of Naive Genius,* ed. Walter Teller. Ayer Co. Pub., 1972, pp. 17-60.

Trachtenberg, Joshua. *Jewish Magic and Superstition: A Study in Folk Religion,* 1939. (Reprint New York: Atheneum, 1970.)

Thrash, Agatha, and Calvin Thrash. *Home Remedies: Hydrotherapy, Massage, Charcoal, and Other Simple Treatments.* Seale, Alabama: Newlifestyle Books, 1981.

Trotter, Robert T. *Curanderismo: Mexican-American Folk Healing.* Second Edition. Athens, Georgia: University of Georgia Press, 1997.

Tyler, Varro. *The Honest Herbal: A Sensible Guide to the Use of Herbs and Related Remedies.* Third Edition. New York: Haworth Press, 1993.

Tyler, Varro. *Herbs of Choice: The Therapeutic Use of Phytomedicinals.* New York: Haworth Press, 1994.

Tyler, Varro. *Hoosier Home Remedies.* West Lafayette, Indiana: Purdue University Press, 1985.

Val Alphen, Jan and Anthony Aris, ed. *Oriental Medicine: An Illustrated Guide to the Asian Arts of Healing.* Boston: Shambhala, 1996.

Vance, Randolph. *Ozark Magic and Folklore,* 1947. (Reprint New York: Dover, 1964.)

Vogel, Virgil. *American Indian Medicine.* Norman, Oklahoma: University of Oklahoma Press, 1970.

von Hausen, Wanja. *Gypsy Folk Medicine.* New York: Sterling Publishing Company, 1992.

Weiss, Rudolf Fritz. *Herbal Medicine.* Beaconsfield, England: Beaconsfield Publishers, 1988. (Translated from: *Lehrbuch der Phytotherapie,* 6th ed. Stuttgart: Hippokrates Verlag, 1985.)

Williams, Phyllis H. *South Italian Folkways in Europe and America.* New Haven, Connecticut: Yale University Press, 1938.

Wood, Matthew. *The Magical Staff: Handing Down the Tradition of Natural Medicine.* Berkeley, California: North Atlantic Books, 1992.

Woodward, Marcus, ed. *Gerard's Herbal.* London, England: Studio Editions, 1994.

Yoffie, Leah Rachel. "Popular Beliefs and Customs among the Yiddish-Speaking Jews of St. Louis, Mo." *Journal of American Folklore,* Vol. 38 (1925), pp. 375-399.

Young, James Harvey. *The Toadstool Millionaires: A Social History of Patent Medicines in America Before Federal Regulation.* Princeton: Princeton University Press, 1961.

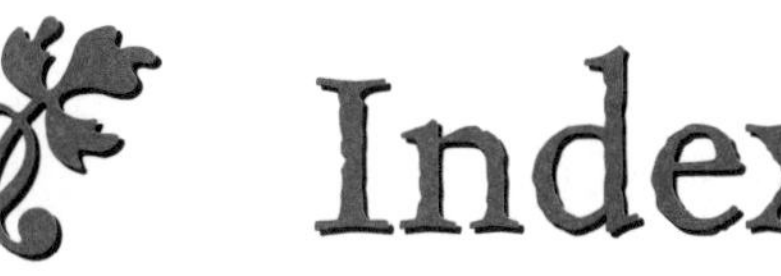
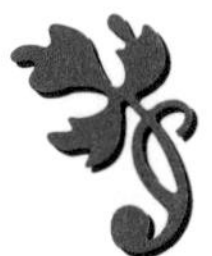

Index

A

acne, 18–21
adaptogens, 168, 211
African American medicine, 254–255, 287, 339
  anxiety remedies, 31–33
  arthritis remedies, 47, 51
  bites and stings remedies, 68–69
  bladder and kidney infection remedies, 78
  chapped skin remedies, 334
  colic remedies, 136
  hives remedies, 25, 29
  indigestion and heartburn remedies, 184–185, 257
  toothache remedies, 293, 296
  wounds and cuts remedies, 361
alcohol
  anxiety and, 31
  arthritis and, 225
  colds and, 129
  depression and, 164
alfalfa, 44, 105
allergies, 22–25, 29–33, 36–38
  asthma and, 53
  ear infections and, 187
  feverfew and, 229
aloe vera
  for athlete's foot, 223
  for burns and sunburn, 108–109
  for hemorrhoids, 244–245
  for itching and rashes, 274
  for poison ivy and poison oak, 322
  for sores and skin ulcers, 354–355
American ginseng, 36, 365
  for arthritis, 46
  for fever, 221
  for indigestion, 177, 179
  for insomnia, 267
Amish medicine
  anxiety remedies, 36–37
  asthma remedies, 54
  bites and stings remedies, 67–68
  bladder and kidney infections remedies, 72, 77
  blood purifiers and blood builders, 83, 91
  breast conditions remedies, 105–106
  burns and sunburns remedies, 109, 111–112
  catarrh remedies, 113, 114
  colds and flu remedies, 121–122, 130–131
  constipation remedies, 142, 146, 147
  cough remedies, 149
  depression remedies, 168–169
  diarrhea remedies, 171–172, 174
  eczema remedies, 194, 195
  eye conditions remedies, 205
  fatigue remedies, 210
  fever remedies, 214–215
  headache remedies, 230–231, 238
  heat rash remedies, 334, 340
  hemorrhoid remedies, 244, 245, 247
  insomnia remedies, 264, 265
  menstruation and, 277, 282, 284, 285
Amish medicine *(continued)*
  pregnancy and, 325
  scar remedies, 337–338
  sore throat remedies, 350
  sores and skin ulcers remedies, 354
  toothache remedies, 290
amulets, 42–43, 74
angelica, 40, 317
animal remedies, 26–28, 114–116, 225
anise seeds, 77, 101, 137
antibiotics, 18–19, 187, 193, 342
anxiety, 30–33, 36–38
aphrodisiacs, 166–167
Appalachian medicine
  allergy remedies, 23, 24, 25
  anxiety remedies, 33, 36–37, 38
  arthritis remedies, 41, 44, 45, 46, 47, 50, 51, 52
  asthma remedies, 56
  bites and stings remedies, 69
  bladder and kidney infections remedies, 73
  blood purifiers and blood builders, 83, 85, 88–90, 91, 98
  boils and carbuncles remedies, 94, 95, 98
  breast conditions remedies, 101
  catarrh remedies, 113, 117
  colds and flu remedies, 123–124, 125, 129
  colic remedies, 135, 136
  constipation remedies, 142–143, 146–147
  cough remedies, 157

Appalachian medicine (continued)
depression remedies, 168–169
diarrhea remedies, 171–172
ear conditions remedies, 192
eczema remedies, 194, 195
eye conditions remedies, 200, 201, 204
fever remedies, 213, 215, 218, 219–220, 221–222
headache remedies, 231, 234, 235, 237–238
indigestion and heartburn remedies, 184–185, 253, 256, 257
indigestion remedies, 176–177, 179
insomnia remedies, 262, 265, 267
itching and rash remedies, 272
muscle strains and sprains remedies, 298–299
pain remedies, 315, 317
poison ivy and poison oak remedies, 318–319, 321–323
skin problems remedies, 332–333
sore throat remedies, 343
sores and skin ulcers remedies, 351–352, 355, 356
toothache remedies, 293, 296
wounds and cuts remedies, 361, 364
Arabic medicine
arthritis remedies, 315
catarrh remedies, 113
ear conditions remedies, 187, 190, 191
eye conditions remedies, 200
fever remedies, 213
headache remedies, 238, 315
indigestion remedies, 176
menstruation and, 275, 277
pain remedies, 315
sore throat remedies, 345
toothache remedies, 290, 292, 296
arnica, 298, 302, 316
aromatherapy, 264
arthralgia. *See* arthritis.
arthritis, 38–41, 44–47, 50–52
asafoetida, 66
for anxiety, 37–38
for colic, 137, 140
for hives, 29
Asian ginseng, 168
arthritis and, 46
for cold feet, 227
for fatigue, 210–212
as stimulant, 177, 179
Asian medicine. *See* Chinese medicine.
aspirin, 40, 41, 119, 228, 230
asthma, 35, 53–57, 60–61
astragalus, 227
astringents, 319
athlete's foot, 222–224, 226–227
Áwachse, 139
Ayurvedic medicine. *See* Indian medicine.

B

bad breath, 293
baking soda, 256
for bites and stings, 68
for burns and sunburns, 108
for eczema, 195
for hives, 29
for itching and rashes, 272
for poison ivy and poison oak, 323
for toothaches, 296
baldness, 294–295
barberry. *See* goldenseal.
barley water, 100–101
basil
for colic, 140–141
for earaches, 187
for hives, 25, 29
for itching and rashes, 269
for menstrual problems, 281–282
bayberry, 107
bearberry, 70
bedsores. *See* sores and skin ulcers.
bedwetting, 266
bee balm, 124
bee stings, 51
beets, 91
bergamot, 21, 117
betony, 207, 210
birth order, 120
bites and stings, 61–63, 67–69
black cohosh
for arthritis, 40, 41, 44
for depression, 169
black haw, 40
for menstrual problems, 285
for pain, 311
black pepper, 151
blackberry root, 171–172
blackheads, 18
bladder and kidney infections, 69–73, 76–79
blankets, 222
bleach, 224
bleeding, 301, 307. *See also* wounds and cuts.
blood purifiers and blood builders, 46, 82–85, 88–92, 333
blue cohosh, 280–281
boils and carbuncles, 93–95, 98–99
boneset
as blood purifiers and blood builders, 89
for colds and flu, 122–123
for constipation, 146–147
for depression, 169
for fever, 215, 218
for headaches, 237
for indigestion, 184
Brazilian medicine, 36–37
bread, 358
breast conditions, 99–101, 105–107
breast milk, 192

breathing techniques, 251–252, 265
buchu, 78–79
buckeyes, 244
burdock
for acne, 19, 20
for bladder and kidney infections, 78
as blood purifiers and blood builders, 83, 98
for boils and carbuncles, 98
for eczema, 194
for hemorrhoids, 246
burns and sunburns, 107–112, 273
butter
for burns and sunburns, 108
for colds and flu, 132
for coughs, 159
B-vitamins, 31, 39, 258

C

caffeine
anxiety and, 30–31
fatigue and, 206
headaches and, 228, 234
for poison ivy and poison oak, 322–323
calcium, 22
calendar and medicine, 188–189
calendula
for hemorrhoids, 244
for minor wounds, 355–356
pus and, 356, 364
for sores and skin ulcers, 355–356
for wounds and cuts, 364–365
California poppy, 164–165
camphor, 62, 65–66
cancer, 242–243
canaigre, 19, 20–21
capsaicin. *See* cayenne peppers.
caraway seeds, 177, 256
carbuncles. *See* boils and carbuncles.
carminatives, 180
carrot bolus, 247
cascara sagrada, 142–143
castor oil, 134, 140, 185–186
cat remedies, 26–27, 59
catarrh, 112–113, 117–118
catnip
for anxiety, 33
for asthma, 60
for colic, 133, 135
for fever, 215
for hives, 25
for indigestion and heartburn, 184–185, 257
for insomnia, 265
for nausea, 308
cayenne peppers
for arthritis, 45–46
as blood purifiers and blood builders, 84–85
for muscle strains and sprains, 297–298
for pain, 310–311
celery, 37, 39–40
chamomile, 178
for boils and carbuncles, 93
for breast conditions, 105, 106–107
for colic, 136–137
for diarrhea, 174
for eczema, 198
for hay fever, 24
for headaches, 239
for hemorrhoids, 244
for indigestion and heartburn, 180, 185, 256–257
for insomnia, 265, 267
for menstrual problems, 281
for nausea, 305–306
chaparral, 47, 354
chapped skin. *See* skin problems.
charcoal
for bites and stings, 68
diarrhea remedies, 172, 174
for oozing pus, 368
for poison ivy and poison oak, 323
charm books, 104
chicken remedies, 27–28
chicken soup, 131
chickweed, 105–106
childbirth, 196–197, 278–279. *See also* pregnancy.
Chinese medicine, 144–145
acne remedies, 19, 20
allergy remedies, 24–25
anxiety remedies, 31, 32, 33, 36, 37–38
arthritis remedies, 40, 44, 45–46
asthma remedies, 54–55, 56
bites and stings remedies, 68
bladder and kidney infections remedies, 71
blood purifiers and blood builders, 84
boils and carbuncles remedies, 98, 99
burns and sunburns remedies, 109, 111–112
cold limb remedies, 226
colds and flu remedies, 123–124, 125, 129, 132
colic remedies, 135–136
constipation remedies, 142, 147
cough remedies, 56, 151, 158, 159
depression remedies, 168
ear conditions remedies, 187, 190
eczema remedies, 195, 198
eye conditions remedies, 200, 204
fatigue remedies, 210–212
fever remedies, 213–214, 220–222
headache remedies, 230–231, 234, 238
heat rash remedies, 340
hives remedies, 25, 29
indigestion and heartburn remedies, 176, 177, 181, 185, 253, 256

Chinese medicine *(continued)*
insomnia remedies, 263–264, 267
itching and rashes remedies, 268–269
liver dysfunction and, 161
menstruation and, 275, 277, 280, 281–282, 286, 288
muscle strains and sprains remedies, 297–299
pain remedies, 310–311, 315, 317
sore throat remedies, 344–345, 348
sores and skin ulcers remedies, 352, 354
toothache remedies, 290, 292
wounds and cuts remedies, 363
chocolate, 19
chrysanthemum flowers, 98, 204
cinnamon, 181, 226–227, 277, 306, 308
clay
for acne, 20
for bites and stings, 68–69
for itching and rashes, 274
for poison ivy and poison oak, 323
for skin problems, 334
for splinters, 359
cleavers, 79, 269, 272
cloves
for earaches, 187, 190
for itching and rashes, 268–269
for nausea, 308
for toothaches, 290
cobwebs, 368
colds and flu, 118–119, 121–125, 129–132, 151
colic, 132–137, 140–141
colitis. *See* diarrhea.
comedones, 18
comfrey, 364
conjunctivitis. *See* eye conditions.
constipation, 141–143, 146–147
copper bracelets, 47, 50, 225
corn silk, 71
cornmeal, 94, 337
cornmint. *See* mints.
cornstarch, 337
corpse remedies, 96–97
corticosteroids, 39
coughs, 56, 148–149, 151–153, 157–159
counterirritants, 48–49, 65–66
arthritis and, 44, 225
for bee stings, 51
muscle strains and sprains and, 297
pain and, 310
cramp bark, 285, 311
cranberry juice, 76
cream, 108, 201
cucumber bark, wild, 52
cupping, 99, 301
curanderismo, 260–261, 313
cuts. *See* wounds and cuts.

D

daisy blossoms, 56
dandelions
as blood purifiers and blood builders, 85
for depression, 165
for eczema, 193–194
for fever, 220–221
for hemorrhoids, 245–246
dang gui, 40, 317
degenerative joint disease (DJD). *See* arthritis.
demulcents, 79, 148, 149, 253
dental problems, 289–290, 292–293, 296
depression, 160–161, 164–165, 168–169
devil babies, 331
devil's dung. *See* asafoetida.
dextromethorphan, 148
diaphoretics, 214, 340
diarrhea, 170–172, 174–175
diet
acne and, 19
allergies and, 22
anxiety and, 30–31, 31
arthritis and, 39
asthma and, 54
colic and, 132–133
dental problems and, 289
depression and, 160
digestion and, 184
fatigue and, 206, 212
fever and, 218
hemorrhoids and, 240
indigestion and, 176
insomnia and, 258
lactation and, 132–133
dill seeds
for breast conditions, 101
for colic, 136
for hiccups, 249
for insomnia, 263–264
diuretics, 50, 69–70
dog remedies, 26, 51, 59, 224
dong quai, 40, 317
dressings, 86, 87

E

ear conditions, 186–187, 190–192
Eastern medicine. *See* Chinese medicine.
echinacea
for bites and stings, 63, 67
as blood purifiers and blood builders, 83–84
for colds and flu, 119, 121
for eczema, 198
for gum infections, 292
for sore throats, 345, 348
for toothaches, 292
Eclectic medicine, 29
allergy remedies, 25
anxiety remedies, 36–37, 38
arthritis remedies, 41, 44
asthma remedies, 56

Eclectic medicine *(continued)*
bladder and kidney infections remedies, 72, 78, 79
blood purifiers and blood builders, 83–84, 91, 98
breast conditions remedies, 101, 105
catarrh remedies, 117–118
colds and flu remedies, 119, 121
depression remedies, 165, 168, 169
indigestion remedies, 181, 184
menstruation and, 276, 277, 280, 284, 285, 288
narcotic poisoning remedies, 56
pain remedies, 311
poison ivy and poison oak remedies, 318–319
skin problems remedies, 336–337
sore throat remedies, 343
sores and skin ulcers remedies, 354
wounds and cuts remedies, 361, 363, 365
eczema, 193–195, 198
edema, 70
eggs
for asthma, 57, 60
for boils and carbuncles, 95
for fatigue, 212
elder flowers and berries
for asthma, 57
as blood purifiers and blood builders, 89
for breast conditions, 105
for colds and flu, 121–122
for fever, 214–215
for flu, 89
elecampane, 159
electrolyte replacement, 170, 172, 306
emetics, 55
English medicine, 346–347
Englishman's Footprint. *See* plantain.
epazote, 90
ephedra, 54–55
Epsom salts
for arthritis, 50–51
for constipation, 143
for muscle strains and sprains, 302
for pain, 316–317
ergot alkaloids, 235
essential oils, 131
evil eye, 202, 219, 236, 261, 301, 362
excrement remedies, 65, 66, 111
exercise
for insomnia, 264
for menstrual problems, 284
during pregnancy, 325, 329
exhaustion. *See* fatigue.
expectorants, 148, 149
eye conditions, 199–201, 203–205, 291
eyebright, 25, 201

F

falling out, 339
fasting, 52, 218
fatigue, 206–207, 210–212
fennel seeds
for breast conditions, 100–101, 101
for colic, 135–136
for indigestion and heartburn, 177, 185, 256
for menstrual problems, 277
fertility, 326–327
fever, 212–215, 218–222, 335
feverfew, 215, 229
fiber, 184
figs, 99, 296
fire doctors, 110
flax seeds and oil
for boils and carbuncles, 94–95
for constipation, 146
for coughs, 149, 151
flaxseed, 205
flu. *See* colds and flu.
folk illnesses, 138–139, 181
food as medicine, 86–87. *See also* diet.
foot problems, 222–224, 226–228
formulas
for asthma, 60–61
for bladder and kidney infections, 78–79
for blood purifiers and blood builders, 92
for constipation, 146
for coughs, 152, 158
for fever, 220
for hemorrhoids, 245
for indigestion and heartburn, 257
for insomnia, 267
for menstrual problems, 288
for pain, 310
for wounds, 357
fringe tree bark, 195

G

gallstones, 328
garden sage, 106
garlic
for asthma, 55, 56
for athlete's foot, 223–224
for bites and stings, 67–68
as blood purifiers and blood builders, 84, 98
for colds and flu, 125
for coughs, 151–152
for ear infections, 190, 191
in folklore, 65, 66
for hemorrhoids, 246
for skin problems, 337
for sore throats, 350
for sores and skin ulcers, 351–352
for wounds and cuts, 361
gentian, 181

German chamomile. *See* chamomile.
ghost sickness, 139
ginger
for colds and flu, 123–124
for coughs, 158
for fever, 213
for indigestion and heartburn, 181, 253, 256
for menstrual problems, 277
for morning sickness, 328
for nausea, 305, 328
for pain, 315
for sores and skin ulcers, 355
for spasms, 315
gold, 39
goldenrod, 71
goldenseal, 88
for catarrh, 113, 117–118
for ear infections, 191
for eye conditions, 201, 203
for gum infections, 292–293
for indigestion, 181, 184
for mouth ulcers and infected gums, 290
for skin problems, 336
for sore throats, 343–344
for sores and skin ulcers, 352
gravel-root, 71–72
greens, 91
gums. *See* dental problems.
gumweed, 321, 336–337, 356–357
Gypsy medicine
acne remedies, 21
anxiety and, 37
anxiety remedies, 32
arthritis remedies, 52
bites and stings remedies, 68
bladder and kidney infections remedies, 70–71, 76–77
boils and carbuncles remedies, 95
burns and sunburns remedies, 109
constipation remedies, 146
depression remedies, 164
Gypsy medicine *(continued)*
diarrhea remedies, 174
eczema remedies, 193–194
fever remedies, 222
hiccups remedies, 249
puffy skin remedies, 338
sore throat remedies, 350
sores and skin ulcers remedies, 351–352
wounds remedies, 357

H

hay fever. *See* allergies.
headaches, 228–231, 233–239
heartburn. *See* indigestion and heartburn.
heat rash. *See* skin problems.
hemorrhoids, 239–241, 244–248
herbalism, 154–156, 238
herbs, 325, 329
hiccups, 248–249, 251–252
Hispanic medicine, 260–261, 362
acne remedies, 20
anxiety remedies, 31–33, 33, 36
arthritis remedies, 45, 46–47, 51
bites and stings remedies, 68–69
bladder and kidney infections remedies, 77–78
blood purifiers and blood builders, 98
boils and carbuncles remedies, 94, 95
burns and sunburns remedies, 109–110
catarrh remedies, 117
chapped skin remedies, 334
cold feet remedies, 226
colic remedies, 133, 135, 137, 140–141
ear conditions remedies, 187, 190
Hispanic medicine *(continued)*
eczema remedies, 198
eye conditions remedies, 200, 204–205
fever remedies, 213, 214–215
headache remedies, 234, 239
hemorrhoid remedies, 241, 244, 245–246
hiccups remedies, 251
indigestion and heartburn remedies, 180–181, 181, 184–185, 257
itching and rashes remedies, 268–269, 272
menstruation and, 281–282, 284, 285–286, 286, 288
morning sickness remedies, 329
muscle strains and sprains remedies, 297–298, 299
pain remedies, 315–316
skin problems remedies, 338, 340
sore throat remedies, 343, 345, 348–349
sores and skin ulcers remedies, 352, 354, 355
toothache remedies, 290, 296
wounds and cuts remedies, 363
hit medicine, 302, 311
hives. *See* allergies.
Hmong medicine, 145
hog remedies, 27, 95, 359, 363
hollyhock flowers, 157–158
homeopathic medicine, 117–118, 316
honey
for asthma, 56–57
as blood purifiers and blood builders, 92
for burns and sunburns, 111–112
for coughs, 56
for eczema, 195, 198
for hiccups, 251
for sores and skin ulcers, 352

hoodoo, 43, 255, 287
hop
for anxiety, 32–33
for arthritis, 46–47
for breast conditions, 101, 102, 105
for headaches, 238–239
for insomnia, 263
horehound, 153, 158–159, 344
horse chestnuts, 244
horse remedies, 28, 87
horsemint, 124, 219–220
horseradish, 23
horsetail, 77–78
hot-cold balance, 173
hydrotherapy. *See* water treatments.

I

impetigo. *See* skin problems.
Indian medicine
catarrh remedies, 113
ear conditions remedies, 191
eye conditions remedies, 200
fever remedies, 213
headache remedies, 238
indigestion remedies, 176
menstruation and, 275
toothache remedies, 290, 292
indigestion and heartburn, 175–177, 179–181, 184–186, 252–253, 256–257
influenza. *See* colds and flu.
infusions, 178
insomnia, 258–259, 262–265, 267
isotretinoin, 19
Italian-American medicine, 300
itching and rashes, 268–269, 272, 274, 318

J

jewelweed, 318–319, 321
Jewish medicine, 216–217
jimsonweed, 57
Joe-Pye weed, 71–72
jojoba oil, 333
juju, 287
juniper
for acne, 21
for bladder and kidney infections, 73
for insomnia, 264
for itching and rashes, 268–269
for menstrual problems, 277
for wounds and cuts, 365

K

kerosene, 49, 69
kidney infections. *See* bladder and kidney infections.
kidney stones, 71, 72

L

lactation. *See also* breast conditions.
bearberry and, 70
boneset and, 123
California poppy and, 164
diet and, 132–133
elder flowers and, 122
goat's rue and, 100
laxatives and, 237
lady slipper, 33
latah, 138
Latino medicine. *See* Hispanic medicine; Southwestern medicine.
laxatives, 235, 237, 245
lemon balm
for colds and flu, 124–125
for colic, 137
for fever, 218–219
for menstrual problems, 282, 284
lemon juice
for colds and flu, 130
for fever, 221
lemon juice *(continued)*
for hiccups, 249, 251
for itching and rashes, 272
for sore throats, 350
licorice
for asthma, 54
for coughs, 158
for indigestion, 185
for sore throats, 344–345
liver disease, 364
liver dysfunction, 161, 164
lockjaw, 358
love potions, 166–167

M

ma huang, 54–55
magical fright, 183
magical healing, 58–59, 74–75, 347
magnesium, 22
mallow, 157–158
marijuana, 45
marking during pregnancy, 330–331
marshmallow root, 157–158
massage, 264–265
measuring health, 34–35
melancholy. *See* depression.
menstruation, 232–233, 275–277, 280–282, 284–286, 288
Mexican medicine. *See* Hispanic medicine.
midwives, 196–197, 278, 279, 324
milk
for ear infections, 192
for eye conditions, 201
for insomnia, 265
for skin problems, 338, 340
milkweed, 322
mints
for bites and stings, 62
for catarrh, 113, 117
for colds and flu, 124

mints *(continued)*
for colic, 135
for fever, 213–214
for hay fever, 24–25
for headaches, 231, 234
for indigestion and heartburn, 176–177, 185, 257
for itching and rashes, 269
for morning sickness, 329
for nausea, 304, 305–306, 329
for sore throats, 348
miscarriage, 276
molasses
for asthma, 57, 60
as blood purifiers and blood builders, 91
for depression, 165
moon phases and medicine, 189
Mormon tea, 54–55
motherwort, 37, 280
mouth problems. *See* dental problems.
mucus, 148. *See also* catarrh.
mullein
asthma remedies, 56–57
for coughs, 153, 157, 158–159
for earaches, 190
for flu, 153, 157
for hemorrhoids, 241, 244
muscle strains and sprains, 297–299, 302
mustard plaster, 45, 48, 130
mustard seeds, 56, 151, 298–299
myrrh gum, 290, 292–293, 349, 356

N

napping, 210
Native American medicine, 126–128
acne remedies, 21
anxiety remedies, 33, 37
arthritis remedies, 40, 41, 44, 45, 46, 47, 50
Native American medicine *(continued)*
asthma remedies, 54–55, 56–57
athlete's foot remedies, 223
bites and stings remedies, 62–63, 67, 68–69, 88
bladder and kidney infections remedies, 70–71, 72, 73, 77–78, 79
blood purifiers and blood builders, 83–85, 89–91, 90–91, 91, 98
boils and carbuncles remedies, 94
burns and sunburns remedies, 109–110, 112
catarrh remedies, 117–118
colds and flu remedies, 119, 121–123, 123, 125, 129
colic remedies, 133, 135
constipation remedies, 142–143, 146–147
cough remedies, 56–57, 149, 153, 157, 158, 159
depression remedies, 165
diarrhea remedies, 171–172, 174–175
ear conditions remedies, 190, 191–192
eczema remedies, 193–194, 198
eye conditions remedies, 200, 201, 203–204
fatigue remedies, 210
fever remedies, 214–215, 218, 219, 220, 221–222
flu remedies, 89
headache remedies, 40, 229–230, 234, 237–239
hemorrhoid remedies, 240–241
indigestion and heartburn remedies, 181, 184–185, 257
insect bites remedies, 333–334
insomnia remedies, 264, 265
itching and rashes remedies, 268–269, 272, 274
Native American medicine *(continued)*
menstruation and, 169, 285–286, 288
minor wounds remedies, 333–334
mouth sores remedies, 293
mouth ulcers and infected gums remedies, 290, 292
muscle strains and sprains remedies, 299, 302
pain remedies, 311, 315, 317
poison ivy and poison oak remedies, 318–319, 321–322
skin problems remedies, 333, 334, 336–337, 340–341
sore throat remedies, 342–345, 348–349
sores and skin ulcers remedies, 352, 354–355, 356–357
splinters remedies, 358, 359
toothache remedies, 293, 296
wounds and cuts remedies, 361, 363–364, 365
nausea and vomiting, 55, 122–123, 303–306, 308
near-death experiences (NDE), 183
nervousness. *See* anxiety.
nettle. *See* stinging nettle.
neurasthenia. *See* depression.
New Age healing, 366–367
New England medicine
allergy remedies, 23
anxiety remedies, 33
arthritis remedies, 50–51
asthma remedies, 56
athlete's foot remedies, 224, 226
bites and stings remedies, 68–69
bladder and kidney infections remedies, 72–73, 76–77
blood purifiers and blood builders, 89–90
boils and carbuncles remedies, 94–95, 98, 99

New England medicine (continued)
breast conditions remedies, 106–107
burns and sunburns remedies, 108–111
chapped skin remedies, 334
colds and flu remedies, 123–124, 125, 129–130, 131, 132
colic remedies, 135–137
constipation remedies, 142–143, 146, 147
cough remedies, 149, 151, 159
dental problems remedies, 296
diarrhea remedies, 171–172, 175
ear conditions remedies, 191, 192
eye conditions remedies, 200, 201
fever remedies, 213, 215, 218, 219, 221–222
headache remedies, 229–230, 235, 241
hemorrhoid remedies, 241, 244, 245, 247
hiccups remedies, 251–252
hives remedies, 29
indigestion and heartburn remedies, 176–177, 180, 181, 184–185, 253, 256–257
insomnia remedies, 262, 265, 267
itching and rashes remedies, 272
menses and, 277, 284–285
muscle strains and sprains remedies, 297–298, 299, 302
pain remedies, 310–311, 315, 316–317
poison ivy and poison oak remedies, 318–319, 321–322, 323
pregnancy and, 325, 328
skin problems remedies, 338, 340
sore throat remedies, 342–343, 349
spasm remedies, 315
splinters remedies, 358, 359
toothache remedies, 290
nightshade vegetables, 39
nipple discomfort. *See* breast conditions.
nonsteroidal anti-inflammatory drugs (NSAIDs), 39, 40, 228, 230
nutmeg, 98

O

oak bark, 344
oatmeal
for breast conditions, 106
for chapped skin, 334
for depression, 165, 168
odors for healing, 64–66
oil, 192
ointments, 240, 338
omega-3 fatty acids, 22, 31
onions
for anxiety, 37
for bites and stings, 67–68
as blood purifiers and blood builders, 84
for boils and carbuncles, 94
for colds and flu, 125, 129
for coughs, 152–153
for fever, 221–222
for hemorrhoids, 247
for sore throats, 349
for sores and skin ulcers, 356
orange peel, 174
Oregon grape root. *See also* goldenseal.
for eczema, 195
for eye conditions, 203–204
for fatigue, 210
for indigestion, 181, 184
for sore throats, 343–344
osha, 153, 340–341, 348–349
osteoarthritis. *See* arthritis.
over-the-counter drugs, 309

P

pain, 309–311, 315–317
parsley, 76–77
passion flower, 36–37, 265
patent medicines, 80–81
Pennsylvania Dutch. *See* Pennsylvania German.
Pennsylvania German medicine, 102–104
blood purifiers and blood builders, 90, 91
eczema remedies, 194
pennyroyal
for asthma, 60
for bites and stings, 62
for headaches, 231
for menstrual problems, 284
toxicity of, 288
pepper, 48–49
peppermint. *See* mints.
Physiomedicalist medicine, 109
arthritis remedies, 41
catarrh remedies, 117–118
gum infection remedies, 292–293
indigestion remedies, 181, 184
menstruation and, 276, 280, 284, 285, 286, 288
muscle strains and sprains remedies, 299
pain remedies, 311, 315–316
poison ivy and poison oak remedies, 318–319
sore throat remedies, 343
piles. *See* hemorrhoids.
pine
for arthritis, 45
for burns and sunburns, 112
for coughs, 153
for insomnia, 264
for sores and skin ulcers, 355

pinkeye. *See* eye conditions.
plantain
  for athlete's foot, 223
  for bites and stings, 67
  for burns and sunburns, 109–110
  for chapped skin, 333–334
  for itching and rashes, 274
  for poison ivy and poison oak, 321–322
  for splinters, 358
  for toothaches, 296
  for wounds and cuts, 363–364
pleurisy root, 117
poison ivy and poison oak, 318–323
poison sumac, 320
poke root, 272
popcorn, 305
possession. *See* depression.
pot marigold. *See* calendula.
potatoes, 110–111, 201, 338
poultices, 86, 87
powwow healing, 102–104, 314
prayer and healing, 162–163, 255, 312–314, 339
pregnancy, 324–325, 327–331
  bearberry and, 70
  boneset and, 123
  California poppy and, 164
  cascara sagrada and, 143
  catnip and, 60
  cinnamon and, 181
  elder flowers and, 122
  fenugreek and, 113
  feverfew and, 229
  hemorrhoids and, 239–240
  isotretinoin and, 19
  laxatives and, 142, 237
  morning sickness and, 250
  parsley juice and, 77
  pennyroyal and, 60
  rosemary and, 231
  yellow dock and, 85, 88
prickly ash, 293, 296
prostate problems, 70, 72–73, 88–89
prunes, 146
psychic surgery, 75
psychotherapy, 168–169
psyllium seeds, 246
pumpkin seeds, 72–73
pus
  calendula and, 356, 364
  charcoal and, 368
  comfrey and, 364

Q

queen of the meadow. *See* Joe-Pye weed.

R

rashes. *See* itching and rashes.
raspberry leaves, 241, 282, 324–325
red clover
  for acne, 19, 21
  as blood purifiers and blood builders, 89
  for hemorrhoids, 245
  for skin problems, 332–333
respiratory sedatives, 148, 149
rheumatism. *See* arthritis.
rheumatoid arthritis. *See* arthritis.
roots, 287
rootwork, 287
rose oil, 21, 264
rosemary
  for anxiety, 33, 36
  for arthritis, 40–41
  for catarrh, 117
  for chapped skin, 337
  for headaches, 230–231
  for muscle strains and sprains, 299
  for pain, 315–316
  for sores and skin ulcers, 355
  for wounds and cuts, 365
roses, 200, 345
rubefacients, 48

S

sage
  for colds and flu, 129–130
  for headaches, 230–231
  for insomnia, 264
  for sore throats, 345
St. Anthony's Fire, 235
St. John's wort, 161, 164
saints, 312–314
saliva, 365, 368
salves, 105, 240, 338
sarsaparilla, 90
sassafras, 89–90
scars, 336
senna, 142
septicemia, 360
sesame seeds, 44, 147
Seventh Day Adventist medicine
  anxiety remedies, 32–33
  arthritis remedies, 51, 52
  asthma remedies, 55, 60
  athlete's foot remedies, 223–224
  bites and stings remedies, 68
  bladder and kidney infections remedies, 72, 76, 79
  burns and sunburns remedies, 108
  colds and flu remedies, 123, 131–132
  depression remedies, 168
  diarrhea remedies, 172, 174
  eczema remedies, 195
  fever remedies, 215
  hemorrhoid remedies, 247–248
  indigestion remedies, 185
  insomnia remedies, 259, 262, 263, 264–265
  itching and rashes remedies, 272, 274
  pain remedies, 317
  poison ivy and poison oak remedies, 322, 323
  skin problems remedies, 334

Seventh Day Adventist medicine *(continued)*
sore throat remedies, 349–350
wounds and cuts remedies, 368
shamans, 127–128, 145
shape-shifting, 209
shepherd's purse, 286, 288
Siberian ginseng, 211–212
signatures, doctrine of, 155, 166
skin problems, 332–334, 336–338, 340–341
skin ulcers. *See* sores and skin ulcers.
skullcap, 33
sleep paralysis, 208–209
slippery elm
for boils and carbuncles, 94
for coughs, 157
for diarrhea, 174–175
for indigestion and heartburn, 253
for sore throats, 342–343
for sores and skin ulcers, 355
snake remedies, 81, 115–116
snakebites. *See* bites and stings.
snakeroot, 63, 67
soap, 359
sore throats, 341–345, 348–350
sores and skin ulcers, 351–353, 354–357
soul loss, 182–183, 208–209
Southwestern medicine. *See also* Hispanic medicine.
anxiety remedies, 32–33
arthritis remedies, 45–47, 51
asthma remedies, 56
athlete's foot remedies, 224, 226
bites and stings remedies, 63, 67–68
blood purifiers and blood builders, 84–85, 90–91
boils and carbuncles remedies, 93, 94, 95, 98
burns and sunburns remedies, 108, 111–112
Southwestern medicine *(continued)*
chapped skin remedies, 333
colds and flu remedies, 125
colic remedies, 136–137, 140–141
constipation remedies, 142–143
cough remedies, 149, 153, 157
diarrhea remedies, 172
ear conditions remedies, 187, 190, 191, 192
eczema remedies, 194–195, 198
fever remedies, 219, 220
headache remedies, 229–230, 234, 237–238
hiccups remedies, 251
indigestion and heartburn remedies, 176–177, 180, 184–185, 253, 256, 257
insomnia remedies, 263, 265, 267
itching and rashes remedies, 268–269, 274
mouth sores remedies, 293
muscle strains and sprains remedies, 299
pain remedies, 310–311, 315
skin problems remedies, 336–337
sores and skin ulcers remedies, 354
toothache remedies, 290
spearmint. *See* mints.
spiderwebs, 368
splinters, 357–359
steroid drugs, 53, 193
sties, 291
stinging nettle
for acne, 21
for arthritis, 51–52, 88–89
for asthma, 57
for bladder and kidney infections, 70–71
as blood purifiers and blood builders, 88–89
stinging nettle *(continued)*
for eczema, 193–194
for nourishment during pregnancy, 325, 328
for prostate problems, 88–89
stings. *See* bites and stings.
strep throat, 341–342, 343
stress
acne and, 18
headaches and, 236
insomnia and, 258, 259
suction, 359
sugar
anxiety and, 31
fatigue and, 206
for hiccups, 251
infections and, 77
for splinters, 359
sulfur, 65
sunburns. *See* burns and sunburns.
suppressants, 148, 149
susto, 139, 182, 261
sweating, 214
for asthma, 60
for fever, 121, 218, 335
for skin conditions, 340
swimmer's ear, 186–187
sympathetic magic, 58, 326
synovitis. *See* arthritis.

T

teas, 175, 178, 200, 267, 306
teeth. *See* dental problems.
thyme
for acne, 21
for catarrh, 117
for colds and flu, 124
for eczema, 198
for fever, 219–220
for hay fever, 23–24
for indigestion, 185
for itching and rashes, 269
tobacco
for bites and stings, 63

tobacco *(continued)*
for burns and sunburns, 110
colic and, 134, 137
for earaches, 191
folk medicine and, 49
toenails, ingrown, 223, 228
tonics, bitter, 179, 207
trachoma. *See* eye conditions.
turpentine, 45, 49

U

urinary tract conditions. *See* bladder and kidney infections.
urine, 65
for athlete's foot, 224, 226
for chapped skin, 334
for ear infections, 192
for eye conditions, 204–205

V

valerian, 31–33, 262
vervain, 36
vinegar
for bites and stings, 68
for burns and sunburns, 108
for chapped skin, 334
for colds and flu, 130
for headaches, 238
for poison ivy and poison oak, 321
for sore throats, 350
vision quests, 128
vitamin C, 22
vitamin E, 39, 258, 336, 337–338
vomiting. *See* nausea and vomiting.
voodoo, 255, 287

W

warts, 270–271
water treatments
for anxiety, 32
for arthritis, 51
water treatments *(continued)*
for asthma, 60
for bladder and kidney infections, 73, 79
for catarrh, 113
for cold feet, 226
for colds and flu, 123, 131–132
for colic, 140
for constipation, 147
for coughs, 159
for dental problems, 296
for depression, 168
for eye conditions, 205
for fever, 222
for headaches, 237
for hemorrhoids, 247–248
for indigestion, 185
for ingrown toenails, 228
for insomnia, 259, 262–263
for menstrual problems, 285
for pain, 317
for sore throats, 348, 349–350
for splinters, 358
watermelon, 72, 340
weather and illness, 283
White Man's Footprint. *See* plantain.
white willow bark, 40
wicca, 197
wild cherry bark, 149
willow bark
for fever, 219
for headaches, 229–230
for menstrual problems, 284–285
for mouth and gum infections, 292
for pain, 311, 315
for sore throats, 348
wintergreen, 40, 41, 299
witch hazel
for eye conditions, 200
for hemorrhoids, 240–241
for muscle strains and sprains, 299, 302
witchcraft, 103, 196–197, 208, 209, 346, 347
worms, 150
wormwood
for depression, 165
for diarrhea, 172
for headaches, 237–238
for indigestion, 180–181
wounds and cuts, 360–361, 363–365, 368

Y

yam, wild, 47
yang, 144–145
yarn, 228
yarrow
for colds and flu, 123
for earaches, 191–192
for eczema, 198
for fever, 220
for headaches, 234
for hemorrhoids, 244
for menstrual problems, 285–286
for nausea, 305
for wounds and cuts, 361, 363
yellow dock
as blood purifiers and blood builders, 85, 88
for eczema, 194–195
for hemorrhoids, 247
yerba mansa
as blood purifiers and blood builders, 90–91, 98
for mouth sores, 293
for sores and skin ulcers, 354
for wounds and cuts, 365
yin, 144–145
yu mi shu, 71
Yunnan Pi Yao, 363

Z

zinc, 19